Drugs and Addictive Behaviour

A GUIDE TO TREATMENT

D1240581

When you can cure by regimen,
avoid having recourse to medicine;
and when you can effect a cure
by means of single medicine,
avoid using a compound one.
Razi (Rhazes)
Persia, 850–922 AD

Drugs and Addictive Behaviour

A GUIDE TO TREATMENT

HAMID GHODSE

MD PhD FRCP FRCPsych DPM

Professor and Director
Psychiatry of Addictive Behaviour
St George's Hospital Medical School
University of London
Honorary Consultant Psychiatrist
St George's and Springfield
University Hospitals

SECOND EDITION

Blackwell
Science

To Barbara, Amir-Hossein, Nassrin and Ali-Reza

© 1989, 1995 by
Blackwell Science Ltd
Editorial Offices:
Osney Mead, Oxford OX2 0EL
25 John Street, London WC1N 2BL
23 Ainslie Place, Edinburgh EH3 6AJ
238 Main Street, Cambridge
  Massachusetts 02142, USA
54 University Street, Carlton
  Victoria 3053, Australia

Other Editorial Offices:
Arnette Blackwell SA
1, rue de Lille, 75007 Paris
France

Blackwell Wissenschafts-Verlag GmbH
Kurfürstendamm 57
10707 Berlin, Germany

Blackwell MZV
Feldgasse 13, A-1238 Wien
Austria

First published 1989
Second edition 1995

Set by EXPO Holdings, Malaysia
Printed and bound in Great Britain
at the University Press, Cambridge

DISTRIBUTORS

Marston Book Services Ltd
PO Box 87
Oxford OX2 0DT
(*Orders*:   Tel: 01865 791155
             Fax: 01865 791927
             Telex : 837515

North America
  Blackwell Science, Inc.
  238 Main Street
  Cambridge, MA 02142
  (*Orders*:   Tel: 800 215-1000
               617 876-7000
               Fax: 617 492-5263)

Australia
  Blackwell Science Pty Ltd
  54 University Street
  Carlton, Victoria, 3053
  (*Orders*: Tel: 03 347-5552)

A catalogue record for this title
is available from the British Library

ISBN 0-86542-608-2
ISBN 0-86542-868-9 (Pbk)

Library of Congress
Cataloging-in-Publication Data

Ghodse, Hamid.
    Drugs and addictive behaviour:
    a guide to treatment/Hamid
    Ghodse – 2nd ed.
        p.   cm.
    Includes bibliographical references
    and index.
    ISBN 0-86542-608-2
    ISBN 0-86542-868-9 (Pbk)
    1. Substance abuse.   I. Title.
    [DNLM: 1.   Substance Abuse – therapy.
    2.   Substance Dependence – therapy.
    WM 270 G427d 1995]
    RC564.G39   1995
    616.86′ 06 — dc20 94-34463

Contents

Preface

Although the structure of the second edition of this book remains
unchanged, there has been significant up-dating and revision throughout.
Every attempt has been made to retain the straightforward approach
adopted in the first edition, so that the contents are easily accessible to a
wide audience and the emphasis, throughout, has been on practical
approaches so that the book is genuinely 'a guide to treatment'.

Naturally, some parts have required a more radical overhaul than
others. In particular, the latest epidemiological statistics are included for the
UK and, reflecting the continuing globalisation of drug use and misuse, a
more detailed account is provided in Chapter 2 of the international drug
scene. Although the same drugs continue to be used and misused, the
growing problem of steroid misuse is described in Chapter 3 where there are
also new sections on over-the-counter medicines, herbal preparations and
the combined use of drugs and alcohol. The important role of the laboratory
in the assessment of drug problems is recognized in Chapter 4, where there
is also a section on drug-screening programmes. Another important addition
to this chapter is the section dealing with the classification of mental and
behavioural disorders due to psychoactive substance use, including descriptions of ICD-10, DSM-III-R and DSM-IV. There is now a more detailed
account of both general and specific measures of intervention and, in
Chapter 7, the accounts of HIV/AIDS and hepatitis in substance misusers
have been substantially changed to reflect current knowledge. The role of
the Accident and Emergency department receives greater emphasis in
Chapter 8, where there is an additional section on substance misusers
detained in police custody. Modern approaches to harm reduction are
discussed in Chapter 10 while in Chapter 11, local (UK) and international control measures are described in more detail than in the earlier
edition.

The references and further reading sections have been substantially
revised so that they offer an up-to-date approach to the literature for the
interested student.

It is impossible to acknowledge all the sources of inspiration and information on which I have drawn while writing this book, but first of all, and above all, I must thank my patients – *all* the patients with drug problems whom I have met over the last 25 years and more. They are the *raison d'être* of the book and the experience I have gained with them and from them is central to it. Additional material has been drawn from the work of the worldwide community of scientists and researchers in the field, and the World Health Organization, the United Nations, the International Narcotics Control Board, ISDD and NIDA have all been valuable sources of information.

I thank, sincerely, my colleagues Gill Tregenza, Carmel Clancy, Megan Jones, Fiona Marshall, Paul Davis and Cynthia Scott for their generous help, and Stuart Taylor of Blackwell Science for his unfailing patience. Health-care students, both undergraduate and postgraduate, of all disciplines, have contributed through their interest and enthusiasm and their enlightening discussions. I also thank the World Health Organization and the American Psychiatric Association for permission to reprint parts of ICD-10 and DSM-III-R and DSM-IV.

Introduction

Drug use of one sort or another has occurred for a very long time – probably ever since the time that early humans, eating plants that grew around them, found that some plants had medicinal properties and that some made them feel different. Since that time, drug use has been part of the human lifestyle, with different societies using different 'natural' intoxicants depending on the indigenous flora. A few of these drugs have become familiar to many, beyond the confines of their original use. Opium, alcohol and cannabis spring immediately to mind; they have been used for centuries and are still widely used today. So too is coffee, which although it is bought in packets and jars as a food, fits all five definitions of the word 'drug' given in Chapter 1.

Coffee is indigenous to Ethiopia where it was first consumed by chewing the beans or infusing the leaves. It was certainly known to the Arabs in the sixth century and its medicinal properties were described by the Persian physicians, Razi (or Rhazes; 850–922) and Ibn-sina (or Avicenna; 980–1037). In the fourteenth century the technique of roasting and grinding coffee beans was developed and only then did coffee drinking become prevalent. By this time, the cultivation and use of coffee had spread to Arabia where its popularity was enhanced because the use of alcohol had been banned by the Koran. Coffee was used medicinally as well as for religious purposes, particularly by the Dervishes to keep themselves awake during long religious rituals. With the increasing popularity of coffee, coffee houses were established which soon became meeting places for intellectuals. The use of coffee in its social setting of the coffee house spread through the Arab world and to Turkey, Persia and beyond. There were many attempts, in different countries, to close down the coffee houses which were seen as centres of sedition and dissent, and to ban the use of coffee altogether. All of these attempts at prohibition eventually failed and coffee was then heavily taxed so that coffee houses became valuable sources of revenue for the authorities. During the seventeenth century, coffee drinking spread to England and other parts of Europe. As in Arabia, it was first used medicinally, and in particular as a cure for drunkenness which was then rife. Coffee houses soon opened and again became important social, political and business centres, attracting opposition, almost from the start, from brewers and others with vested interests in the sale of alcohol. Taxes were imposed and provided considerable revenue, but despite this, attempts were made in England to close the coffee houses that were once again seen as centres of radicalism and political dissent. As in Arabia these attempts failed and heavier taxes were imposed instead. Gradually in the latter part of the eighteenth century, the clientele of the coffee houses started to join clubs and the heyday of coffee houses was over, this change being accelerated by the importation of tea by the British East India Company and the acceptance of tea (which also contains caffeine) as the national drink.

From this necessarily brief history of coffee it is possible to identify certain themes that crop up repeatedly when modern drugs of abuse and dependence are considered. For example, many of these drugs were first used, like coffee, for medicinal purposes even though they are now considered to have minimal or no therapeutic value; alcohol, tobacco, cannabis and LSD (lysergic acid diethylamide) all fit into this category. In the case of the first three drugs, all of which have a long history, it is easy to imagine them as the 'wonder drugs' of their time, being prescribed enthusiastically for a variety of conditions. Modern sophisticated research produces many such drugs, and many have psychoactive properties. Some of these have already repeated the cycle from apparently safe therapeutic agent to drug of misuse or dependence, and undoubtedly more will do so in the future. Apart from their medicinal value, many drugs (e.g., opium, cannabis, cocaine and mescaline) have been used, as coffee was, in religious rituals, and the use of alcohol in this way continues today in two of the world's three monotheistic religions. It is of interest that the third and youngest religion, Islam, bans its use altogether.

A third way in which drugs are used, is for social and recreational purposes and it was this use of coffee that provoked so much controversy and opposition just as it does today for the other drugs. All of the 'old' drugs (those with a long history, e.g., opium, cannabis and alcohol) were used in this way and drug use was often the whole reason for a group coming together; the drug became the very substance of communication, the dynamic of the group activity. Alcohol continues in this role today, in public houses, night clubs, cocktail parties and so on, and for some drugs, notably cannabis and other psychedelic drugs, taken specifically by those interested in mysticism and exploration of the inner world, the setting in which the drug is taken and the shared group experience remain important. As far as illicit drug use is concerned, the very fact that the drug is forbidden encourages the formation of a group (and often of a whole sub-culture) concerned, among other things, with obtaining the drug and concealing its use from the authorities.

The story of coffee also illustrates the significance of technological innovation in drug use. Only when the techniques of roasting and grinding the coffee beans became prevalent, did the use of coffee become popular and spread widely and become perceived as problematic. Similarly the use of alcohol was profoundly affected by Razi's discovery of the process of distillation which made it easier to transport alcohol and to become drunk. Later the identification of the active alkaloids of opium and the subsequent development of the process of acetylation by which morphine is converted to heroin changed the whole pattern of opiate use, not only in the West where this discovery was made, but also in the East, where the parent drug originated. The extraction of cocaine from the leaf of the cocoa plant and more recently, the ability to prepare pure cocaine 'free-base' ('crack') have had equally profound effects, and now the process has gone one stage further, with new 'designer' drugs being manufactured for the sole purpose of abuse.

It is often assumed that the spread of drug use from one country to another is a new problem brought about by modern, rapid means of transport. The story of coffee, or indeed of any of the 'old' drugs, suggests that this is not so. For centuries there has been travel not only from one country to another, but also from one continent to another, and humans on their travels have taken drugs with them. There is no doubt, however, that modern methods of travel and communication have had a profound effect on drug use and abuse because the physical transportation of drugs is so much easier and speedier. In addition, the rapid movement of large numbers of people means that many more people are exposed to the drug-taking practices of another culture. This exposure is increased still further by the effect of the media, so that no drug or drug-taking practice can remain localized. They are bound to spread and in so doing there is usually a loss of the traditional constraints upon drug use imposed by the family and society as a whole. This means that new drugs and new ways of taking them gain acceptance much more easily than when drug use was under strict, local, sociocultural control.

Despite traditional methods of control, the drug scene has never been static. Five hundred years ago in Arabia the use of coffee superseded that of alcohol; this was partly because of the prohibition of alcohol by the Koran, but also occurred because of the availability of coffee. In England too, coffee drinking in the seventeenth century reduced the popularity of alcohol, but in turn gave way to tea. Similar changes in the pattern and fashions of drug use have occurred in the past and continue today, the availability of the particular drug often playing a crucial role.

Governments have long been concerned in controlling drug availability. Centuries ago, in Arabia, there were attempts at prohibiting coffee and when these failed, high taxes were imposed, ostensibly to discourage its use. However, this resulted in such high revenues that it then became economically almost impossible to pursue definitive policies to reduce coffee consumption. This cycle of events was repeated when coffee drinking spread to England and has also occurred with alcohol and tobacco – both of which now occupy entrenched positions within the economy of most countries.

Many other parallels can be drawn between what has happened to coffee in the past and what is happening to many drugs of abuse and dependence today. Recognition of this fact is not a counsel of despair. It is not meant to imply that heroin will ever be available on the shelves of the supermarket, as coffee is today. But the generality of the themes that have emerged over centuries of drug use does suggest that problems of drug abuse and of dependence on different types of drugs have commonalities that transcend substance-specific problems. This in turn suggests that it is the nature of drug abuse and dependence that are important rather than the specific drug that is causing concern at that particular time. However threatening, however modern, however unique present problems appear, it is undoubtedly true that their similarities to what has arisen before are more striking than differences which are more likely to be quantitative than qualitative.

Unfortunately, this quantitative difference, the enormous scale of modern drug abuse and drug dependence, has caused particular problems. Nowadays, so many people have drug-related problems that their care can no longer be left to a small band of interested specialists. All health-care professionals come into contact with drug abusers and drug-dependent individuals, as do probation officers and the police and others involved with the law, as well as those concerned with welfare services. All of these people require a basic understanding of the problems of drug abuse and dependence if their interventions are to be effective, and this book attempts to convey the general knowledge about drug abuse and dependence that is essential for that understanding.

In addition to general knowledge, however, there is a need for clear and practical advice on what to do in particular situations. Despite a wealth of research literature and a plethora of weighty tomes on drug dependence, it is difficult to find such advice. This book attempts to fill that gap, with chapters on how to assess individuals with drug-related problems and how to go about helping them. Although the emphasis is first on general measures of intervention, specific treatment programmes are also described so that the non-specialist, armed with a general understanding of the nature of the problem, is able to make intelligent decisions and to initiate treatment. Here the emphasis is on flexibility and a variety of treatment options are described and discussed, from acupuncture to intravenous heroin maintenance. Obviously it is not possible to cover every eventuality but many problems and problematic situations are included such as the management of an intoxicated, psychotic patient in the accident and emergency department; the care of children of drug-abusing parents; the question of whether drug-dependent individuals are eligible for driving licences; the management of drug-abusing health-care professionals, and so on.

Although drug-dependent individuals and drug abusers need help and it is essential that there are sufficient trained people to provide it, local responses to particular individual drug problems will never be enough. The final chapters of the book therefore examine the problem from a wider perspective, describing and explaining national and international control measures. Most important of all, perhaps, is the chapter on prevention which emphasizes the personal responsibility of every individual to develop more thoughtful attitudes towards drug taking.

In a book of this size it is only possible to cover a small fraction of the topics related to drug abuse and drug dependence. For example, problems associated with alcohol and tobacco are not included. Their omission is not intended to imply that because use of these drugs is widespread and socially acceptable, dependence on them is unimportant. Rather the magnitude and complexity of these two legal (in most countries) recreational drugs is such that they cannot be adequately dealt with in one small general book such as this. The interested reader should consult one of the many specialist books on these drugs.

The choice of topics covered by this book has been influenced by their practical relevance, but sufficient background information has been included to enable understanding of basic principles. It is hoped that it will encourage those who are inexperienced and unfamiliar with the field to become involved. In the past, many professionals have taken avoiding action when faced by a drug-abusing or drug-dependent individual, preferring to shunt the person off to another agency. They often justified their action by the belief that nothing could be done to help the person anyway, but such responses usually concealed underlying anxiety about their own ability to respond effectively.

A few references have been included at the end of each chapter for those readers who are stimulated to follow up particular aspects. Included are some references that have been used as source material although the list is by no means comprehensive and some references, although mentioned only once, have a bearing on more than one chapter. A list of general background reading is given below.

References and further reading

Advisory Committee on Drug Dependence (1968). *Cannabis. The Wootton Report.* HMSO, London.

Advisory Council on the Misuse of Drugs (1982). *Report of the Expert Group on the Effects of Cannabis Use.* Home Office, London.

Anderson P, Cremona A, Paton A, Turner C & Wallace P (1993). The risk of alcohol. *Addiction,* **88,** 1493–1508.

Austin GA (1978). *Perspective on the History of Psychoactive Substance Use.* National Institute of Drug Abuse, Rockville.

Banks A & Waller TAN (1988). *Drug Misuse: A Practical Handbook for GPs.* Blackwell Scientific Publications, Oxford.

Berridge V & Edwards G (1987). *Opium and the People: Opiate Use in Nineteenth Century England.* Yale University Press, New Haven.

British Journal of Addiction (1987). Psychology and addiction (Special Issue). *British Journal of Addiction,* **82,** 329–449.

Bucknell P & Ghodse AH (1991). *Misuse of Drugs,* 2nd edn. Waterlow, London. First supplement to the 2nd edn, 1993, Sweet & Maxwell, London.

Dupont RI, Goldstein A & O'Donnell J (eds) (1979). *Handbook on Drug Abuse.* National Institute of Drug Abuse, Washington DC.

Edwards G & Arif A (eds) (1980). *Drug Problem in the Sociocultural Context: A Basis for Policies and Programme Planning,* Public Health Papers No. 73. WHO, Geneva.

Edwards G & Busch C (eds) (1981). *Drug Problems in Britain: A Review of Ten Years.* Academic Press, London.

Edwards G & Lader M (eds) (1990). *The Nature of Drug Dependence.* Oxford University Press, Oxford.

Ghodse AH & Maxwell D (eds) (1990). *Substance Abuse and Dependence: an Introduction for the Caring Professions.* Macmillan Press, London.

Ghodse AH (ed.) (1994). Substance misuse. *Current Opinion in Psychiatry,* **7, No. 3,** 249–294.

Glatt MM (1974). *A Guide to Addiction and its Treatment.* Medical & Technical Publishing Co, Lancaster.

Herrington RG, Jacobson GR & Benzer DG (eds) (1987). *Alcohol and Drug Abuse Handbook.* Warren H Green, Inc, Missouri.

International Review of Psychiatry (1989). Special double issue: Psychiatry and the Addictions. *International Review of Psychiatry,* **1,** 1–190.

Jaffe J, Petersen R & Hodgson R (1980). *Addiction Issues and Answers.* Harper & Row, London.

Lowinson LH & Ruiz P (eds) (1981). *Substance Abuse. Clinical Problems and Perspectives..* Williams & Wilkins, Baltimore.

Madden JS (1984). *A Guide to Alcohol and Drug Dependence,* 2nd edn. Wright, Bristol.

Madden JS & Schuster CR (eds) (1993). *Current Opinion in Psychiatry.* **6, No. 3,** Current Science, 379–429.

Murray R, Ghodse AH, Harris C, Williams D & Williams P (eds) (1981). *The Misuse of Psychotropic Drugs*. Gaskell, Royal College of Psychiatrists, London.

Orford J (1985). *Excessive Appetites: A Psychological View of Addiction*. Wiley, Chichester.

Platt JJ (1986). *Heroin Addiction: Theory, Research and Treatment*, 2nd edn. Robert E. Krieger, Malabar.

Richmond RL & Anderson P (1994). Research in General Practice for smokers and excessive drinkers in Australia and the UK. *Addiction*, **89**, 35–62.

Royal College of Psychiatrists (1987). *Drug Scenes*. Gaskell, London.

Senay EC (1983). *Substance Abuse Disorders in Clinical Practice*. John Wright, Boston.

West R & Grunberg NE (eds) (1991). Future directions in tobacco research (Special Issue). *British Journal of Addiction*, **86**, 483–666.

Whitaker B (1987). *The Global Connection. The Crisis of Drug Addiction*. Jonathan Cape, London.

Wilford BB (1981). *Drug Abuse for the Primary Care Physician*. American Medical Association, Chicago.

World Health Organization (1993). *WHO Expert Committee on Drug Dependence. Twenty-Eighth Report*. WHO Technical Report Series 836. WHO, Geneva.

1

Drugs, addiction and behaviour

What is a 'drug'?

There are several possible definitions, as the examples below will show, but all have their limitations.

1 'A substance which, when injected into a rat, produces a scientific paper' – facetious, certainly, but probably accurate.

2 'A substance used as a medicine in the treatment of diagnosed mental or physical illness'. This definition is based on the shifting sands of therapeutic efficacy; coffee, cannabis and tobacco were used in times gone by for their medicinal properties and, accordingly, would then have been classified as drugs. Nowadays, however, all would escape that definition, a decision that would make most people uneasy, certainly as far as cannabis is concerned, and perhaps for tobacco and coffee too.

3 'Any chemical substance, other than a food that affects the structure of a living thing'. This too is unsatisfactory because there are a few substances generally considered to be drugs which are also consumed as foods. Alcohol is the obvious example, but there are others – some mushrooms would be 'food' while others would be drugs; caffeine, obtained in coffee jars from the supermarket, is perceived as a food, whereas in tablet form from the chemist, it is considered a drug.

4 'Any psychoactive substance' – that is any substance that affects the central nervous system and alters mood, perception or consciousness. Most of this book will, in fact, be concerned with psychoactive substances, their effects and the problems related to their use, but this definition ignores the fact that non-psychoactive substances may, on occasion, give rise to very similar problems. This is of theoretical, if not numerical, importance because it emphasizes the point that the drug-related problems with which this book deals, are not solely due to the particular properties of psychoactive drugs, but are also due to qualities of the individual concerned and of society.

5 A drug is 'any substance, other than those required for the mainte-

nance of normal health, that, when taken into the living organism, may modify one or more of its functions'.

This chosen definition is deliberately broad. It has the added advantage that having been developed by the World Health Organization (WHO), it is used and understood internationally.

What is drug misuse?

At first it seems easy to define misuse: 'To use or employ wrongly or improperly', according to the *Shorter Oxford English Dictionary*. However, when 'misuse' refers to drug misuse, definitions again become elusive. The term carries implications, according to the drug concerned, of social unacceptability, of illegality or of harmfulness. Sometimes it seems to mean that the drug is being used without medical approval, sometimes that it is being used excessively. Because of such ambiguities, and because the term suggest value judgements, that say more about the attitudes of the observer than they do about the way in which the drug is taken, it is often avoided altogether. The term 'drug use' is substituted, qualified by an appropriate adjective, such as illegal drug use, unsanctioned use (when the use of a particular drug is not sanctioned by society or a group within society), hazardous use (probably leading to harmful consequences for the user), dysfunctional use (leading to impaired social or psychological functioning), non-medical drug use (not in accordance with recommended medical practice), etc. Obviously this format begs the question of what constitutes misuse, but it can give a more precise picture of the way in which a particular drug is taken.

Drug abuse; harmful use

Drug abuse is an alternative phrase, although it too is often used imprecisely and is considered by many to be value laden. It has the advantage of an international (WHO) definition, utilized in the international conventions for drug control: 'Persistent or sporadic excessive use inconsistent with or unrelated to acceptable medical practice'. This is an uncomfortable definition for those who smoke tobacco and for many of those who drink alcohol, forcing them to face up to the nature of their own drug-taking behaviour. It also emphasizes the close relationship between socially acceptable drug-taking behaviour and the range of drug-related problems with which this book is largely concerned.

More recently, the WHO Expert Committee on Drug Dependence introduced the term 'harmful use': a pattern of psychoactive drug use that causes damage to health, either mental or physical. The Committee also noted that the harmful use of a drug by an individual often has adverse effects on the drug user's family, the community and society in general.

Drug dependence

The difficulties of defining the essential characteristics of drug dependence are illustrated by the changes that have taken place in the last 30 years. At one time, drug addiction and drug habituation were recognized as separate entities, with the former being more severe than the latter and distinguished on such grounds as the intensity of desire to take the drug, the tendency to increase the dose and the detrimental effect on the individual and/or society. Thus some drugs were described as habituating and others as addictive, and one individual might be considered addicted to a drug whereas another was merely habituated to the same drug. Such terms were impractical, particularly for international application and a new term, drug dependence, was introduced: 'a state, psychic and sometimes also physical, resulting from the interaction between a living organism and a drug, characterized by behavioural and other responses that always include a compulsion to take the drug on a continuous or periodic basis in order to experience psychic effects, and sometimes to avoid the discomfort of its absence. Tolerance may or may not be present'.

Within this definition are two components of very different importance – psychological dependence, without which the state of dependence cannot be said to exist, and physical dependence which may or may not be present. Thus an individual may be dependent on a drug without manifesting any physical dependence and, conversely, an individual taking drugs that cause physical but not psychological dependence, is correctly described as physically dependent, but not as drug dependent.

Because of the overwhelming importance of psychological dependence in diagnosing drug dependence, another more modern definition has been proposed: 'A cluster of physiological, behavioural and cognitive phenomena of variable intensity in which the use of a psychoactive drug (or drugs) takes on a high priority. The necessary descriptive characteristics are preoccupation with a desire to obtain and take the drug and persistent drug-taking behaviour. Determinants and the problematic consequences of drug dependence may be biological, psychological, or social, and usually interact'.

It can now be appreciated that drug abuse may occur without causing physical or psychological dependence. LSD, for example, is a common and dangerous drug of abuse, but does not induce physical or psychological dependence; indeed the sporadic abuse of most drugs is not likely to cause dependence.

Psychological dependence

It will be perceived that at the core of the definition of drug dependence lies psychic or psychological dependence upon the drug. This is a 'feeling of satisfaction and a psychic drive that requires periodic or continuous administration of the drug to produce pleasure or to avoid discomfort'. This precise but dry definition conveys nothing of what it is like to be severely psychologically dependent upon a drug. Eloquently described by those experiencing it as 'the drug calling to them' or as 'always a little geyser in there, hammering away at you to take it', the psychic drive to obtain and to take the drug is often dismissed by those who have not experienced it as a manifestation of 'weak will' or as evidence of a lack of motivation to stop. Nothing could be further from the truth; psychological dependence is an overriding compulsion to take the drug, even in the certain knowledge that it is harmful and whatever the consequences of the method of obtaining it.

Physical dependence and the withdrawal syndrome

Physical dependence is 'an adaptive state manifested by intense physical disturbances when the drug is withdrawn'. Many, but not all drugs cause physical dependence and of those that do, not all are drugs of abuse. Chlorpromazine, for example, causes physical dependence but is not usually abused. The development of physical dependence depends on the drug being administered regularly, in sufficient dosage over a period of time; the necessary dose and duration of administration depend on the particular drug and may also vary from person to person.

In the condition of physical dependence, the body becomes so 'used' or accustomed or adapted to the drug that there is little, if any, evidence that the person concerned is taking it. However, sudden drug withdrawal is followed by a specific array of symptoms and signs collectively known as the withdrawal or abstinence syndrome. The nature of the withdrawal syndrome is characteristic of each drug type, and the symptoms and signs tend to be opposite in nature to the effects of the drug when it is acutely administered. Thus, physical dependence on a stimulant drug such as amphetamine is manifested by drowsiness, apathy and depression when drug administration ceases, whereas physical dependence on a sedative drug such as a barbiturate leads to a very different type of withdrawal syndrome with hallucinations and convulsions as evidence of stimulation in certain parts of the brain. However, as sudden drug withdrawal is intensely stressful for a physically dependent individual, all the body's responses to stress are called into play and the clinical picture becomes blurred by the activity of the autonomic (involuntary) nervous system.

Although partial symptomatic relief of some of the manifestations of the withdrawal syndrome is possible using a variety of measures, the condition can be treated effectively only by administration of the drug concerned, or one of similar type. Thus, the symptoms of the opiate withdrawal syndrome are relieved only by opiates, of the amphetamine withdrawal syndrome only by amphetamines and so on. Many of the common drugs of abuse cause physical dependence and it can be readily understood that the unpleasant nature of the withdrawal syndrome – or fear of it – can increase the intensity of drug-seeking behaviour because of the need to avoid or relieve withdrawal discomfort. Sometimes, the physiological changes may be of sufficient severity to require medical treatment.

Tolerance

Tolerance is 'a state of reduced responsiveness to the effects of a drug caused by its previous administration'. Increased doses are required to produce the same magnitude of effect previously produced by a smaller dose. Many drugs, including some that are abused, induce tolerance, and therefore those who take them regularly can consume, without intoxication, far larger doses than can be tolerated by those without prior exposure. For tolerance to develop and to be maintained, the drug must be taken regularly and in sufficient dosage. If drug administration is interrupted for any reason, tolerance is lost and the high dose that was previously tolerated without adverse effect becomes as toxic as it is for the drug-naive individual. This situation arises not infrequently when a drug-dependent individual resumes drug taking after a period of abstinence – in hospital or in prison for example – and the high dose of drug that he or she had previously been taking regularly and safely may then have fatal consequences.

Tolerance does not necessarily develop equally or at the same rate to all the effects of a drug. For example, a very high degree of tolerance develops to the actions of opiates that cause analgesia, mental clouding and respiratory depression (slow and shallow breathing) so that these effects of opiates are not apparent even when the individual is consuming a very high daily dose – as long as that dose level has been reached gradually. However, little or no tolerance develops to the action of opiates on the pupil of the eye or on the bowel so that the same individual usually displays a typically constricted pupil and suffers from constipation.

Although tolerance to most of the effects of opiates is apparently open ended (the dose can be gradually increased to any level), this is not true for all drugs. A barbiturate-tolerant individual, for example, can take a dose of barbiturate that would render a non-tolerant individual comatose; there comes a point, however, when a further increase of dose will lead to severe toxicity or death even for someone who is barbiturate tolerant. In this case tolerance can be said to have reached a 'ceiling'. Tolerance is not completely drug specific. If an individual has become tolerant to the effects of heroin, for example, he or she can take large doses of any other opiate (but not of other classes of drugs). If heroin is withdrawn, the resulting abstinence syndrome can be relieved by the administration of any opiate (but not by any other type of drug). This phenomenon is known as cross-tolerance.

Mechanisms of tolerance

The mechanisms of tolerance are not fully understood and undoubtedly differ for different drugs. Changes in absorption, metabolism, distribution and excretion might all, theoretically, affect the serum concentration of a drug and consequently its effect upon target cells. For example, tolerance to barbiturates is partly due to the induction (switching on) of special enzymes in the liver (hepatic microsomal enzymes) by the barbiturates themselves. These enzymes then metabolize (breakdown) the barbiturates, which can therefore be said to speed their own destruction. An increased dose is then needed to maintain the original effect. Pharmacodynamic tolerance also occurs resulting from adaptive changes within the nervous system so that the response to the drug is reduced in the presence of the same concentration. It is likely that these changes occur at the neuronal synapses – the junction areas between different nerve cells – affecting either neurotransmitter release from one cell, or the receptors on which the neurotransmitter acts.

Relationship between tolerance and physical dependence

The nature of the relationship between tolerance and physical dependence is not clear. Some of the drugs to which tolerance develops also cause physical dependence and the drugs of abuse and dependence with which this book is mostly concerned are in this group. For these drugs, physical dependence, with unpleasant symptoms on drug withdrawal, leads to the need to take the drug regularly. This is, of course, a necessary condition for tolerance to develop, which in turn leads to escalating doses, greater physical dependence and so on. Because of this parallel development it has been suggested that a common mechanism is responsible for both phenomena.

This hypothesis probably emerged because the drugs which have been studied the longest and most intensively are the opiates, drugs to which open-ended tolerance develops rapidly and on which physical dependence is severe and easily recognizable. Similarly tolerance develops to some of the effects of alcohol, barbiturates and other sedatives, and physical dependence on these drugs is again well known. From observations such as these grew the belief that tolerance and physical dependence are both manifestations of a single, as yet unknown neural mechanism. However, tolerance is a very general phenomenon, observed with many drugs. It is after all very common in medical practice to start with a small dose of a drug and to increase it gradually as the patient becomes tolerant of the side effects, and physical dependence does not develop in every situation in which tolerance develops.

Perhaps the best way to understand the relationship between tolerance and physical dependence is to say that the existence of tolerance, by permitting the administration of large doses of the drug, enables or enhances the development of severe physical dependence, if the drug has a dependence-producing liability as well. Undoubtedly, the two conditions, of tolerance and physical dependence, occur after chronic administration of a wide range of drugs (including tricyclic antidepressants, phenothiazines and anticholinergics) that are not self-administered by animals or usually abused by humans. This serves to emphasize the point that neither tolerance nor physical dependence, separately or together, are sufficient to cause a true state of dependence on a drug. For that, the psychological element, the inner compulsion, must always be present.

Types of drug dependence

The definition of drug dependence used in this chapter is broad-based and embraces dependence on a very wide range of drugs, some of which are used medically (e.g., opiates, sedative hypnotics) while others (khat, hallucinogens) are not. It is perhaps not surprising that the characteristics of the dependent state vary according to the type of drug. Some drugs cause marked physical dependence with a correspondingly severe withdrawal syndrome, others cause less physical dependence but profound psychological dependence. The extent to which tolerance develops also varies with different classes of drugs. Caffeine, consumed as it is by most people in tea or coffee, produces a limited degree of psychological dependence sometimes manifested as 'I can't get going in the morning without my cup of tea', and a mild state of physical dependence with headaches on drug withdrawal. This degree of dependence is not particularly harmful either to the individual or to society, although it should be noted that a more severe degree of dependence on caffeine (often in cola-type drinks) may sometimes arise.

However, several classes of dependence-producing drugs affect the central nervous system profoundly, producing stimulation or depression and disturbances in perception, mood, thinking, behaviour or motor function. The use of these drugs may produce individual, public health and social problems and is, therefore, a justifiable cause for concern.

There is no wholly satisfactory way of classifying drugs of abuse and dependence because drugs with similar pharmacological effects may produce quite different types of dependence. Cannabis, for example, has both sedative and hallucinogenic effects but the pattern of its abuse, by millions of people worldwide, is quite different to the abuse of barbiturates which are sedatives, and LSD which is a hallucinogen.

The Tenth Revision of the International Classification of Diseases (ICD-10) recognizes the psychoactive drugs or drug classes listed in Table 1.1, the self-administration of which may produce mental and behavioural disorders, including dependence (see Chapter 4).

Abuse and dependence on a wide range of other drugs also occurs. For example, abuse of minor analgesics, such as aspirin, is so widespread that it has been estimated that there may be as many as a quarter of a million analgesic abusers in Britain alone. This problem is frequently ignored in studies of drug abuse and dependence, firstly because it involves drugs over which there are no legal controls (or only very limited ones) and which may be easily obtained from outlets such as newsagents, supermarkets and even slot-machines, as well as from pharmacists. Secondly, it is easy to dismiss it as uninformed self-medication by a group ignorant of the dangers of excessive use of these drugs. In many ways, however, those who abuse minor analgesics (and other drugs not included on the above list) resemble those who abuse illicit or restricted drugs: they often deny their drug-taking and may go to considerable lengths to conceal it; they often admit that they take the drugs for the feeling of well-being that they induce and, in the case of aspirin, specifically to experience the dangerous state of salicylism (aspirin intoxication) that they find pleasurable. Above all, they are psychologically dependent on these drugs – showing craving, drug-seeking behaviour and an inability to stop taking them.

In addition to the drugs already discussed, there are many other drugs each of which is abused by just a few people who may then become dependent on them. Some, such as the antiparkinsonian anticholinergic, drugs, may be taken for their psychic effects. Others, such as purgatives or anticoagulants, may be taken to produce fictitious disease, with those who abuse

Table 1.1 Drugs recognized by the ICD-10

Alcohol

Opioids: including naturally occurring opiates (e.g., opium, morphine, codeine), synthetic or semisynthetic opiates (e.g., methadone, pethidine, dipipanone, dextromoramide) and opiate agonist–antagonists (e.g., pentazocine, buprenorphine)

Cannabinoids: preparations of cannabis sativa (e.g., marijuana, ganja, hashish)

Sedative hypnotics: including barbiturates, non-barbiturate sedatives (e.g., chloral, methaqualone, glutethimide, meprobamate) and benzodiazepines

Cocaine

Other stimulants: including amphetamines and similar stimulants (e.g., methylphenidate, phenmetrazine), anorectic agents, (e.g., diethylpropion, phentermine) and khat (preparations of *Catha edulis*)

Hallucinogens: including LSD, mescaline, psilocybin

Tobacco

Volatile solvents: including substances, such as toluene, acetone, carbon tetrachloride

Multiple drug use and other psychoactive substances

them often concealing this fact, and seeking and apparently enjoying repeated, intensive medical investigation and care. Finally, some drugs prescribed for somatic disease may be taken excessively, primarily to avoid unpleasant withdrawal symptoms although eventually a true dependent state may develop. For example, increasing doses of ergotamine, prescribed for migraine, may be consumed to avoid withdrawal headaches, and increasing doses of steroids may be taken to avoid unpleasant psychological effects on drug withdrawal. The family, friends and colleagues of doctors as well as doctors themselves, may be vulnerable to this type of drug abuse if their powers of persuasion overcome normal professional prescribing practices.

These, much less common types of drug dependence have been introduced into the discussion because their existence illustrates and emphasizes a very important point – that abuse and dependence do not only occur with 'dangerous' psychoactive drugs. In other words, dependence is not just a manifestation of a specific drug effect, but is a behaviour profoundly influenced by the individual personality and the environment, as well as by the specific drugs that are available. As a behaviour, drug dependence is similar to compulsive gambling and compulsive eating, and what all have in common is an overwhelming psychic drive to behave in a certain way. A better understanding of this compulsion will enable us to reach out towards a better understanding of drug dependence and a whole range of similar human behaviours.

Causes of drug dependence

The cause or causes of drug dependence are not known. More specifically, it is not known why some people but not others in the same situation start experimenting with drugs, or why some, but not others, then continue to take them and, finally, why some but not all become dependent on drugs.

When seeking causes it is easy to limit the scenario to that of the local problems which receive so much publicity – poverty, unemployment, break-up of local communities, drug pushers, organized crime, breakdown of parental authority. These often repeated phrases spring to mind and they may well be contributory factors, as far as the European and North American drug scene is involved, in the ever increasing number of people abusing or dependent on drugs – but they are not the causes of drug dependence.

It must never be forgotten that drug dependence is not a new phenomenon; the use of drugs is probably as old as man himself and dependence has been recognized for thousands of years. It occurs in every culture and any theory of drug dependence should be sufficiently general to encompass the vast range of dependent behaviour that exists today – for example, the young drug abuser, taking a wide range of drugs, the housewife dependent on benzodiazepines, the adolescent sniffing glue, the Middle Eastern opium smoker, a Jamaican cannabis smoker, the American free-basing cocaine, the Yemeni khat chewer, the mystic seeking truth with LSD, the doctor injecting himself with pentazocine, to describe just a few. It is perhaps not surprising, therefore, that there are almost as many theories about dependence and its causes as there are types of dependence behaviour. While recognizing that very different situations may share hidden commonalities, it is fair to comment that many theories seem to say more about the viewpoint of the investigator than about the dependent state they attempt to describe, and, as such, they are not helpful in getting to grips with the phenomenon of drug dependence.

It is generally accepted that drug-related behaviour is the consequence of interaction between the drug, the individual and society – and the keyword in this well-worn phrase must be 'interaction'. None of the component factors alone is sufficient to cause drug dependence and their relative importance varies in different circumstances.

The drug

The availability of the drug is obviously a prerequisite for abuse and dependence, and the rapid transport methods of the modern world ensure that most drugs are obtainable everywhere. Transportation of drugs is not, of course, a recent occurrence – opium was moved half-way round the world centuries ago – but modern communications have greatly increased the speed and volume of this traffic. It is easy to be misled by reports in the media of vast quantities of illicit drugs coming into developed countries and to believe that the traffic is entirely one way. Going in the opposite direction, however, are equally vast quantities of alcohol and manufactured drugs which pose problems of their own to the countries that import them, and which are as vital to the economies of the exporting countries as the highly profitable cash crops of illicit drugs are to their producers.

In addition to the availability of a drug, the form in which it is available is very important. Modern chemical techniques permit the extraction of highly purified and very potent forms of drugs, making them easier to transport and smuggle, and because of their greater potency, much more efficient at causing dependence. For example, one can only conjecture how long it would take a South American Indian to chew sufficient coca leaves to obtain the same dose of cocaine as that in a single vial of 'crack', the purified version of cocaine currently in vogue in the USA; and it is unlikely that the Indian ever achieves blood levels (or nervous system levels) of cocaine sufficient to cause serious dependence. Again, this is nothing new: the ability to distil alcohol must have had equally dramatic effects when it was first discovered. Similarly, it can be understood that the invention and dispersal of the syringe and needle has had a profound effect upon drug abuse and dependence, by virtue of the ability to deliver large doses of dependence-producing drugs, straight into the bloodstream and thence to the brain.

Although a few people become dependent upon apparently extraordinary drugs, such as laxatives, most drug dependence is concerned with just a few types of psychoactive substances. The question arises therefore as to how these drugs produce dependence. What is it that they have in common? It is immediately apparent that they have very different chemical and pharmacological properties. For example, cocaine and amphetamine are central nervous stimulants while opiates and sedative hypnotic drugs are depressants. Although the effects of cocaine and amphetamine are in some ways remarkably similar, there is no cross-tolerance so that the abstinence syndrome of one is not relieved by the other. Cocaine too has local anaesthetic properties, which amphetamine does not, but other local anaesthetic drugs do not cause dependence. Equally obvious pharmacological differences exist between the different classes of abused drugs but the one factor that all drugs with a strong dependence potential share, is a rewarding or reinforcing property. This is best demonstrated in a laboratory situation where an animal (usually a rat or a monkey) obtains a dose of a drug, such as cocaine, by pressing a lever. Thereafter the animal will press the lever repeatedly to obtain more cocaine, and as it receives more, will press the lever more and more rapidly. In other words, cocaine increases – or reinforces – behaviour resulting in its own administration, and is said to be a primary reinforcer and to have primary reinforcing properties. Not all drugs possess this property; those that do and which are administered by animals in a laboratory situation are the same as those commonly abused by humans. They include stimulants (amphetamine, cocaine), opiates, sedative hypnotics, alcohol and some, but not all hallucinogens (e.g., phencyclidine). Of these, cocaine and heroin stand out as the most powerful reinforcers, as defined by the rapidity of acquisition of self-administration.

It is not known why drugs with such different pharmacological properties should share the property of primary reinforcement, and the underlying neural mechanisms are not fully understood. They are, however, the subject of intense research, and it has been suggested that reinforcement works by centrally activating endogenous reward circuits which evolved, not for the sake of cocaine or opiates, but to reward behaviour such as obtaining food, water, warmth and shelter – all essential to survival. It has been found, for example, that stimulating particular sites in the brain via electrodes is positively reinforcing, particularly at the lateral hypothalamic level of the medial mid-brain bundle and in the ventral tegmentum. Several lines of evidence suggest that dopaminergic pathways* are implicated within this ventral tegmental reward system, with the main site of action being the nucleus accumbens. Dependence-producing drugs, it is suggested, activate this reward system, 'switching on' the circuits at different points. Stimulants and cocaine, for example, lead to a functional increase in the levels of dopamine and other neurotransmitters within the nucleus accumbens, while opiates and alcohol increase the activity of cells in the ventral tegmental area.

It seems, therefore, that psychological dependence, which is central to any concept of drug dependence, is the real life manifestation of the reinforcing property of a drug, demonstrable by laboratory animals. Of course, there is a difference between a rat or monkey pressing a lever to get

*Neural pathways within the brain with dopamine as the main neurotransmitter.

a dose of drug and an individual's overwhelming craving for it. There are, however, certain similarities between the two conditions: the monkey will press the lever thousands of times just to get a dose of a powerfully reinforcing drug and, given unlimited access to it, may stop eating food altogether and will increase its intake of drug to the point of severe toxicity and death. There are obvious parallels with human drug-seeking behaviour so intense that it disrupts all normal activities and sometimes so self-destructive that the individual dies as a consequence.

It should therefore be understood that the reinforcing drug does not necessarily produce a pleasurable state and, if it does, it is not exclusively the pleasurable state that leads to drug-seeking behaviour. In other words, the monkey, or the human, is not just (if at all) taking the drug for enjoyment, but because it (or he or she) has to. Many drugs of abuse also cause physical dependence and the rigours of the abstinence syndrome, or fear of it, are another reason for continuing to take the drug. Although many opiate-dependent individuals claim that this is why they cannot stop taking opiates, it is not the only reason. Even if they are provided with sufficient opiate to prevent the onset of withdrawal symptoms, drug-seeking behaviour often persists – a manifestation of the powerful reinforcing properties of opiates.

Psychological dependence on a drug can therefore be presented as a direct effect of a drug; some drugs cause psychological dependence, some do not. If those that do are abused, they are likely to cause dependence – the 'drive to take the drug on a continuous or periodic basis to experience psychic effects'. Some drugs of abuse, particularly cocaine and heroin, cause intense psychological dependence; others (e.g., cannabis) are much less potent in this respect.

The people who take drugs also vary tremendously in their response to drugs, from those who are very sensitive to a particular drug, requiring only a small dose to experience its effects, to those who require a large dose. This is true for all classes of drugs and is particularly apparent in the case of psychoactive substances where the suggested therapeutic dose range may be very wide. It does not seem surprising, therefore, that a drug that is known to cause psychological dependence may do so rapidly in some individuals and slowly or negligibly in others, and it is possible to reconcile apparently conflicting accounts of 'being hooked after the first dose' with stories of long-term, occasional, non-compulsive use of the same drug.

Individual personality

The underlying reason for such differing vulnerabilities is very interesting, or would be if it were understood. There have been many attempts to define the psychological characteristics of a dependence-prone personality and even to demonstrate that certain personality types develop substance-specific dependence – in other words, that alcoholics are a different 'type' to those dependent on heroin, who in turn are different to those dependent on cocaine.

Many studies have shown that there is indeed an increased incidence of personality disorder among drug addicts. For example, application of the Minnesota Multiphasic Personality Inventory to opiate users showed that they scored higher than expected for psychopathic deviance. However, when the Eysenck Personality Inventory was applied to opiate users, they scored higher on neuroticism than normals (but lower than neurotic or alcoholic patients) but did not score highly on extroversion. They did not therefore fit Eysenck's definition of 'psychopathic'. Another study asserted that 73–90% of opiate addicts were diagnosed as having some sort of personality disorder, although this must mean that up to a quarter did not, which itself is an important and interesting observation. It has also been shown that there is a higher incidence of drug abuse among those with personality disorder than in those without. Therefore, while it is fair to conclude that there is an epidemiological association between drug abuse and personality disorder, no deductions can be made about causality. Most studies have compared drug-dependent with non-dependent individuals and it would be just as reasonable to conclude that prolonged drug taking had affected the results of personality testing as to assume that personality disorder had caused the drug dependence. Thus, behaviour such as crime or prostitution, often perceived as maladaptive behaviour and evidence of underlying personality disorder, may in fact be highly adaptive behaviour, carried out in an attempt to get money to sustain an ever-growing, irresistible drug habit.

Another problem is that any one study usually concentrates on a particular, highly selected sub-group of drug-dependent subjects, such as those in prison or in hospital, who are probably unrepresentative of the drug-dependent population as a whole. In addition, institutionalization and other factors may affect the results of personality testing. Clearly, what is needed is knowledge of the personality before drug taking started, but prospective personality testing, with a waiting period to see who later becomes a drug abuser, is very difficult to carry out. Retrospective personality assessment, by asking about early relationships, school records, truancy, employment, etc., before drug abuse started is notoriously difficult to assess and very unreliable.

Bearing all these limitations in mind, the conclusion of many investigators is that drug-dependent individuals have 'personality disorders' in excess of their prevalence in the general population, and the terms often used to describe them include 'immature', 'unable to delay gratification', 'difficulty forming stable relationships', and so on. There are also indications that they show more 'neuroticism' and 'hostility' than non-users. This seems a long way from a description of dependence-prone personality, although there may be personality traits which change the likelihood of an individual becoming dependent on drugs.

Those who abuse drugs undoubtedly do so for many different reasons both stated and unconscious. It is a behaviour in industrialized countries that often starts in adolescence or young adulthood, and research indicates that the single personality dimension most closely linked with drug abuse by this age group is lack of traditional values. This may be manifested by rebelliousness, resistance to social structures, disregard of social expectations and a willingness to participate in deviant activities. It is therefore not surprising that those who abuse drugs also show other patterns of deviant behaviour, such as truanting from school and sexual promiscuity, and that drugs may be abused as an expression of independence and sometimes of overt hostility. Such behaviour is often perceived by the young as adult and sophisticated and may be one way of gaining peer approval and acceptance into a group when conventional family groups and social values are being rejected.

Another motivation for abusing drugs is often curiosity – curiosity about their effects combined with a desire for new, pleasurable, thrilling and even dangerous experiences.

These two factors, curiosity and rebelliousness, both common and normal in adolescence, probably account for the high incidence of drug abuse in this age group. Such curiosity is closely related to 'novelty-seeking', one of three personality traits identified by Cloninger in his neurobiological learning model for drug dependence. The other traits are harm avoidance and reward dependence. According to Cloninger, these heritable tendencies reflect activity in specific neural pathways and are associated with particular types of dependence behaviour. 'Novelty seeking' individuals, with enhanced activity in the dopaminergic ventral tegmental reward system, find the use of opiates, stimulants and alcohol reinforcing. Harm avoidance is associated with serotonergic neurones in the septohippocampal system, and benzodiazepines act on this system by enhancing γ-aminobutyric acid (GABA) inhibition of serotonergic neurones. Reward dependence involves noradrenergic neurones, particularly in the locus coeruleus. Such biological differences may explain why some, but not all, adolescents succumb. Of course, the development of adolescent personality is heavily dependent on both inheritance and childhood experience. Loss of a parent, parental conflict, lack of appropriate affection and guidance, and the type of parental behaviour to which the child is exposed, appear to be important environmental factors in personality development and, therefore, albeit indirectly, in potential drug-taking behaviour.

Satisfactory family relationships and climate, emotional support, and moderation in the use of alcohol are influences that appear to delay or diminish adolescent initiation into drug use. These are influences that are developed over a long period of time and attempts to make up for their absence by measures such as a sharp increase in parental control of the adolescent's behaviour may lead to increased rather than diminished drug abuse. It is interesting that while parental use of alcohol seems to be a strong interpersonal predictor of adolescent alcohol use, peer cannabis use appears to be the strongest interpersonal predictor of cannabis use, and family/best friend's use of other illicit drugs appear to be among the better interpersonal predictors of adolescent use of these substances.

Other reasons for the initiation of drug abuse may be of greater importance at different ages and in different cultures. For example, the consumption of sedatives and tranquillizers by older people may begin as self-medication, or as treatment prescribed by a doctor for anxiety or insomnia. Drugs may be taken to overcome hunger or fatigue, to enhance sexual performance or for religious purposes – as an aid to meditation or to induce mystical states.

The reasons for continuing to use a drug may or may not be the same as those that led to its original consumption. If, for example, the anxiety-provoking situation that made tranquillizers necessary persists, it is not surprising if their use continues. If drug use which started out of curiosity leads to acceptance within an attractive peer group, it too is likely to continue. Again, if drug use produces feelings of ease and relaxation or provides escape from immediate problems, there is every reason to expect it to persist. It is obvious, therefore, that in addition to the primary reinforcing properties of the drug itself, non-pharmacological consequences may be rewarding and thus function as reinforcers too. In other words, repetitive and persistent drug taking can be seen as a learned behaviour, and more specifically as an operant behaviour, established and maintained by its own consequences. For a drug that induces physical dependence, the instant relief of the symptoms of withdrawal brought about by drug administration is instantly rewarding and it can be argued that in this case drug taking is under the control of aversive stimuli and is continued to avoid the unpleasant experience of the abstinence syndrome. Environmental stimuli associated with drug taking may also assume importance in the maintenance of drug-taking behaviour. For intravenous drug abusers, for example, the

syringe and needle may become secondary reinforcers because of their association with the rewards of the drug itself; measures aimed at the extinction
of such secondary reinforcers may make a significant contribution to the
treatment of drug dependence.

The importance of the individual personality interacting with the effect
of the drug is emphasized and illustrated by two descriptions of somewhat
different types of drug-taking behaviour. The first is the individual prescribed opiates for severe pain; if the prescriptions continue for some time,
the patient becomes physically dependent on opiates and, were they to be
suddenly stopped, the symptoms and signs of the withdrawal syndrome
would be manifest. In practice, this rarely if ever occurs because the most
common situation for prolonged prescription of opiates is in terminal
disease and prescription continues until death. Usually, therefore, neither
doctor nor patient is aware of the existence of physical dependence. It is
interesting that tolerance does not always develop, or at any rate, not to
the level that is common with recreational use, and continuing escalation
of dose is rarely necessary to control pain. It is also puzzling that there is
usually no evidence of psychological dependence either – no craving, or
demands for drugs or for increasing doses although this behaviour is
common in 'recreational' opiate-dependent individuals even when they are
receiving a regular prescription. These observations show that opiates,
despite their powerful reinforcing properties, do not necessarily or always
cause dependence. Psychological dependence does develop in some individuals treated with opiates, usually those being treated for chronic pain, often
of indeterminate origin. Such patients are described as 'therapeutic addicts'
and although they may be regarded as the innocent 'victims' of medical
treatment, their behaviour is similar in many ways to that of the much
more common non-therapeutic addicts. The second example is of those who
are dependent on 'unusual' drugs, which do not have primary reinforcing
properties and which are not abused by animals in a laboratory situation.
The personality of the people who do abuse them seems to be the 'cause' of
the behaviour in this case, rather than any innate property of the drug.

It is, of course, of considerable interest to know whether individual
factors contributing to drug dependence can be inherited. Most research
has focused on alcohol abuse which, it has been noted, tends to 'run in
families' and the question then arises as to whether this is due to 'nature'
or 'nurture'. The finding in many studies is that alcoholism in the biological
family predicts alcoholism in children reared away from home, while the
converse is not true. This suggests an inherited, and therefore genetic, basis
for at least some types of alcoholism and this is supported by biological
research on the enzyme aldehyde dehydrogenase. This enzyme metabolizes

alcohol in the liver, but some individuals possess it only as an inactive variant; consumption of alcohol then leads on to an accumulation of acetaldehyde and an unpleasant, toxic reaction which discourages further consumption. There is a low incidence of alcoholism among this population, supporting genetic theories for the basis of alcoholism. It must be remembered, however, that this is a quite specific example and cannot be extrapolated to a general theory on hereditary factors in drug dependence.

Society

What then of society? What is the role of society in the triple interaction that leads to drug abuse behaviour? It is quite understandable that environmental factors should be blamed for drug abuse, particularly when its prevalence starts to rise sharply, and in Western urban society, poverty and unemployment are the usual candidates for blame. They may indeed be relevant, although it must be remembered that not everyone in a particular environment – however deprived – abuses or becomes dependent on drugs. Equally, there are frequent stories which often receive even greater attention in the media, of abuse and dependence among the affluent, educated, employed, etc. Ultimately, of course, environmental factors such as these are local and inapplicable to general and global theories of drug abuse. Undoubtedly, however, society does play a significant role in the development and control of drug-abuse problems and there are various sociological theories of addiction, seeking to find causes in the way that individuals intereact with society as a whole. However, no theory provides a satisfactory explanation for the wide range of addictive behaviours that exists. Instead, they tend to focus on causes of addiction in urban, deprived youth. The important theory of 'anomie', for example, describes the goals, the culture, the norms to achieve these goals, and the 'institutionalized means' which is the distribution of opportunities available for achieving the goals. If there is marked disjunction between these factors, socially structured strain occurs that can be dealt with in various ways. One way is to reject the goals and to 'retreat'. Alternatively, goals such as status and influence may be achieved by illegal methods. According to this theory, drug use becomes a way of life in its own right, giving the user a sense of identity and a clearer role. Another theory is that of deviancy classification, according to which, controls introduced by society in response to deviant behaviour, increase the deviancy, leading to further controls and so on. Believers in this theory would support the legalisation/decriminalisation of drug use although there is no clear evidence that introducing 'controls' does, in fact, increase consumption.

Psychoactive substances have been known and available to humans for thousands of years. For most of that time their use was geographically restricted and under societal constraints, and (with the exception of distilled alcohol) the drugs themselves were available only as crude plant products which contained only small quantities of the active drug.

Within the last few decades several changes have taken place simultaneously, which together have had a profound influence on drug-taking behaviour. Firstly, as already mentioned, highly potent psychoactive substances are widely available way beyond their societies of origin and therefore without the cultural traditions that might naturally restrict their use and abuse. In the case of manufactured psychoactive drugs, these are of such recent origin that cultural traditions controlling their use are as yet rudimentary or non-existent. More important, however, than availability is a general attitude to drugs and drug taking, an attitude which has become so widespread that it can probably be described as truly global. For example, in nearly all countries, two drugs – alcohol and tobacco – are recognized as legal, recreational drugs, and even though the former is prohibited in Islamic countries, few people would care to guarantee that it is not consumed there. Of course, there is nothing new about this situation, both alcohol and tobacco have been widely used for centuries, but what has been happening over those centuries is their gradual absorption into the fabric of society. They have become incorporated into every aspect of daily life – they are widely advertised, they are seen being consumed on films and television, they are present at sports events. The cost of an average 'habit' of these drugs forms part of the cost of the living index. Revenue from their taxation is so enormous that few governments would care to do without it. They affect the employment of millions. Consumption of these two drugs is therefore, by any standard, perceived as 'normal' and ordinary.

More recently, over decades rather than centuries, many other psychoactive substances have been attaining a similar status. A vast number of psychoactive drugs are now manufactured for the treatment of psychiatric illness, and indeed they are so effective that many patients who would once have been confined to mental hospitals for life can now live within the community. Much of the fear of mental illness has been allayed and there is less stigma attached to it. It has become correspondingly easier for people to admit to symptoms of mental stress, knowing that effective and acceptable treatment is available. Often these symptoms are attributable not to illness, but to personal and interpersonal problems, and whereas they would once have been dealt with or suffered within the community, pharmacological solutions are now sought and provided. Gradually, these manufactured drugs are being incorporated into daily life, in the same way as tobacco and alcohol, although not yet to the same extent. Already, however, they are shared and borrowed like cigarettes (can you lend me a sleeping pill?'); they are taken like alcohol, and sometimes together with alcohol, to achieve a relaxed mental state; they are mentioned casually in books and on television. Everyone by now knows what Valium is. The pharmaceutical industry that manufactures them makes significant contributions to employment and the economy. Many of these drugs, like alcohol and tobacco, cause psychological dependence and their widespread abuse in the form of drug overdoses has become virtually endemic in some places.

Thus we find ourselves in a society that is drug orientated to a degree previously unknown, at a time when very pure and potent forms of drugs, such as heroin and cocaine with a severe dependence liability, are widely available. When seen in this context, the illicit use of drugs by young people who have grown up surrounded by drug-taking behaviour – albeit legal drug taking – is perhaps an understandable, if undesirable behaviour. It is further reinforced by the influence of the peer group, which may be another important determinant among the young who are normally introduced to drug taking by friends. Participating in this activity permits entry to a group and the drug taking in turn reinforces the identity of the group, becoming a ritualized behaviour. It has also been found that as a drug becomes freely available and acceptable in society, those using it heavily and becoming dependent on it are less likely to show evidence of pre-existing personality disorders. These psychologically 'normal' individuals are often able to stop their drug use if their sociocultural environment alters, and the drug is no longer available and acceptable. Personality variables associated with drug users in college tend to be those for the age group as a whole. In other words, the more normal drug taking becomes, the more normal are the drug abusers.

Clearly it is a much smaller step into drug abuse and dependence now than it was when psychoactive drugs were medicines that were unfamiliar to the general population and taken, if at all, only for the treatment of specified illness. It is this total background acceptance of drug-taking behaviour that is the most significant change that has taken place in society in recent years and it has set the scene for new problems of abuse and dependence.

References and further reading

Cami J, Bigelow GE, Griffiths RR & Drummond DC (eds) (1991). Clinical testing of drug abuse liability (Special issue). *British Journal of Addiction*, **86**, 1525–1652.
Craig RJ (1982). Personality characteristics of heroin addicts: a review of empirical research 1976–79. *International Journal of Addiction*, **17**, 227–248.

Comparative Analysis of Illicit Drug Strategy (1992). Monograph series No. 18. Australian Government Publishing Service, Canberra.

Hammersley R (1994). A digest of memory phenomena for addiction research. *Addiction*, **89**, 283–293.

International Narcotics Control Board (1992). *Report of the INCB for 1992. (E/INCB/1992/1)*. United Nations Publication, New York.

Johns A (1990). Identifying the problem. In: Ghodse AH & Maxwell D (eds). *Substance Abuse and Dependence*, 5–29. Macmillan Press, London.

Khantzian EJ & Treece CJ (1977). Psychodynamics of drug dependence: an overview. In: Blaine JD & Julius DA (eds). *Psychodynamics of Drug Dependence*. NIDA Research Monograph 12. National Institute of Drug Abuse, Rockville.

Nelson JE, Pearson HW, Sayers M & Glynn TJ (eds) (1982). *Guide to Drug Abuse Research Terminology*. NIDA Research Issues 26. Department of Health & Human Services, Rockville.

Nurco DN (1987). Drug addiction and crime: a complicated issue. *British Journal of Addiction*, **82**, 7–9.

Nutt DJ (1993). Neurochemistry of drugs other than alcohol. *Current Opinion in Psychiatry*, **3**, 395–402.

Oyefeso A (1994). Sociocultural aspects of substance use and misuse. *Current Opinion in Psychiatry*, **7**, **No. 3**, 273–277.

West R (1989). The Psychological basis of addiction. *International Review of Psychiatry*, **1**, 71–79.

Widiger TA & Smith GT (1994). Substance use disorder: abuse, dependence and dyscontrol. *Addiction*, **89**, 267–282.

Wikler A (1971). Some implications of conditioning theory for problems of drug abuse. *Behavioural Science*, **16**, 92.

Wise RA (1984). Neural mechanisms of the reinforcing action of cocaine. In: Grabowski J (ed.) *Cocaine: Pharmacology, Effects and Treatment of Abuse*, 15–33. NIDA Research Monograph 50. Department of Health & Human Services, Rockville.

World Health Organization (1974). *WHO Expert Committee on Drug Dependence. Twentieth Report*.WHO Technical Report Series No. 551. WHO, Geneva.

World Health Organization (1975). *Evaluation of Dependence Liability and Dependence Potential of Drugs*. WHO Technical Report Series No. 577. WHO, Geneva.

World Health Organization (1981). Nomenclature and classification of drug and alcohol-related problems: a WHO memorandum. *Bulletin of the World Health Organization*, **59**, 225–242.

World Health Organization (1993). *WHO Expert Committee on Drug Dependence. Twenty-Eight Report*. WHO Technical Report Series 836. WHO, Geneva.

2

Drug dependence in the UK
– and elsewhere

In the midst of current concern about drug-related problems and of endless dialogue about what should or should not be 'done' about them, it is interesting and valuable to consider the historical background to the present situation: interesting because it increases our understanding about how present policies have evolved, and useful because of the possibility of learning from previous experience.

Drug dependence in the UK

It is perhaps surprising to learn that opium was widely used in Britain during most of the nineteenth century – so widely used, so ordinary that it aroused little interest or concern. It was available in a variety of patent medicines, obtainable from any sort of shop without any legal restriction, and crude opium was sold for eating or smoking. The first attempts to restrict its sale were probably more for the sake of pharmacists trying to obtain a monopoly of this profitable trade, than because of concern about the effects of opiates. Medical interest in the topic became keener with the introduction of the hypodermic syringe and the concept of 'morphinomania' emerged. Despite an awareness of the addictive properties of opiates no prescription was necessary to obtain opium or its preparations. These could be purchased from a pharmacist by anyone known or personally introduced to the pharmacist, as long as the Poisons Register was signed.

Growing international concern about opiate use led to the First Opium Convention in the Hague in 1912 and Britain, as one of the signatories, agreed to the principle of adopting controls over opium, morphine and cocaine. However no legislation was passed until concern about the use of cocaine by members of the armed forces led to the Defence of the Realm Regulations (1916) which made it an offence to give or sell cocaine to soldiers. Subsequently the Regulations were changed so that only authorized people (members of the medical profession and those receiving a prescription) were allowed to be in possession of cocaine.

After the First World War, the 1920 and 1923 Dangerous Drugs Acts were passed and for the first time a doctor's prescription was necessary to obtain opium and its derivatives and cocaine. In the first year of operation there were only 67 prosecutions of which 58 were for cocaine, and in 1927 there were only two cocaine prosecutions. Thus it was possible for Britain to say with pride – and some complacency – that drug addiction was not prevalent.

The birth of the 'British system'

The problem then arose about whether the prescription of opiates to addicts constituted legitimate medical treatment. In the USA, for example, the 1914 Harrison Act had decided that it did not; the right of doctors to prescribe opiates was severely restricted and their prescription to regular users was illegal unless it was part of an attempt to cure (detoxify) the habit.

In Britain the Ministry of Health set up a committee to examine this question. The Rolleston Committee as it came to be known after its chairman, Sir Humphrey Rolleston, was composed of members of the medical profession anxious, no doubt, to safeguard their valued clinical freedom to prescribe whatever they thought fit for any patient for whom they considered it necessary. At the time that the committee was deliberating, many addicts, probably the majority, were either members of the medical or nursing professions ('professional' addicts), who had easy access to drugs, or those who had become addicted during the course of treatment with opiates ('therapeutic' addicts). There were also a few non-therapeutic addicts in London, obtaining their heroin largely by trips to the continent. In general these people were of 'good' social standing and did not form any sort of criminal network. It is not surprising that the equally respectable members of the Rolleston Committee did not perceive these addicts as criminals and thought that they should continue to be treated as patients. The report (1926) therefore recommended that heroin could be prescribed to addicts if, after every effort had been made to cure them, complete withdrawal produced serious symptoms which could not be satisfactorily treated, or if the patient, while capable of leading a useful and normal life so long as he/she took the drug of addiction, ceased to be able to do so if it were withdrawn. In other words, maintenance – the legal supply of a daily dose of opiate to an opiate-dependent individual – was permitted.

With the Rolleston Report arose the so-called 'British system' for dealing with addiction. A system was never planned or even visualized, but the idea that addicts were patients and not criminals and could receive drugs on prescription contrasted sharply with the situation in the USA. There, where opiate maintenance had been banned, drug addiction increased rapidly and was associated with major crime, while in the UK the drug scene remained small and stable. This was attributed, complacently, to the correctness of the British approach which was promoted into a 'system'.

From about 1950, however, it became apparent that there was an increasing interest in drugs by young people. This was shown by the sharply increasing number of prosecutions for cannabis offences. At first this largely involved West End jazz clubs and seamen, but it spread from different sea ports to many parts of the country. At this time too, occurred the first serious cases of drug trafficking involving heroin, cocaine and morphine stolen from pharmacies.

An awareness of the changing drug scene prompted the Ministry of Health to convene an Interdepartmental Committee on Drug Addiction, chaired by Sir Russell Brain. As a result of enquiries made in 1958–59, the Brain Committee came to the conclusion that the problem of addiction was static and that no special measures needed to be taken. This first report (1961) was soon overtaken by events as the number of heroin addicts known to the Home Office began to increase rapidly, approximately doubling every 2 years, from 94 in 1960 to 175 in 1962 and to 342 in 1964. At this time, it should be emphasized, there was no compulsory notification of addicts to the Home Office and statistics were complied from an inspection of pharmacists' records and from doctors, police, prisons and hospitals.

An important cause of the increasing number of addicts identified in the early 1960s was over-prescribing of heroin and cocaine by a few doctors who soon achieved notoriety and who provided surplus heroin for addicts to peddle on the black market. If it seems an exaggeration to claim that over-prescribing could precipitate such a crisis, it should be noted that one doctor alone prescribed 600 000 tablets, equivalent to 6 kg of heroin, in the course of 1 year. Even today, in a much larger drug scene, a seizure of 6 kg of pure heroin would be regarded as a major haul. As a result of this situation, Canadian addicts came to Britain because of the ease with which they could obtain heroin here: as a group of experienced drug users with a large daily habit, they brought with them knowledge and experience of an organized black market and undoubtedly contributed to its organization here.

The Dangerous Drugs Act 1967

By 1964 it was apparent that the situation was worsening rapidly and the Brain Committee was hurriedly reconvened. Its second report, published in

1965, formed the basis of the Dangerous Drugs Act of 1967. The most important features of it were:

1   compulsory notification of addicts to the Home Office;
2   the limitation of the right to prescribe heroin and cocaine to addicts to those doctors holding a special licence from the Home Office;
3   the setting up of special clinics to treat drug addicts.

Central to the recommendations of the Brain Committee was the belief that the British system of legal prescription of drugs to addicts had been responsible for the fairly low and static addiction figures between 1926 and 1960. Undercutting the illegal supplier had apparently prevented the development of an organized criminal black market, whereas in the USA where drugs were not prescribed there was a highly organized black market and the prevalence of addiction had increased rapidly. The comfortable situation in Britain seemed to have changed only because of irresponsible prescribing by some doctors and it was believed that the resumption of 'sensible' prescribing policies would restore the status quo. To prevent this problem recurring, only specially licensed doctors, usually working in the new treatment clinics, would be allowed to prescribe to addicts and the compulsory notification of addicts would permit ongoing monitoring of the situation.

In retrospect this interpretation of the rising addiction rate was an oversimplification. It is far more likely that between 1926 and 1960, because of the prevailing social conditions and the generally low availability of drugs, Britain had only a small addiction problem which could be satisfactorily managed by the policy of legal prescription. However, by the early 1960s social changes had accelerated and the demand for drugs grew and unscrupulous doctors took advantage of the liberal system to respond to this demand.

Home Office statistics show that the total number of known addicts increased rapidly between 1961 and 1967. The numbers taking morphine and pethidine, many of whom were therapeutic addicts, remained more or less static and the big increase was due almost entirely to an increased number of young non-therapeutic, recreational heroin and cocaine users.

At the end of 1967 and during 1968, the new treatment clinics recommended by the 1967 Act started to open. They were faced with a large number of patients who could no longer obtain heroin and cocaine from general practitioners (GPs) who did not have the necessary licence to prescribe to them. The addicts, many of whom had drug habits too large to support on the black market, had no choice but to present to the clinics. This brought to light many who were previously unknown and this accounts for the increase in the number of known addicts from 1729 in 1967 to 2782 in 1968.

Originally it was believed that somehow the clinics would prescribe just the 'right' amount of drug for each patient, sufficient to prevent them supplementing it from the black market, but with no surplus to sell. However, the initial response of the clinics, most of whose staff lacked experience, was very much an emergency response. Initially, prescriptions were often for the drug and dose that the patient had been receiving from their GP, and doses of heroin of 300–400 mg were not unusual; cocaine was also prescribed to some patients.

With growing experience, the requirements of individual patients were assessed more critically, the doses prescribed became smaller and the price of black market heroin rose sharply – a clear indication of its reduced availability. Heroin withdrawal was attempted by methadone substitution, a change that was strongly resisted by many patients who preferred heroin, and it was not uncommon for part of the maintenance dose of opiate to be prescribed as heroin and part as methadone. By the end of the 1960s new patients were presenting with primary methadone dependence, confirming the continuing diversion of prescribed drugs to the black market. This accelerated the trend away from prescribing injectable drugs which had, and still have, a high black market value, in favour of the less desirable oral preparation – in practice, oral methadone.

Polydrug abuse

The changes in opiate abuse and dependence that occurred during the 1960s did not occur in isolation, but were only a part, albeit a very important part, of the growing drug scene. The increasing interest of young people in cannabis has already been mentioned and this interest has persisted. Nowadays, although it is difficult to obtain accurate data about the prevalence of cannabis use, smoking cannabis seems to be commonplace behaviour. A survey carried out in 1982 of people aged 15–21 years revealed that 17% had used this drug.

Lysergic acid diethylamide (LSD) also became popular, particularly during the 1960s, and especially among those interested in mysticism and exploration of the inner world. Its use was part of the hippie culture at that time and was much in evidence at pop music festivals.

More important than the hallucinogens, however, is the explosion that has taken place in the use and abuse of prescribed psychoactive drugs. Since the 1950s more and more have been synthesized and prescribed for symptoms such as anxiety, insomnia and depression – symptoms which everyone experiences at one time or another and which may be due to real psychiatric illness or to personal or interpersonal problems.

These drugs have contributed substantially to a pool (a lake?, an ocean?) of easily available psychoactive substances. The sheer scale of their availability may not be readily appreciated but in 1975, for example, it was estimated that there were 47 500 000 prescriptions for these psychotropic drugs in the UK – an increase of 19% over the previous 5 years.

The disadvantages and side-effects of some of the drugs became apparent only gradually. Many were found to have a dependence liability. Barbiturates, for example, were first introduced into clinical practice in 1903, but nearly 50 years elapsed before dependence on them was described. In the early 1960s, therefore, when about 15 000 000 prescriptions were being issued annually for barbiturate hypnotics, it seems likely that there must have been a good number of people who had become dependent on their nightly drug. At that time, a 'typical' barbiturate-dependent individual was a middle-aged woman obtaining her drugs on prescription from her GP, probably with neither of them recognizing or acknowledging her dependence status.

Amphetamines, too, caused problems: first introduced for the treatment of asthma and as a nasal congestant, they became popular by virtue by their stimulant and appetite-suppressant properties. A survey carried out in Newcastle in the 1950s suggested that as many as 1% of the population were then receiving amphetamine on prescription, but it was only in the late 1950s that the phenomenon of amphetamine dependence and its serious consequences was described. Middle-aged women, receiving amphetamine on prescription for the treatment of depression or obesity, again formed a sizeable proportion of the dependent population. Since then other new drugs, both sedative (meprobamate, methaqualone, benzodiazepines, etc.) and stimulant (e.g., methylphenidate, phenmetrazine, etc.), have been introduced, often with confident claims that they lack the dependence-producing properties of their predecessors. The passage of time has all too often revealed their abuse potential with reports of escalating dose, drug-seeking behaviour and characteristic withdrawal syndromes. These drugs have been widely prescribed as a medicopharmacological response to a variety of problems. Often this response involves more than one drug – one psychoactive drug for insomnia, another for symptoms of anxiety, and perhaps another for depressive symptoms, to give an extreme example. As the pool of psychoactive drugs increased, their use in incidents of self-poisoning increased too, a problem which is now of epidemic or even endemic proportions. In this form of drug abuse too it is possible to detect the trend towards multiple drug use.

At a time when many young people were becoming interested in drugs and their effects, this ever-growing pool of psychoactive substances did not remain untapped. Illicit drug taking, using exactly these drugs, became very common and for many youngsters it was and is a convivial social activity and part of their general leisure behaviour. Drugs are taken like alcohol, purely for their psychic effects and indeed are often taken together with alcohol as a cheap way of becoming intoxicated. Polydrug abuse (i.e., the abuse of more than one drug at a time), in a search for heightened and different effects has become part of this recreational activity despite its risks. During the 1960s, for example, amphetamines became an important part of the multiple drugs scene, often being taken in conjunction with barbiturates. The majority of young abusers started their illicit use at weekends and this gradually spread through the week to counteract the withdrawal, depression and irritability induced by amphetamines. Such was the concern about the scale of abuse of amphetamines that there was a voluntary ban on their prescription by many doctors.

Those who abused or were dependent on opiates did not remain aloof from the more ordinary psychoactive drugs. For them multiple drug abuse was not a new phenomenon. Before the clinics opened, many heroin-using individuals had also used cocaine, often administering it in the same syringe to counteract the sedative effect of the opiate. When the right to prescribe cocaine to addicts was restricted, some doctors prescribed methylamphetamine as a substitute; an epidemic of methylamphetamine abuse was curtailed only when the drug was withdrawn from retail pharmacies.

Following the establishment of the drug-dependence treatment clinics, it became apparent that multiple drug use by their patients was very common. The adoption by the clinics of a frugal prescribing policy prevented, or at any rate reduced, overspill to the black market which, for a time, suffered a shortage of heroin and cocaine. Their scarcity, coupled with the wealth of other psychoactive drugs available, contributed to the addicts' willingness to experiment. In particular, it became common in the 1970s for barbiturates and other drugs manufactured for oral use to be crushed and injected, a highly dangerous practice that can cause serious systemic and local complications. Indeed, a significant proportion of addicts known to the Home Office because they were dependent on a notifiable drug died not from this drug but from barbiturate abuse. It should be emphasized, however, that it was not just opiate-dependent individuals who were involved in barbiturate and polydrug abuse – many young people abused a variety of drugs including opiates and barbiturates and became dependent on one or more of them.

Such were the problems caused by barbiturate abuse that there was a general trend in the 1970s towards prescribing newer and apparently safer sedative hypnotics instead. This trend was accelerated by the Campaign for the Use and Restriction of Barbiturates (CURB) and the number of prescriptions for barbiturates fell sharply. Their place in therapeutics was taken over by the benzodiazepines which were widely prescribed for their anxiolytic and hypnotic properties. Once again, however, an apparently safe group of drugs was found to have dependence and abuse potential and again, like the barbiturates before them, it took years for the significance of this observation to be fully appreciated.

The Misuse of Drugs Act 1971 was the response to the increasingly complex and rapidly changing drug scene. It replaced earlier legislation and provided a more rational and comprehensive framework for all aspects of drug control. It is discussed in more detail in Chapter 11.

The 1980s

Initial complacency that problems of opiate dependence had been satisfactorily dealt with by setting up the clinics was soon threatened by the new complexity of drug-abuse problems. The clinics became increasingly irrelevant to the totality of drug abuse in the whole community, offering treatment only to those dependent on opiates while excluding others who were not physically dependent on opiates but who were still abusing the same range of drugs. However, the clinics set up to deal with opiate (and cocaine) dependence were overstretched and did not have sufficient resources to deal with a huge number of other drug problems. An unforeseen difficulty was that instead of the majority of patients being rapidly withdrawn from opiates as originally envisaged, many remained on long-term oral methadone maintenance and often continued to attend the clinics for years. Long waiting lists developed at some clinics and some drug abusers preferred to approach, often privately, non-clinic doctors. As these doctors were not licensed to prescribe heroin, they often prescribed other opiates such as dipipanone or dextromoramide, and stimulants such as methylphenidate.

Although manufactured for oral use, dipipanone and dextromoramide tablets were crushed and injected in a search for heightened effect and some were sold on the black market. This was reflected in an increasing number of cases of primary dependence on them and by the early 1980s the situation was reminiscent of the mid-1960s, before the clinics opened. For this reason, the prescription of dipipanone, which was causing the most problems, was made subject to the same restrictions as heroin and cocaine.

There were calls to extend the licensing restrictions to more drugs, but the relative importance of prescribed opiates in causing dependence declined in the face of a flood of illicit heroin, often of a high degree of purity, reaching the UK from different parts of the world – South East Asia, the Middle East and the Indian Subcontinent. Its price on the black market became as low, relatively, as it had been in the 1960s, reflecting its easy availability. Instead of injecting, it became common for it to be taken by 'chasing the dragon' – a small amount is heated in a spoon or on a piece of foil and the resultant fumes are inhaled. This method attracts many who dislike, at least at first, the idea of injecting themselves and who believe that inhaling heroin is somehow less addictive. Perhaps for this reason, the number of heroin-dependent individuals has increased very rapidly in the last few years and inevitably a proportion of them have become injectors, with all the attendant hazards. This, coupled with the increased abuse of cocaine and fears of large scale importation of 'crack' (a very pure and potent form of cocaine), has again concentrated attention on the 'traditional' drugs of dependence, heroin and cocaine. Anxiety has been exacerbated because both heroin and cocaine have in the past been drugs that were frequently injected. In the face of the impending AIDS (acquired immune deficiency syndrome) epidemic, the existence of a large population of drug injectors, who habitually share syringes and needles, significantly increases the risk of transmission of AIDS into the general population. These fears have tended to divert public attention away from the more 'mundane' problems of abuse of prescribed psychoactive drugs. Nevertheless, they remain a constant backdrop to the changing drug scene and important because of the millions of people who have become inadvertently dependent during the course of treatment.

Organization of treatment services in the UK

Primary health care

Individuals resident in the UK are entitled to free medical care under the National Health Service (NHS). Most register with a local GP, the primary health-care physician, whom they consult free of charge whenever they wish. The GP maintains a record of such consultations and of the treatment that is prescribed and, if necessary, may refer the patient for a specialist opinion. Reports from specialists together with results of laboratory investigations are retained by the GP who thus maintains a comprehensive record of the patient's health and treatment status. This record is passed on if the patient transfers to the care of another GP, for example, on moving house.

A drug-related problem, such as drug dependence, is therefore just one among a huge range of problems for which the GP may be consulted. In practice, some GPs do not 'like' drug-dependent individuals and may refuse to accept them as patients; in other cases a GP may refuse to see a particular patient who has been especially troublesome in the past. In this situation a patient may apply to the local Family Health Services Authority who will then allocate the patient to a GP.

The management of a patient with a drug-related problem lies with the GP. Usually, patients with serious problems are referred to a specialized drug-dependence treatment unit (DDTU). However, the explosion of drug-related problems in recent years, involving opiates as well as a wide range of psychotropic drugs, has led to a realization that GPs should become more involved in the management of these patients. There have been considerable efforts to offer additional training to interested GPs and attempts are being made on the part of the specialized treatment centres to reach out into the community and to work from local venues in conjunction with GPs. It is hoped in this way to be able to offer a prompter and more appropriate response to more patients presenting with drug-related problems so that an opportunity for intervention while the patient is motivated is not lost. This involvement by specialist drug workers in primary-care settings has the advantages that GPs supported in this way feel more confident about managing complex cases themselves and, with greater experience, gain in knowledge and skill.

Some patients prefer to consult a medical practitioner privately, paying for the consultation and the full cost of any prescribed drugs. Drug-dependent individuals sometimes do this to obtain larger supplies of the drug of dependence and may then sell some of it to finance the cost of the consultation and prescription. It is also not unknown for such patients to attend and/or register with more than one GP, perhaps using an alias in an attempt to obtain several prescriptions. It is in fact an offence to make a false statement to obtain a prescription or to obtain a prescription for controlled drugs from one doctor without disclosing that another doctor has also prescribed them.

DDTUs

The DDTUs were set up in 1967 to deal with the growing problem of heroin (and cocaine) abuse. At that time most clinics were in or near London usually in or attached to a general hospital, but as the drug-abuse problem has grown numerically and spread geographically, other clinics have opened. In its 1982 report on Treatment and Rehabilitation, the Advisory Council on the Misuse of Drugs recommended that each of the Regional Health Authorities should establish a multidisciplinary Regional Drug Problem Team, with an identifiable base, usually a designated treatment clinic or another existing specialist service. This would ensure a geographical spread of specialist services within the UK. If a specialized unit is not available, a general psychiatrist may take responsibility for patients with drug-related problems, either because of personal interest in this area or in response to the pressure of referrals.

DDTUs are multidisciplinary units under the overall charge of the consultant psychiatrist, who is usually licensed by the Home Office to prescribe heroin and cocaine to addicts if this is appropriate. The number and disciplines of supporting staff, which may include junior doctors, nurses, social workers, clinical psychologists and clerical administrative staff, vary from clinic to clinic and this may significantly affect the orientation of the clinic.

As it is usually the nurse who has first contact with prospective patients it is his/her responsibility to adequately engage them in assessment and treatment.

The nurse is also responsible for maintaining a high standard of clinical nursing care and, in particular, for preventing the spread of infection between patients and from patient to staff.

The social worker assesses the patients' social functioning, social networks (including family involvement) and accommodation. He/she can offer help with social problems, such as housing, welfare rights and financial difficulties, and can liaise with outside agencies, such as the probation service, with which the patient may have been in contact. The social worker may work with the family of a patient and also has a statutory responsibility for the interests and safety of the children of drug-abusing parents. He/she has a particular role in advising and supporting patients who are considering undertaking a period of residential rehabilitation following drug withdrawal.

The psychologist uses an established repertoire of techniques from cognitive/behavioural and other branches of psychology, either as the sole form of treatment or in conjunction with other interventions, to meet identified treatment or management goals. For example, relaxation training, anxiety and anger management, desensitization, social skill training and cognitive restructuring are some of the special techniques available to psychologists in the treatment of drug-related and other problems. Similarly psychologists working in collaboration with community and voluntary agencies can deploy psychological processes to facilitate rehabilitation.

Patients referred to a DDTU will be assessed by different members of the multidisciplinary team. Findings and opinions are shared at a team meeting and a management plan is worked out. Although individual team members may each have a case load of patients for whom they are specially responsible, all patients are under the care of the consultant psychiatrist in charge of the unit, and it is of course only the medical staff who can prescribe medication for the patients. Although they may be licensed to prescribe heroin and cocaine to those dependent upon them, cocaine prescription has virtually ceased, and heroin is prescribed less often than before, and rarely to new patients.

Patients may be referred to the local clinic by their GP or another doctor, or by a social worker, probation officer or other agency. Some drug-dependent individuals refer themselves, often because a fellow addict is or has been a patient, although some units insist on a formal referral letter from another doctor.

Because the specialist units were initially set up to deal with opiate (and cocaine) abuse, this has always been their primary responsibility. Permanently understaffed and underresourced, they have, in the past, been unwilling and unable to deal with other types of drug abuse and dependence. The modern trend towards viewing substance abuse as a whole, rather than in terms of individual drugs, is however bringing about changes in the role of the specialist units and their policies. Many units will now see patients with other drug-abuse problems, such as solvent sniffing or sedative hypnotic dependence, if the GP feels that these patients have particular problems that require specialist intervention. These sessions are usually separate to those attended by opiate-dependent individuals. This, coupled with a strategy of greater community involvement will, it is hoped, enable the DDTUs to be perceived as a more ordinary place to seek help for all types of drug-related problems, rather than as the 'end of the road' for long-term opiate-dependent individuals.

Community Drug Teams (CDTs)

The changing nature of substance dependence in the UK, and in particular the ever-growing number of people who misuse drugs and the problems that have developed in relation to AIDS, have led to changes in the way that services are provided for these individuals. While the importance of hospital-based, specialist DDTUs is undisputed, there is also an acknowledged need for CDTs which have now been established in many areas.

Although the structure and activities of different CDTs may vary, they are usually multidisciplinary with input from a variety of professionals, such as psychologist, nurse, social worker, etc. Their purpose is to extend the specialist expertise of the hospital-based unit into the community so that more patients can benefit from this expertise, and to improve the quality of care by broadening the range of available treatment options and enabling patients to be seen in the setting most appropriate to their particular

circumstances. To achieve this, CDTs may participate in a number of different and complementary activities:

1   providing a telephone advisory service to encourage those who may not
otherwise approach any agency for help, to make contact through a
confidential and anonymous service;

2   providing clinical services in community-based settings thereby engaging those individuals who, for one reason or another, do not wish to attend
hospital, or for whom treatment in the community may be a more appropriate intervention;

3   increasing services for drug misusers by providing training for other
professional groups who can then offer more appropriate support for their
clients who are misusing drugs;

4   monitoring the extent and nature of drug misuse in the local area and
evaluating existing services;

5   preparing and maintaining a directory of local services for drug misusers for them and their families and also for all workers involved with this
client group, so that, when onward referral is necessary, it is appropriate to
the needs of the individual concerned.

In-patient units

In-patient facilities specifically for the treatment of drug dependence are very
limited, although when the clinics opened it was envisaged that in-patient
care would be an important component of treatment. It was hoped that
regular attendance at the out-patient clinic would lead to a therapeutic relationship between the clinic staff and the patient, who would then feel able to
accept in-patient detoxification and long-term rehabilitation. In practice, in-
patient units have not played a numerically important role in the management of drug dependence although it is not clear if this is due to reluctance
on the part of the patients, the availability and quality of facilities, or a belief
on the part of doctors that out-patient withdrawal is preferable.

Because most DDTUs do not have their own in-patient unit, those that
do have this facility extend its use to patients from other areas. In-patient
care may therefore necessitate patients being treated in a hospital at some
distance from home and by staff whom they do not know. This is more
helpful if effective arrangements for after-care are made prior to admission,
because a brief period of in-patient treatment on its own is unlikely to bring
about lasting change in long-term problems such as drug dependence.

Patients may be admitted to hospital for assessment of a drug-abuse
problem, for stabilization of the dose of their drugs, for detoxification, for
treatment of the complications of drug abuse, or for a general sorting out of

the chaos brought about by their lifestyle. They may remain in hospital for weeks to months for rehabilitation which may be on or off drugs.

Rehabilitation and after-care

Drug withdrawal is only the first phase of a treatment programme which must be completed by a much longer term response known as rehabilitation – the process of integrating the drug abuser into society so that he/she can cope without drugs and can be restored to the best possible level of functioning. Sometimes, however, it has to be accepted that an individual cannot cope without drugs and rehabilitation has to take place in the context of continuing, although controlled, drug use.

In the UK, 'treatment', usually meaning drug withdrawal, is the responsibility of the NHS, while rehabilitation is the statutory responsibility of social service departments. This administrative dichotomy has reinforced the separation of the two components of the treatment process which ideally should occur concurrently with long-term counselling, psychotherapy and social work support, starting as soon as the drug-dependent individual presents for treatment. In practice, and perhaps because, drug withdrawal is the easier component of the package as far as provision of services is concerned, much more emphasis has been placed on facilities for drug withdrawal and much less on long-term facilities for rehabilitation and after-care.

Religious and other charitable organizations have perceived these deficiencies in services for rehabilitation and have set out over many years to remedy them. In doing so they have gained skills and experience that now cannot be matched by statutory services, so that the Government's role in the provision of rehabilitation has largely become confined to providing funding for the work of the voluntary agencies. The Standing Conference on Drug Abuse (SCODA), a voluntary body funded by the DH, acts as a coordinating body for all voluntary services dealing with drug abusers.

Because rehabilitation services have developed from the activities of voluntary organizations, they have done so in an unplanned and often haphazard fashion according to local needs, local interests, local skills and available funding, rather than in a comprehensive country-wide plan. A number of residential establishments exist, most of which insist that prospective entrants must be 'off' drugs before admission. They try to detach residents from their previous environment and to teach them to lead their life without recourse to drugs. In contrast a London hostel, ROMA (Rehabilitation of Metropolitan Addicts), helps addicts achieve a stable lifestyle but does not require them to give up drugs.

In recent years, the voluntary agencies have increasingly extended their activities outside the field of rehabilitation and now offer a variety of services for drug abusers at any stage of a drug-taking career. These include day centres, walk-in counselling services, telephone advisory services, self help groups and parents' support groups in all parts of the country.

Prison medical service

Because of the high incidence of drug-related crime many people admitted to prison either on remand or as convicted prisoners may be dependent on drugs or have a drug-related problem. In fact, their dependent state may come to light for the first time in this situation, which would seem to be an excellent opportunity for intervention and treatment. Prison medical officers are experienced at dealing with drug withdrawal and may admit drug-dependent prisoners to the prison hospital, temporarily, so that dose reduction can be supervised more closely. Unfortunately, after drug withdrawal, when abstinence has been achieved, there are no special treatment facilities for drug-dependent patients so that the essential components of rehabilitation are lacking. It is perhaps not surprising therefore that compulsory 'treatment' in prison consisting only of detoxification appears to have little long-term effect after the prisoner is released.

Sources of epidemiological information

International audit

One way of finding out about patterns of drug use is to investigate the supply situation by obtaining information about the production of drugs and their importation and exportation. In practice, reliable data can only be obtained about licit sources of supply, but a global overview of the situation is maintained by the International Narcotics Control Board (Chapter 11) which collects statistics on drug production and consumption from many countries and collates this with information about illicit drug activity internationally. Analysis of this data provides information on the development of new trends in drug consumption and can give early warning of rapidly increasing use that might suggest abuse.

Drug seizures

More locally, information about illicit drugs can be obtained from figures about drug seizures and purchases made on the black market for investigation purposes. These data give some idea of the availability and purity of individual drugs. In the UK, the Home Office publishes data on seizures of all controlled drugs, thereby providing information on a wide range of substances, as well as information on drug-related offences. While changes in seizures and offenders do not necessarily imply changes in the prevalence of the misuse of controlled drugs, they may reflect changed demand for these substances. It is acknowledged, however, that other factors such as changes in the direction and effectiveness of enforcement effort, and changes in recording and reporting procedures may be significant.

In 1992, the number of drug seizures increased by 3%, a much smaller rate of increase than in recent years (30% in 1989; 16% in 1990 and 1991). As in earlier years, the vast majority of seizures were of cannabis (Fig. 2.1). Table 2.1 shows how the number of heroin seizures soared during the early 1980s from 985 in 1982 to nearly 3200 in 1985. Since then there have been slight reductions followed by compensatory increases, so that in 1992, there were nearly 3000 heroin seizures. In terms of the quantity, more heroin was seized in 1992 (547 kg) than in any of the previous 10 years, except for 1990 (603 kg).

The number of cocaine seizures rose to nearly 2400 in 1992, a new peak, and it is of particular interest that the number of crack cocaine seizures has increased dramatically over the past few years, from 30 in 1988, to 140 in 1989, and 880 in 1992. In view of this increase in the number of seizures, it is not surprising that the quantity of cocaine seized is

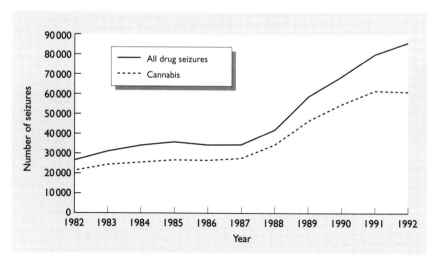

Fig. 2.1 Number of cannabis seizures compared with total number of drug seizures, UK 1982–92. (Source: Home Office.)

Table 2.1 Heroin, cocaine and amphetamine seizures 1982–92. (Source: Home Office)

	Number of seizures each year										
	1982	1983	1984	1985	1986	1987	1988	1989	1990	1991	1992
Heroin	985	1940	2995	3176	2828	2058	2197	2728	2593	2640	2968
Cocaine	389	684	889	662	635	717	829	2045	1805	1984	2365
Amphetamines	1653	2333	2834	3471	3047	2852	3277	3322	4629	6821	10570

	Quantity seized (nearest whole kg)										
Heroin	196	236	362	366	223	236	236	351	603	493	547
Cocaine	19	80	66	85	103	407	323	499	611	1078	2248
Amphetamines	14	35	59	77	116	152	137	108	304	421	569

also at record levels. Indeed, the 2248 kg seized in 1992 was more than twice as much as the 1991 figure, itself a record.

Among the wealth of information available on drug seizures, the following points are of particular interest.

1 In 30% of police forces, MDMA (Ecstasy) was the most frequently seized class A drug (see Chapter 11) In 1992, 550 000 doses were seized, compared with about 44 000 in 1990. Similarly, for 50% of police forces LSD was the most frequently seized class A drug, again with more than half a million doses seized.

2 In 1992 there were 900 seizures involving class C drugs, mainly benzodiazepines, milder stimulants and less potent analgesics; of these, 480 were for benzodiazepines and 340 for buprenorphine.

Persons dealt with for drug offences

The number of persons dealt with for drug offences is yet another indicator of the prevalence of illicit drug misuse, although the figures need careful analysis and interpretation. In summary, the number of drug offenders has continued to rise, and the total number reported to the Home Office in 1992 was 56 500, 5% more than in 1991. Unlawful possession remains the most common offence, with the majority of offenders being found in possession of cannabis (Figs 2.2 and 2.3).

Prescription audit

Another way of investigating patterns of drug use is to assess drug distribution by means of prescriptions. This can provide information on individual

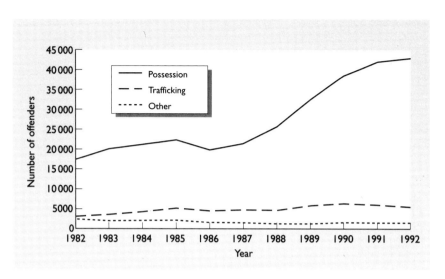

Fig. 2.2 Drug offenders by type of offence, UK 1982–92. (Source: Home Office.)

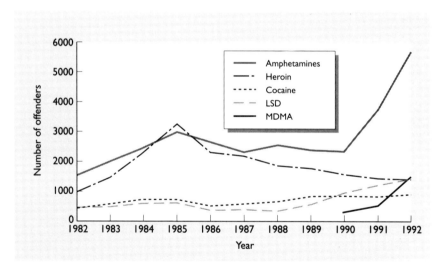

Fig. 2.3 Number of offenders by type of drug, UK, 1982–92 (excluding cannabis). (Source: Home Office.)

drugs or drug classes prescribed either for the total population or for selected populations. It also, of course, allows trends and patterns of pre-scribing practices to be studied.

Thus it can be seen from Table 2.2 and Fig. 2.4, that the total number of prescriptions issued by GPs increased steadily over the period 1980–90

Table 2.2 Total number of prescriptions and number of prescriptions of preparations acting on the nervous system, by selected therapeutic sub-groups, UK 1980–90. (Source: Department of Health)

	Millions of prescriptions										Percentage change	
	1980	1982	1983	1984	1985	1986	1987	1988	1989	1990	1980–90	1970–80
All classes	361	370	376	382	380	384	400	413	421	431	19	22
Central nervous system	84	84	81	82	76	77	80	81	81	85	2	4
Hypnotics	17	17	16	16	16	16	17	16	15	15	−12	−27
Sedatives and tranquillizers	22	21	18	16	14	14	13	12	11	10	−54	19
Anticonvulsants	4	4	4	4	5	5	5	5	5	5	22	14
Antiparkinsonism drugs	2	2	2	2	2	2	2	2	2	2	33	*
Analgesics major	4	5	5	5	5	5	6	6	6	6	41	328
Analgesics minor	21	21	20	22	20	20	23	25	26	28	33	7
Antidepressants	7	7	7	7	7	8	8	8	9	9	30	5

*Category not classified in earlier years.

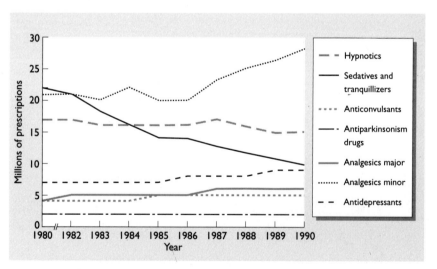

Fig. 2.4 Number of prescriptions for certain therapeutic sub-groups acting on the nervous system. (Source: Department of Health.)

and that the number of prescriptions for drugs that act on the nervous system, after dipping in the mid-1980s, has been increasing since 1987. Within the overall total, there has been an encouragingly steady decline in the number of prescriptions for sedatives and tranquillizers. Although there has also been a reduction in the number of prescriptions for hypnotic drugs, this has been a more gradual and more fluctuating trend. Perhaps the most striking feature, however, is the steady increase, over the last 6 years, in the number of prescriptions for minor analgesics; in 1990, for example, there were 28 million prescriptions for these drugs, compared with 21 million in 1980. Although not generally perceived as dependence producing, these drugs are a frequent substance of misuse, and rising prescription figures, such as those shown in Table 2.2, can act as an early warning system if abuse is becoming widespread. The increased prescription of antidepressants over this time period may be a reflection of the introduction of a large number of new drugs which have fewer and more tolerable side-effects than earlier drugs.

Of course it is possible to analyse prescription data in more detail – even by individual drugs. This shows for example that within the large number of prescriptions for benzodiazepines, there have been more prescriptions for shorter-acting drugs such as temazepam and lorazepam, which have become popular because, when taken as hypnotics, they have less 'hangover' effect and, when taken through the day as anxiolytics there is much less drug accumulation in the body. However, it now appears that dependence on these drugs is more severe and that withdrawal is correspondingly more difficult from these shorter-acting drugs.

Although the information obtained from prescription audit is fascinating, great care needs to be taken in its interpretation, because the method has obvious limitations. For example, a proportion of people who receive prescriptions do not get them dispensed (and are therefore not included in an audit of retail pharmacists) and a proportion of people who have their prescriptions dispensed do not take (all of) their drugs. In other words, it must not be forgotten that the sampling unit is a prescription and not a patient. Furthermore, changes in prescribing may be misrepresented; for example changing from the practice of giving long-term prescriptions for large amounts of a drug to giving short-term prescriptions for small amounts would appear in the statistics as an increase in the total number of prescriptions, even if the amount prescribed is the same or less.

Home Office index

The main source of information in the UK has been the Home Office index of addicts. Before 1968, it was based on a system of voluntary notification by medical practitioners and of inspecting the books of dispensing pharmacists. Since 1968, however, doctors have had a statutory duty to notify the Home

Office of any patient whom they consider to be dependent on certain controlled drugs (cocaine and a number of opiate drugs, see p. 343). The current
index of addicts is derived from these notifications and annual statistics are
published giving the total number of notified addicts at the end of each year,
their sex and age, the number of new (i.e., notified for the first time) and
renotified addicts, the drugs reported to be used at notification and so on.

However, as many addicts obtain drugs illicitly and are intent on con-
cealment from any authority, the official statistics can only represent a proportion, and probably a changing proportion of the total number who are
actually addicted. Furthermore, at any time there are many people misusing the same drugs who are not (yet) addicted to them. A further disadvantage is that notification is not required for a large number of controlled
drugs, such as amphetamines and barbiturates, which are misused and can
cause dependence, and, of course, doctors do not always fulfil their statutory obligation to notify. Thus, although the primary function of the Index
– to reduce the possibility of an individual receiving certain drugs from
more than one doctor simultaneously – is largely achieved, the data it provides are of limited value, because those who are notified are probably only
a small proportion of regular users. Nevertheless, even these data are
generally considered useful for picking up trends and for illustrating general
patterns within a restricted group of drug users.

Source of notification

Altogether, GPs accounted for 37% of first notifications of both new and re-
notified addicts in 1993 while hospitals and treatment centres notified 45%,
prison medical officers notified 13% and police surgeons about 5%.

Number of addicts

The Home Office figures show that there has been a steady, almost relent-
less increase in the number of notified addicts since 1987, with a year-on-
year increase of 17–20% since 1988. Thus the total number of addicts
notified to the Home Office increased from 14 785 at the end of 1989 to
20 800 in 1991 and 27 976 by the end of 1993, a total increase of 89%.
Within this huge increase in 1993, there were 11 561 new notifications,
the highest number of new addicts ever recorded in a single year, and 20%
more than in the previous year (Fig. 2.5). Altogether, new notifications
accounted for 41% of the total.

It has been suggested that some of this increase may have been the
result of efforts to attract more addicts into treatment because of fear of

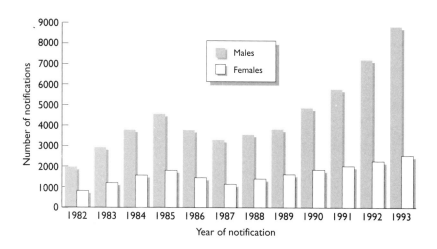

Fig. 2.5 New drug addicts notified to the Home Office, UK 1982–93. (Source: Home Office.)

AIDS. There may also be greater awareness of notification procedures and obligations as a result of the establishment of Regional Substance Misuse Databases (see below) by Health Authorities.

Age and sex (Table 2.3 and Fig. 2.6)

The age of new addicts remained relatively stable during the 1980s, with the average age varying between 25.4 and 27.3 years. However, the number in the under-21 years age group, which fell in 1989, has risen since then. In 1993, 73% of new addicts were under the age of 30 years and 18% were less than 21 years old. Nevertheless, the average age of all addicts (not just new addicts) has risen steadily since the mid-1980s.

Although the number of new female addicts has been increasing, they now form a smaller proportion of the total than previously. In 1993, for example, 22% of new addicts were female, compared with 28% in 1990. It can be seen from Table 2.3 and Fig. 2.5 that the majority of new addicts are men aged between 21 and 34 years of age.

Drugs of addiction (Table 2.4 and Figs 2.7 and 2.8)

The common drugs to which addiction is reported are, in order of frequency, heroin, methadone, cocaine, dipipanone and morphine. A fifth of notified addicts were reported to be polydrug addicts.

Table 2.3 Age and sex of new addicts, UK 1982–93. (Source: Home Office)

Age group in years	1982	1983	1984	1985	1986	1987	1988	1989	1990	1991	1992	1993
Under 21	489	879	1204	1531	1261	975	1063	982	1178	1225	1698	2051
21–24	768	1150	1546	1932	1460	1386	1464	1598	1949	2194	2760	3202
25–29	826	1081	1362	1459	1262	1063	1324	1576	1946	2293	2701	3141
30–34	436	590	776	808	705	618	696	767	964	1128	1253	1639
35–49	159	251	320	394	374	373	478	561	732	943	1080	1218
Over 50	28	56	41	39	41	33	35	44	39	67	81	89
Not recorded	87	179	166	246	222	145	152	111	115	157	90	221
Total	2793	4186	5415	6409	5325	4593	5212	5639	6923	8007	9663	11561
Percentage new addicts under 21 years	18	22	23	25	25	22	21	18	17	16	18	18
Average age of new addicts	26.5	26.2	25.9	25.4	25.8	26.1	26.3	26.8	26.9	27.3	26.9	26.9
Males	1976	2979	3840	4586	3837	3372	3723	3952	4991	5899	7342	8981
Females	817	1207	1575	1823	1488	1221	1489	1687	1932	2108	2321	2580
Total	2793	4186	5415	6409	5325	4593	5212	5639	6923	8007	9663	11561

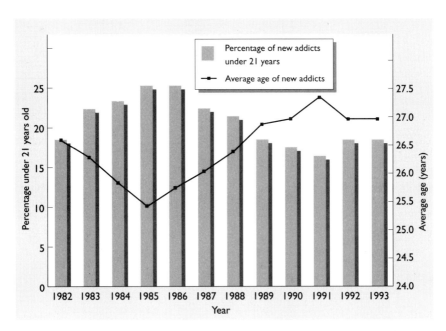

Fig. 2.6 Average age of new addicts and percentage under 21 years, UK 1982–93.
(Source: Home Office.)

Heroin was the most common drug of addiction for new addicts in the 1980s, with the proportion increasing from 72% in 1980 to 93% in 1985, perhaps reflecting ease of availability at that time. In 1993, 9063 new heroin addicts were notified, an increase of 1405 on new notifications in 1992. However, the number of new methadone addicts increased by 48% in 1991, by 14% in 1992 and then by 34% to 3362 in 1993. This increase probably reflects the fact that more new addicts are being treated with methadone.

The number of new cocaine addicts increased in 1993 to 1375, an increase of 22% over the 1992 figure. Nevertheless, despite very large seizures of cocaine, its misuse has, so far, not created a significant demand for medical treatment.

The number notified as addicted to dipipanone fell slightly in 1993, from 320 to 283, continuing the downward trend of recent years. The total is now substantially less than in the early 1980s, suggesting that the stricter controls placed on its prescription have been successful in controlling availability.

Among re-notified addicts, heroin and methadone remained the most common drugs of addiction in 1993, with 9856 addicted to heroin and

Table 2.4 New drug addicts and type of drug to which addiction reported, UK 1982–93. (Source: Home Office)

	1982	1983	1984	1985	1986	1987	1988	1989	1990	1991	1992	1993
Cocaine	214	345	471	490	520	431	462	527	633	882	1131	1375
Methadone	473	633	686	669	659	627	576	682	1469	2180	2493	3362
Heroin	2117	3559	4926	5930	4855	4082	4630	4883	5819	6328	7658	9063
Other	1077	1050	817	709	616	523	471	495	585	479	449	379
Total number of new addicts*	2793	4186	5415	6409	5325	4593	5212	5639	6923	8007	9663	11561

*NB An addict may be reported as addicted to more than one drug.

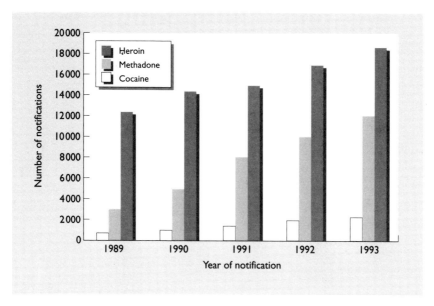

Fig. 2.7 Drugs to which addiction reported: all notifications for UK 1989–93. (Source: Home Office.)

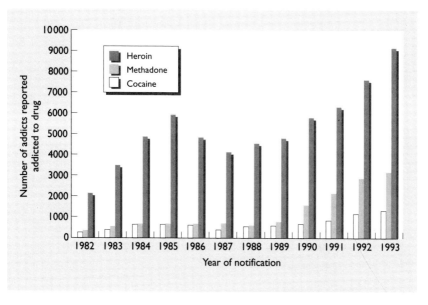

Fig. 2.8 New drug addicts by drug to which addition is reported, UK 1982–93. NB Addicts may be reported as addicted to more than one drug. (Source: Home Office.)

8867 addicted to methadone, 17% more than in 1992. As with new addicts, the increase in the proportion addicted to methadone is substantial, rising to 54% in 1993. Altogether, notifiable drugs were prescribed to 5742 new addicts and 11 803 re-notified addicts at their first notification in 1992, with 70% being prescribed methadone, either alone or in combination with another drug.

Injecting status

Because of concern about the spread of HIV/AIDS, whether or not drug abusers inject their drugs is of the greatest importance. Table 2.5 shows that in 1993, more than half of all addicts whose injecting status was known, were injecting their drugs.

Regional Substance Misuse Databases

Until recently, the only national figures available relating to the nature and extent of drug use were contained within the Home Office's Addict Index. The inadequacies of this system as an epidemiological tool have been outlined above and it has been recognized that more comprehensive information on a wider range of substance misuse was essential for effective service development and policy-making at both local and national level. Since 1989 all Regional Health Authorities have therefore been required to establish databases to monitor trends in drug abuse and the use of drug abuse services, and nationally collated information (October 1992 to March 1993) is now available (for England).

These databases collect information on all forms of drug misuse (not just notifiable drugs) and from a wide variety of sources. For example, the large majority of reports made to the Drug Misuse Databases (DMD) have come from CDTs (44%), with non-statutory, non-residential agencies

Table 2.5 All drug addicts notified to the Home Office by latest injecting status and sex, UK 1993. (Source: Home Office)

| | Percentage injecting* | | |
	New addicts	Re-notified addicts	Total addicts
Males	60	56	58
Females	55	50	52
Total	59	55	56

*Percentages based on total number of addicts for whom injecting status in known.

accounting for 12%, GPs for 11% and out-patient DDTUs for 10%. Nevertheless, in many respects and although they cover a much wider range of drugs, DMD figures broadly confirm the picture produced by analysis of the Home Office Index, that most drug users presenting to services are men in their twenties and early thirties. In total, 65% of individuals reported to the DMD were using opiate drugs as their main drug (heroin 47% and methadone 15%) and 60% of those using heroin were known to be injecting it.

Mortality studies

Mortality studies by definition focus on the most serious forms of drug abuse – those from which the patient has died. Causes of death are numerous, they include overdose (suicidal, accidental or homicidal), side-effects of drugs, complications of non-sterile self-injection and functional impairment that increases the risk of serious accident. Because there are so many possible causes of death and because many are not exclusively due to drug abuse, those that are may be very difficult to identify among a large number of similar deaths that have nothing to do with drugs.

However, the problem of mortality due to drug abuse can be tackled in at least four ways:
1   by analysing a series of forensically examined cases;
2   by analysing national cause of death statistics;
3   by cause of death surveys;
4   by epidemiological studies on the mortality of drug consumers.

Clear differences exist in the indications, objectives, expense and amount of information obtained by these different methods. In most industrialized countries, cause of death statistics are the main source of data about drug overdose deaths and are often used for international comparisons. They are valuable because they are representative but they are always out of date because of delay in publication. In addition, as they are not substance specific, they cannot provide any evidence of new trends of drug abuse. This can be remedied to a certain degree by forensic toxicological analysis which can give an early indication of any increase in the number of deaths due to a specific drug. In the UK, for example, coroners' courts have proved to be a useful source of information about addict deaths. Since the coroner must be informed of any death arising from the use of drugs, whether occurring during treatment or as a result of mishap, abuse or addiction, a survey of coroners' courts' records provides accurate information on the number of addicts who die in a given period and whose death is in any way related to drug taking.

In the UK, a further source of information about addicts' deaths is, once again, the Home Office which keeps a separate list of those addicts removed from the current index by reason of death. By definition, the information refers only to addicts known to the Home Office in the first place and as we have seen, this list is by no means complete anyway. However, the Home Office statistics now also include national statistics of deaths where the underlying cause is drug dependence or non-dependent use of drugs, or the use of controlled drugs (Table 2.6 and Figs 2.9 and 2.10).

Although the Home Office information is incomplete it can be useful in the analysis of trends in addiction both for national and international comparisons. For example, in 1992, there were 345 deaths where the underlying cause was described as drug dependence or the non-dependent abuse of drugs. This was a slight increase on the 1991 figure of 307 (of whom only 69 were previously notified addicts) and continues the upward trend of recent years. Of all addicts who died during 1986–91, about 11% were originally notified less than 12 months before death, 34% within 2 years of death, 34% within 2 years and 62% within 5 years. The most common cause of death was overdose and, where the drugs used were recorded, opiates and opioids were involved in about three-quarters of cases.

Figures published by the Office of Population Censuses and Surveys for England and Wales and by the General Register Offices for the rest of the UK, are another source of mortality data, classified using the Ninth Revision of the International Classification of Diseases (ICD-9). In 1992 there were 1421 deaths involving controlled drugs; in addition to the 345 attributed to drug dependence, 1001 were classified as due to accidental death or suicide, while 75 were due to AIDS. The total number of deaths in which drug dependence/abuse was considered to be an underlying cause more than quadrupled between 1981 and 1991, with the use of volatile substances (solvents) accounting for 40% of the increase.

Accident and emergency (A & E) departments

As psychoactive drugs such as hypnotics, anxiolytics and antidepressants have been prescribed more widely, the morbidity associated with their use has become apparent. Undoubtedly, the most important morbidity in terms of sheer number is that of drug overdose. Such is its frequency that the margin of safety between the therapeutic dose of a psychoactive drug and the dose required for serious overdose or death is at times a property with commercial significance.

The majority of cases of drug overdoses are seen in hospital A & E departments which are, therefore, excellent places to study this particular

Table 2.6 Deaths with underlying cause described as drug dependence or non-dependent abuse of drugs by type of drug, UK 1981–92. (Source: Home Office)

	1981	1982	1983	1984	1985	1986	1987	1988	1989	1990	1991	1992
Morphine type	33	63	69	56	62	70	65	64	77	91	97	155
Cocaine	0	1	1	1	0	2	1	2	2	3	0	0
Cannabis	0	0	0	0	1	2	0	0	1	0	0	0
Hallucinogens	0	0	0	1	0	0	1	0	0	0	1	2
Amphetamine type	0	3	0	3	3	2	1	0	2	2	5	7
Barbiturate type	12	10	7	13	7	14	10	7	15	7	16	6
Volatile substances	6	27	7	12	54	46	76	89	84	112	87	68
Morphine with other	4	15	14	12	4	7	12	10	14	15	18	29
Combinations excluding morphine	0	2	1	0	2	0	1	2	3	1	4	3
Unspecified drug dependence	14	24	21	19	22	21	24	19	27	24	31	26
Antidepressants	0	0	0	0	0	3	8	4	3	4	2	4
Other, mixed, unspecified, non-dependent	2	6	3	16	35	28	29	24	17	35	46	45
Total	71	151	123	133	190	195	228	221	245	294	307	345

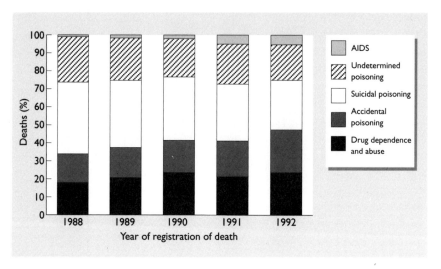

Fig. 2.9 Drug-related deaths by year of registration of death, UK 1988–92. (Source: Home Office.)

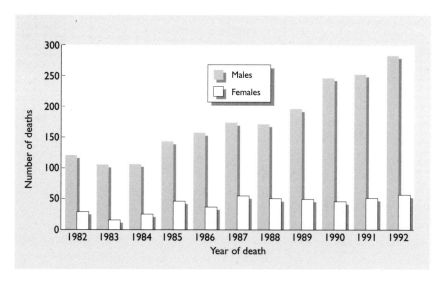

Fig. 2.10 Deaths with underlying cause described as drug dependence or non-dependent abuse of drugs by sex, UK 1982–92. (Source: Home Office.)

morbidity, to monitor the whole range of drug problems and, by including all who attend with a drug-related problem, to identify trends in drug abuse in the general population. These departments offer several advantages for undertaking this kind of epidemiological research. Perhaps most important of all is the fact that although administration and organization may vary, some sort of emergency facility exists in all health-care systems so that there is a ready-made, cost-effective set-up available, worldwide, ready to monitor drug-related problems. Another advantage of A & E departments is that they are 'neutral' ground for those with drug-related problems. For those who have taken a drug overdose, for example, the underlying psychosocial reasons are ignored, at least temporarily while the acute consequences of the overdose are treated by a medical team. It is probable that patients seen in this 'neutral', comparatively non-judgemental situation are more representative than those in more highly selective situations such as specialist drug treatment units, prisons or remand homes. The value of A & E departments as a neutral ground is enhanced by an awareness of medical confidentiality which facilitates the gathering of accurate data on sensitive issues. Nevertheless, it must be noted that studies in these departments, while providing valuable information about drug taking in society as a whole, say little about individual patterns.

If A & E departments are to be utilized on a large scale for this type of research, the monitoring procedure must be planned very carefully. All studies must be prospective in nature because notes taken during an emergency situation are rarely sufficiently detailed for comprehensive data to be gleaned from them retrospectively. However, any prospective study must be aware of the busy conditions prevailing in A & E departments and the questionnaire, designed to elicit maximum information, should also be brief and simple so that the staff of the department, whose main responsibility is to the patient and not to research, can complete it easily.

An important decision to be made when planning the investigation is whether to study incidents or individuals. When individual patients are identified, valuable information is obtained about the comparatively small group of individuals who attend A & E departments repeatedly. They are important partly because they generate a lot of work and also because the health-care response they initiate is clearly inappropriate to their needs, suggesting that an alternative response should be sought. However, having information that positively identifies patients poses difficult problems of confidentiality while that information is being processed.

The largest survey of A & E departments, both geographically and in terms of duration, is that being carried out in the USA by the Drug Abuse Warning Network (DAWN). This receives reports from hospital emergency rooms, medical examiners (i.e., coroners) and crisis intervention centres, which provide some indications of drug-abuse trends in large urban populations. A specially trained reporter recruited from the staff of each hospital and located in the A & E department is responsible for identifying patients with a drug-related problem and for completing the DAWN questionnaire. This focuses on two main issues: the drug(s) used and the drug user. As more than one drug may be used in a particular incident, more drug 'mentions' are recorded than drug-related incidents; no identifying information about the patients is collected.

In contrast, a survey carried out in June 1975 in 62 A & E departments and again in 1982 in 10 A & E departments in London specifically identified patients with drug-related problems by recording their name, date of birth and address so that they could be traced if they presented to hospital on more than one occasion during the period of the survey. Information was also elicited about the drug(s) of abuse and self-poisoning, the underlying reason for the drug overdose, the source of supply of drugs, their method of administration and any history of drug overdoses taken in the 12 months prior to the survey.

Comparison of the 1982 findings with those obtained in the same 10 hospitals 7 years earlier showed that the rate of drug-related attendance in the adult (15 years and over) casualty population fell from 20.1 per 1000 in 1975 to 15.4 per 1000 in 1982, although there were only minor differences between the two surveys in terms of the age and sex of the patients (Table 2.7). Applying these monthly rates to the whole year, and taking the catchment area populations into account, gives a yearly incidence rate for drug-related problems of 3.8 per 1000 and 3.1 per 1000 in 1975 and 1982, respectively. Altogether there were 435 drug-related incidents in July 1975 and 337 incidents in the corresponding period in 1982, 413 (95%) incidents in 1975 and 311 (92%) in 1982 were episodes of self-poisoning (Table 2.8). The drugs used for self-poisoning are shown in Table 2.9 and it is immediately apparent that there was a striking reduction in the use of barbiturate and non-barbiturate hypnotics between 1975 and 1982. Polydrug abuse was common in both years of the survey (Table 2.10), but there was a significant reduction in the percentage of patients who had taken one or

Table 2.7 Age and sex with drug-related problems

Age	1975			1982		
	Male (no.)	Female (no.)	Total (%)	Male (no.)	Female (no.)	Total (%)
15–29	107	135	56	86	92	53
30–49	58	54	26	41	58	30
50+	24	25	11	20	23	13
Not known	14	17	7	10	5	4
Total	203	231	100	157	178	100

Table 2.8 Nature of self-poisoning episodes

Nature of self-poisoning	1975 No.	(%)	1982 No.	(%)
Suicide attempt/gesture	226	(66)	191	(72)
Overdose in the course of addiction	72	(21)	27	(10)
Accidental	43	(13)	49	(18)
Total known	341	(83)	267	(86)
Not known	72	(17)	44	(14)
Total	413	(100)	311	(100)

Percentages of each nature of episode are based on known cases only.

Table 2.9 Agent self-poisoning

Drug	1975 (%) (n = 393)	1982 (%) (n = 300)
Barbiturates	27	7
Minor tranquilizers	28	38
Non-barbiturate hypnotics	18	4
Other psychotropics	19	17
Opiates	8	10
Alcohol	26	29
Minor analgesics	22	29

Percentages do not sum to 100% because of multiple drug use.

Table 2.10 Polydrug use

No. of drugs used	1975 No.	(%)	1982 No.	(%)
1	207	(53)	165	(55)
2	149	(38)	97	(32)
3	31	(8)	32	(11)
4 or more	6	(2)	6	(2)
Cases where drugs identified	393	(95)	300	(96)
Cases where drugs not identified	20	(5)	11	(4)
Total cases	413	(100)	311	(100)
Total drugs used	623		479	
Mean drugs/case	1.59		1.60	

Percentages for each number of drugs used are based on the number of cases where drugs were identified.

more drug overdoses during the previous year (Table 2.11). It is also interesting that the number of drug-dependent individuals attending in 1982
was significantly smaller than in 1975 (Table 2.12). Both of these changes
are probably related to reduced abuse of barbiturates. CURB was launched
in 1975, although the dangers of these drugs had long been recognized and
their prescription had been falling since 1965. Thus by 1982 barbiturates
were much less easily available and the consequences of this reduced availability were reflected in the results of the 1982 survey.

A reduction in the use of one psychotropic drug by a population is
usually associated with an increase in the use of another. Indeed, the

Table 2.11 Previous overdoses

	1975		1982	
Overdoses in previous year	No.	(%)	No.	(%)
0	168	(56)	148	(68)
1	40	(13)	27	(12)
2	22	(7)	15	(7)
3	14	(5)	8	(4)
4 or more	57	(19)	19	(9)
Total known	301	(73)	217	(70)
Not known	112	(27)	94	(30)
Total	413	(100)	311	(100)

Percentages of each number of previous overdoses are based on known cases only.

Table 2.12 Drug-related status of patient attending accident and emergency
departments with a drug-related problem

	1975				1982			
			Total				Total	
Dependence status	Male (no.)	Female (no.)	No.	(%)	Male (no.)	Female (no.)	No.	(%)
Definite	53	30	83	(23)	32	11	43	(15)
Probable	32	26	58	(16)	22	10	32	(11)
Not dependent	84	139	224*	(61)	79	134	215*	(74)
Total known	169	195	365	(84)	133	155	290	(86)
Not known	34	36	70	(16)	24	23	47	(14)
Total	203	231	435	(100)	157	178	337	(100)

Percentages for each status are based on known cases only.
*Numbers do not sum to the total as the sex of three patients was not known.

reduced prescription of barbiturates was partly due to the availability of safer alternative hypnotics. The reduction in the proportion of overdoses involving non-barbiturate (benzodiazepine) hypnotics was therefore unexpected, although compensated for, to a certain extent, by the increased use of minor tranquillizers (also benzodiazepines) in overdoses.

Of course the picture in A & E departments today might be quite different to that in 1975 and 1982, but the survey and comparisons described illustrate the type of information that can be collected in A & E departments and therefore shed light on drug-taking practices. They show a picture of drug abuse quite different to that of the Home Office statistics which rely mainly on information from the drug-treatment clinics and which can only, therefore, present an incomplete picture of drug dependence of those who regularly use mainly opiates. This is an important group of people suffering from a very severe form of drug dependence, but it is not the totality of drug dependence in the UK, let alone the totality of drug abuse. A & E departments can play an important role in providing information about a much wider spectrum of drug problems in a polydrug abusing community, but the essential point is not whether one epidemiological approach is better than another; different methods provide complementary information and complementary views of the problem and only when all the different information has been incorporated and amalgamated, does the whole picture begin to emerge.

Because the picture is constantly changing it is essential for epidemiological research to be regular and in some situations continuous. In A & E departments, for example, ongoing research could form a sensible early warning system to identify new drugs of abuse so that responses could be swift and appropriate. Ideally such research should be taken in several centres, even internationally, but then great care must be taken about the data that are recorded. Soft data, such as the dependence status of the patient or the motivation of an overdose, are difficult to categorize even with careful operational definitions so that there are always a large 'unknown' group. In contrast, hard data on age, sex and drug(s) taken are easy to elicit and record. However, even with hard data a uniform system of tabulating results must be decided in advance if valid comparisons are to be made. For example, uniform age- and drug-classification systems are essential if research done in one department is ever to relate to that done in another.

Other epidemiological approaches

There are many other potential sources of information about drug abuse. Individually, they often deal with highly selective groups of the population

and provide unrepresentative information. Together, however, they contribute to a more complete picture about the trends in drug use and drug
abuse.

Possible sources of information are.

1   *Drug-dependence treatment services, rehabilitation centres and voluntary
agencies.* Various types of surveys in these places can provide information
about the characteristics of clients, treatment and outcome.

2   *Toxicology laboratories.* Now that reliable methods have been developed
for the qualitative and quantitative measurement of drugs in body tissues
and fluids, toxicological analysis is playing an increasingly important role
in providing firm data about drug use. Where this is done, it is a good,
cost-effective method of gathering data on drug-related health problems.

3   *Drug-related disease.* One way of finding out about drug-related problems
is to monitor public health data on the frequency of reports of various types
of pathology such as HIV/AIDS, viral hepatitis, fetal damage, etc., on the
assumption that these problems are sufficiently closely linked to drug consumption to be reasonable indicators. The advantage of this method is its
simplicity and low cost, and if data are gathered promptly and routinely it
should provide early information about the extent of drug abuse. However,
the simplicity and economy are offset by the lack of the specificity of a particular morbidity for psychoactive drug abuse. To give an extreme example,
it would be hopeless to try and monitor drug abuse by reports of skin
rashes – many drugs can cause rashes as can a variety of infections and
allergic conditions. It follows that the disease of disturbance must be relatively specific for the drug in question and that the majority of cases must
be due to that drug.

Another difficulty is that monitoring of public health data depends on
the identification of cases in different centres with an epidemiological
picture being built up by multicentre reporting of fairly low frequencies.
Case definition and case recognition will probably vary from centre to
centre and may vary in time with changing medical awareness. Other
factors also combine to make morbidity an unreliable indicator of drug
abuse: the proportion of casualties presenting to medical agencies may vary
at different times and at different centres and the percentage of those who
take drugs and sustain a particular complication may also vary from time
to time. Hepatitis, for example, used to be a reliable indicator of heroin
dependence, but for a variety of reasons, now seems a much less certain
marker.

Because of difficulties such as these, attempts to design indirect indices
of drug misuse similar to those designed for alcohol are unlikely to succeed,
although specific morbidities can be useful in providing an early warning of

new drugs being misused, of geographical spread to new areas and of involvement of new population groups.

The international drug scene

The problems of drug abuse that have preoccupied the UK during the last 30 years have not been confined to this country. There is a worldwide concern about all aspects of drug abuse, although specific drug problems may be of greater importance in some areas than in others. In much of Europe, the changes in the patterns of drug abuse have been very similar to those in the UK during the same period. Cannabis, for example, became popular in the 1960s in much of Western Europe as did LSD, although to a much smaller extent. Elsewhere, especially in Sweden, amphetamines were the preferred drugs and their intravenous use has become common and remains a problem today. The influx of illicit heroin into Europe first from South East Asia, and later from South West Asia, caused serious problems of opiate dependence in many countries. In Poland, however, the problem was with home-grown heroin, prepared from the straw of opium poppies which were grown quite legally to provide the poppy seeds found in so many Polish dishes.

Other notable trends in drug abuse have been the rapid spread of cocaine and solvent abuse and changes in the pattern of barbiturate abuse. The latter drugs, once the cause of serious problems in several countries, have become less important as they are now prescribed less and heroin has become so easily available. More recently, as in the UK, benzodiazepines have largely taken their place as drugs of abuse often used in combination with other drugs, particularly alcohol.

Information on the seizures of drugs, worldwide, illustrates the changing nature of the global drug problem over the past decade (Figs 2.11–2.17). For example, the quantity of cannabis resin seized nearly trebled from 1984 to 1993, with an increasing proportion of the seizures being made in Europe. In contrast, most of the increasing quantity of cocaine seizures related to the Americas. Although there were fluctuations in the quantities of opium reported seized over this period, the quantity of morphine that was seized increased dramatically.

Demand and supply of opiates for medical and scientific purposes

While focusing on the abuse of drugs, it should not be forgotten that many have legitimate and important medical uses. Not least among these are the opiates, which are widely used for the treatment of severe pain,

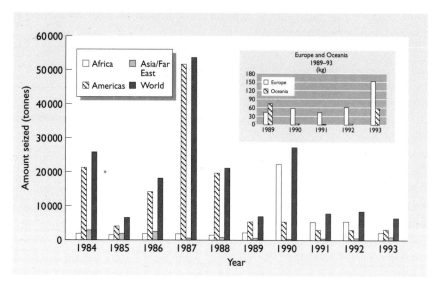

Fig. 2.11 Cannabis herb/plants: quantities reported seized 1984–93. (Source: UNDCP.)

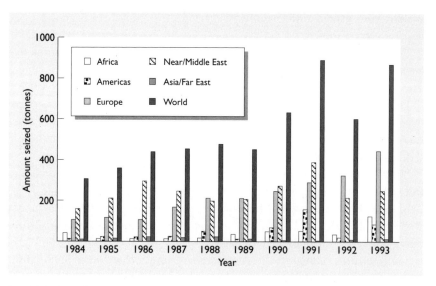

Fig. 2.12 Cannabis resin: quantities reported seized 1984–93. (Source: UNDCP.)

particularly in cancer patients. Despite the increasing use of morphine for this purpose, the annual worldwide consumption of opiates has remained fairly steady over the last 20 years at about 200 tonnes of morphine-equivalent annually, with a moderate increase in 1993 to 223 tonnes; codeine accounted for 177 tonnes of this in 1993. Total global production

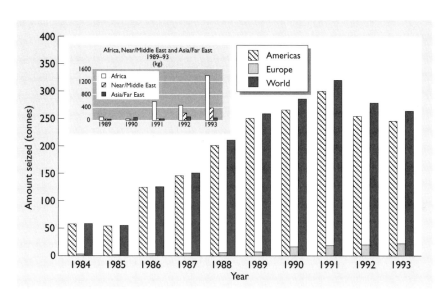

Fig. 2.13 Cocaine: quantities reported seized 1984–93. (Source: UNDCP.)

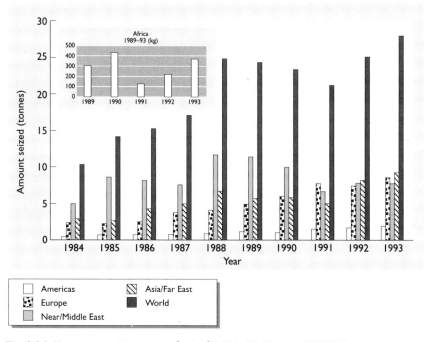

Fig. 2.14 Heroin: quantities reported seized 1984–93. (Source: UNDCP.)

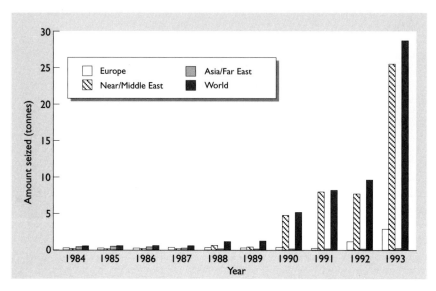

Fig. 2.15 Morphine: quantities reported seized 1984–93. (Source: UNDCP.)

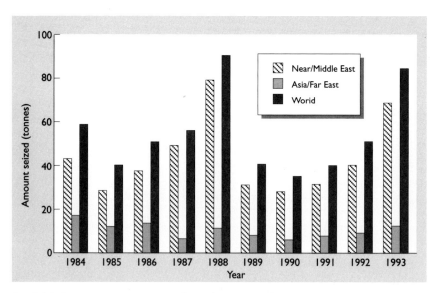

Fig. 2.16 Opium: quantities reported seized 1984–93. (Source: UNDCP.)

fluctuates from year to year, according to climatic and social and political conditions and in 1991 and 1992 production exceeded consumption. In 1993 and 1994, however, production was less than consumption. The main producer countries in 1994 were Australia (78 tonnes morphine-

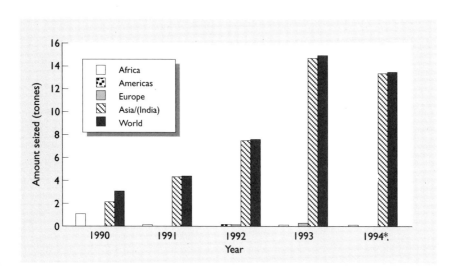

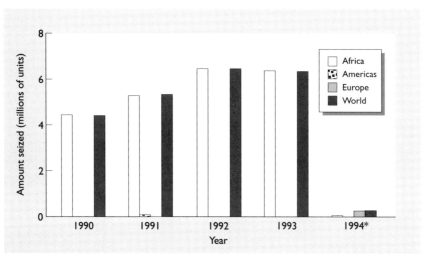

Fig. 2.17 Methaqualone: quantities reported seized 1990–94 by weight and millions of units (preliminary figures for 1994). (Source: UNDCP.)

equivalent), India (41tonnes), Turkey (38 tonnes), France (27 tonnes) and Spain (12 tonnes). The USA was the largest importer of opium in 1992 (36 tonnes).

It is important that a balance between production and licit requirements is maintained because this controls the amount of this highly prized drug that is available for diversion to the black market. In fact, the amount of such diversion is small in comparison with the volume of illicit transactions, indicating that international control measures are largely effective for this group of substances.

The diversion of psychotropic substances

The control of psychotropic drugs under the international conventions has been less successful, resulting in large diversions of these drugs into the illicit market. This has frequently involved drugs such as stimulants, sedative-hypnotics and tranquillizers, mainly in developing countries, and suggests that current control mechanisms are inadequate. Moreover, for several years, some parties to the 1971 Convention on Psychotropic Substances (see Chapter 11), have failed to bring some of these drugs under the control of national legislation, enabling traffickers to exploit these gaps. Despite these setbacks, the worldwide reduction in stocks of methaqualone in line with declining medical requirements is an example of how the system can work well, and there has been a similar reduction in stocks of the stimulant fenetylline.

Global drug problems

A brief description of drug problems in other parts of the world is helpful in putting the UK's problems into an international perspective.

Africa

Cannabis is the most commonly abused drug in Africa and in many countries abuse can be described as endemic. There is already large scale cultivation in Morocco, both for domestic consumption and for smuggling to Europe, but there is evidence that cannabis is now widely grown in other countries too.

The abuse of stimulants remains a major problem in many countries in Africa, with the bulk of drugs being smuggled in from Europe. Pemoline continues to be a feature of illicit stimulant abuse, while large amounts of other psychotropic substances (particularly methaqualone) are also diverted from licit sources as well as being manufactured in clandestine laboratories. It is believed, however, that India is the main source of illicit methaqualone found in Africa.

In the Horn of Africa, khat (*Catha edulis*) poses a different problem. Its trade and consumption are not prohibited or controlled by international treaties, and it is grown in Ethiopia, Kenya and Yemen. Although most is consumed locally, freeze-dried and vacuum-packed leaves are shipped to Europe and some countries have introduced national control measures to prevent its importation.

In addition to domestic drug problems, African transit routes and couriers from West Africa are heavily involved in the transport of heroin and cocaine into Europe. This transit activity has a spillover effect on illicit markets and there is now evidence of opiate abuse in some countries. In view of the popularity of stimulant drugs in Africa, an increase in the availability of cocaine could lead to a very sharp increase in cocaine abuse in Africa.

Central America and the Caribbean

The strategic location of the Caribbean region has led to its being an important transit area for cannabis and cocaine being imported into North America and, to a lesser extent, into Europe. Indeed, transit traffic in cocaine constitutes the greatest drug problem in the region and this has led to domestic drug problems too, with an associated increase in drug-related deaths. There is a long history of cannabis cultivation in the region and this continues today; most is intended for local use although some is smuggled into the USA and Canada.

North America

Cannabis is the most commonly abused drug in North America; in Canada, for example, the national annual prevalence of cannabis abuse was reported to be 5%. Although substantial amounts of the drug are smuggled in, domestic cultivation is becoming an increasingly important source of supply. The latest technology is being applied to all stages of the process with the result that the THC (tetrahydrocannabinol) content of cannabis is now much higher than previously.

Heroin abuse remains a significant cause for concern; heroin seizures increased in 1993 and the purity level of heroin seems to be 10 times that of a decade ago. However, there is no doubt that cocaine (particularly in the form of 'crack') abuse is a major problem and the major challenge to drug law enforcement. Nevertheless, it may be a hopeful sign that, in the USA, the estimated number of cocaine abusers actually fell from 6 million in 1991 to 5 million in 1992, with an associated decrease in the number of frequent cocaine abusers, particularly among young people in middle-income, suburban areas.

The extent of money-laundering in North America is an indication of the extent of their drug problem.

South America

The illicit production, manufacture, traffic and abuse of cocaine is the cause of serious economic and social problems in several South American countries. Peru is the largest producer of coca leaf in the world, although Colombia and Bolivia also have tens of thousands of hectares under coca bush cultivation. In Bolivia and Peru, the leaves are processed into coca paste which is then smuggled into Colombia for conversion into cocaine hydrochloride. However, it appears that increasingly, the manufacture of the final product is being undertaken in clandestine laboratories in the producer countries. The drug law enforcement authorities have a particularly difficult task because they have to deal not only with illicit crop growers and traffickers, but with terrorist guerrillas who derive income from taxes on illicit plantations and trafficking routes. Powerful drug cartels in Colombia appear to be expanding their influence in other South American countries, which are increasingly being used for the transshipment of cocaine to other parts of the world. Although the traditional practice of chewing coca leaves appears to be declining in Bolivia and Peru, the abuse of coca paste is common.

Drug problems in South America are not confined to cocaine. Cannabis is cultivated in most countries, mostly for domestic consumption and, in addition, illicit poppy cultivation has been introduced because the associated profits are higher than those from growing cocaine. Solvent abuse poses major problems particularly among the large population of street children in the urban slums.

East and South East Asia

South East Asia continues to be a major producer of illicit opium, with poppy cultivation taking place mainly in Myanmar and in the Lao People's Democratic Republic. The area under opium poppy cultivation has, however, been successfully reduced in China and in the northern provinces of Viet Nam. Illicit heroin production still continues in the clandestine laboratories in the Golden Triangle – particularly along the Myanmar and Thai borders. Countries such as China, Hong Kong, Japan, Malaysia, Philippines, Republic of Korea, Thailand and Viet Nam are increasingly being used as transit points for illicit consignments of heroin bound for North America and Australia. Sadly, this is contributing to the substitution of heroin abuse for the more traditional opium abuse in these countries. In particular, China has been experiencing an upsurge in heroin abuse especially in Yunnan province where an increase in HIV/AIDS has been attributed to increased drug abuse by injection.

Stimulant abuse is common in several countries, most notably, Japan, the Republic of Korea and Thailand, where the abuse of amphetamine has been implicated as a cause of road traffic accidents. Against this background popularity of stimulants, it is feared that the recent increase in the number of seizures of cocaine may herald a major outbreak of cocaine abuse; concern is heightened by reports that South American cartels may have developed links with Japanese criminal organizations.

South Asia

The opium poppy is cultivated legally in India, and although small quantities are diverted into illicit channels, far greater problems are posed in this region by transit traffic in heroin from South West and South East Asia. The number of heroin seizures in India doubled between 1992 and 1993 and there is growing evidence of abuse of this drug, both in the major cities and beyond; this has been accompanied by increased evidence of HIV infection. Heroin abuse is also a serious problem in Nepal and Sri Lanka, and has also been reported in urban slums in Bangladesh. Buprenorphine, which is licitly manufactured in India, is increasingly being abused in Bangladesh, India and Nepal.

There is large scale cannabis cultivation in parts of Sri Lanka while Nepal remains an important source of cannabis resin for countries in Europe as well as India.

Growing abuse of psychotropic substances has been reported by every country in the region, but the increasing illicit manufacture of methaqualone constitutes a major problem in India; the bulk of it is destined for South Africa but methaqualone abuse has also started to spread in those African countries that serve as transit points.

West Asia

Afghanistan and neighbouring parts of Pakistan appear to be the main sources of large quantities of cannabis resin that is smuggled into Europe along various trafficking routes. There is also considerable illicit traffic in cannabis in CIS member states, and it has been reported that cannabis grows wild on about 140 000 hectares in Kazakhstan. Unofficial estimates suggest that at least 500 000 people (1% of total population) in the five CIS member states in Central Asia are occasional or regular drug abusers. As well as being involved in the production of cannabis, Afghanistan is also one of the largest producers of illicit opium in the world – not least because of the inaccessible nature of the terrain. Much of the opium processing is carried out in the border area with Pakistan, where there are believed to be about 100 illicit heroin laboratories. Major seizures of opium and morphine base have been made by the Iranian authorities, mostly along their border with Afghanistan and intended for onward shipment to the Western market. Much of the illicit traffic to Europe follows the Balkan route (Turkey → Bulgaria → Former Yugoslavia → Austria → Germany), but substantial quantities are used locally, with reports of 500 tonnes of opium being consumed by abusers in Pakistan.

Illicit traffic in fenetylline from European countries, mainly Bulgaria, to countries in the Arab Peninsula has continued, with more than 4 million tablets (original and counterfeit) being seized in 1992.

Europe

Cannabis remains the main drug of abuse in Europe, with huge quantities being smuggled in from Africa and West Asia. There is also a more local source in the Netherlands, where varieties of cannabis with a very high THC content are cultivated.

The cultivation of poppy for culinary purposes has been traditional in countries such as Poland and some of the CIS republics; a recent development is the use of poppy straw to prepare an abusable extract of opium. However, West Asia is the major source of illicit heroin in Europe where the turmoil in the former Yugoslavia and the opening of borders of former socialist countries has led to considerable diversification in trafficking routes.

A newer problem is the increasing traffic in and abuse of cocaine in Europe, most of it originating in Colombia. Although the traditional entry points have been in Spain and Portugal, bulk shipments also arrive at seaports and airports in Belgium and the Netherlands; more recently airports in eastern and Central European countries have been used as transit points with the cocaine couriers continuing their journey by rail and road, across the newly opened borders, to their destinations in Western Europe. Increasingly, cocaine hydrochloride is converted to cocaine base (crack) in clandestine laboratories in Europe, although crack itself is being imported directly into the UK from the Caribbean.

Other important drug problems in Europe include the illicit manufacture of amphetamines and of hallucinogenic amphetamines (e.g., Ecstasy). There has been a drastic increase in the abuse of the latter drugs, which are being used by young adults in nightclubs and all-night parties.

Finally, it should be noted that the long-standing drug problems in Europe have been compounded by the political changes there. The relaxation of border controls, both in Western and Eastern Europe; growing international trade with CIS countries, which frequently lack appropriate drug control mechanisms and where drug-associated crime is increasing at a formidable rate; the war in former Yugoslavia and the consequent political instability – all of these factors make the traffic in illicit drugs much easier to conduct than formerly. New developments in the CIS member states include the appearance on illicit markets of heroin from Afghanistan, buprenorphine from India and cocaine from countries in Latin America.

Oceania

Although substance misuse does not constitute a major problem in this region, Pacific islands are increasingly being used as transit points. Cannabis is cultivated in Australia and New Zealand but in addition to this, some is smuggled in from Papua New Guinea and from South East Asia. Heroin also comes in from Asia while cocaine originates in South America. Stimulants such as amphetamine are manufactured illicitly, mostly for markets in Australia and New Zealand, while hallucinogenic amphetamine abuse is becoming more common, mostly under the control of gangs of motorcyclists.

Summary

The global picture of drug abuse seems to have two major components which used to be quite distinct, but which now appear to be merging. There is the traditional form of drug abuse using crude plant material which contains only a low concentration of active drug. This type of abuse by adults of opium, coca and cannabis has been going on for centuries and continues today in the areas where the plant is grown. In addition, there is the abuse of highly potent, synthetic or semisynthetic substances mostly by young people in industrialized countries who often abuse several different types of drugs. It is this latter type of drug abuse that has been spreading rapidly worldwide and that has been given back to the countries where the traditional use of the drug originated. Thus Thailand and Pakistan now have a major problem with heroin abuse and Bolivia with cocaine abuse.

It is also apparent that the distinctions that used to be made between supplier and consumer countries no longer have any meaning. Consumer countries are simultaneously suppliers of other drugs, while those that supply the world markets themselves import drugs. The notion of transit countries is also somewhat out of date as they too are often involved in both supply and consumption. Underlying this 'globalization' of the drug abuse problem, is the internationalization of and cooperation between the powerful drug cartels. They are skilled at identifying the weak links in the international drug control measures – countries that are not parties to the international drug control treaties (see Chapter 11) and those that have not fully implemented their provisions – and they take advantage of countries that, because of political unrest, terrorist activities or civil war, are unable to ensure governmental control over some parts of their territories and to maintain adequate law enforcement, customs and pharmaceutical control.

Certainly as drug abuse spreads throughout the world, the target population is definitely the young. At first it was predominantly young males that became involved – often students – and drug use often became associated with protest movements. It soon spread, however, to involve those from deprived social backgrounds as well, and to involve nearly as many females as males.

When these broad trends in the patterns of drug abuse are considered against a background of global demographic trends, it is possible to make some guesses about what will happen to drug abuse in the future. It seems likely, for example, in industrialized countries, with a falling birth rate and an ageing population, that there will be an increase in drug abuse by the elderly, which is most likely to involve prescribed drugs. In contrast, in many poor countries with an exploding birth rate, there will be a massive increase in the juvenile and young adult population just at the time when illicit drug abuse is becoming entrenched. Never has there been a greater need for effective, preventive action.

References and further reading

Advisory Council on the Misuse of Drugs (1982). *Treatment and Rehabilitation*. HMSO, London.

Das Gupta S (1990). Identifying the problem. In: Ghodse AH & Maxwell D (eds). *Substance Abuse and Dependence*, 53–79. Macmillan Press, London.

Ghodse AH (1977). Casualty department and the monitoring of drug dependence. *British Medical Journal*, 1, 1381–1382.

Ghodse AH, Sheehan M, Stevens B, Taylor C & Edwards G (1978). Mortality among addicts in Greater London. *British Medical Journal*, 2, 1742–1744.

Ghodse AH, Sheehan M, Taylor C & Edwards G (1985). Death of drug addicts in the United Kingdom 1967–1981. *British Medical Journal*, 290, 425–428.

Ghodse AH, Stapleton J, Edwards G, Bewley T & A-Samarrai M (1986). A comparison of drug-related problems in London Accident and Emergency Departments, 1975–1982. *British Journal of Psychiatry*, 148, 658–662.

Home Office (1994). *Statistics on the Misuse of Drugs in the United Kingdom*. Home Office, London.

Idanpaan-Heikkila J, Ghodse AH & Khan I (eds) (1987). *Psychoactive Drugs and Health Problems*. National Board of Health, Helsinki.

International Narcotics Control Board (1993). *Narcotic Drugs: Estimated World Requirements for 1994; statistics for 1992. (E/INCB/1993/2).* United Nations Publication, Vienna.

International Narcotics Control Board (1993). *Report of the INCB for 1993. (E/INCB/1993/1).* United Nations Publication, New York.

International Narcotics Control Board (1993). *Psychotropic Substances: Statistics for 1992; Assessment of Medical and Scientific Requirements for Substances in Schedule, II, III & IV; Requirements of Import Authorizations for Substances in Schedule III & IV (E/INCB/1993/4).* United Nations Publication, Vienna.

Plant MA, Peck DF & Samuel E (1985). *Alcohol, Drugs and School Leavers.* Tavistock, London

Rootman I & Hughes PH (1980). *Drug Abuse Reporting Systems.* WHO Offset Publication No.55. WHO, Geneva.

Wagstaff A & Maynard A (1988). *Economic Aspects of the Illicit Drug Market and Drug Enforcement Policies in the United Kingdom.* Home Office Research Study No. 95. HMSO, London.

3

Drugs of abuse and dependence

Opiates

The parent drug of this class is opium, and the term 'opiates' is used here to include those drugs that are structurally similar to opium and have similar properties. It includes naturally occurring substances, their semisynthetic derivatives and newer, wholly synthetic drugs; this last group is sometimes known collectively as the opioids.

Opium itself is obtained from the opium poppy, *Papaver somniferum*, which grows in large areas of South East Asia and the Middle East (Turkey, Iran, Afghanistan, Pakistan, Myanmar, Thailand, etc.), as well as in other parts of the world (e.g., Poland). After the poppies have bloomed, the unripe seed capsules are incised with a knife and the milky exudate that oozes out is allowed to dry. It becomes a brown, gummy mass which is scraped by hand from the seed capsule. This, dried further and then powdered, is crude opium which may be smoked in special pipes, chewed, or inserted as small pellets into cigarettes. 'Prepared' opium is a boiled down aqueous solution of raw opium, prepared for opium smokers by repeated boiling and filtration to extract all possible opium and to remove all impurities. The final boiling leaves a thick, sticky paste.

Crude opium contains a number of chemical compounds called alkaloids which possess the same or similar properties as opium. The major alkaloids obtained from opium include morphine (10% by weight) and codeine.

Effects

The outstanding property of opiate drugs is their ability to relieve pain. It was this that inspired Thomas Sydenham in 1680 to say, 'Among the remedies which it has pleased Almighty God to give to man to relieve his sufferings, none is so universal and so efficacious as opium', and it is this property that continues to set opiates among the most useful therapeutic agents available today.

The analgesic action of opiates is probably due not only to their direct action at one or more sites within the nervous system, but also to the way in which they make pain seem more tolerable. This in turn is related to the euphoriant effect of opiates – their ability to induce a state of mental detachment and of extreme well being. In some individuals, some opiates induce not euphoria, but the opposite mental state of dysphoria.

Opiates also have a sedative effect on the nervous system causing inability to concentrate, drowsiness and sleep. In addition they depress the respiratory centre, the part of the brain that controls breathing, so that respiration becomes progressively slower and more shallow. Higher doses causes respiratory arrest (breathing stops), unconsciousness and death. Opiates also control cough by suppression of the cough reflex.

A stimulant effect on specific areas of the brain may cause nausea and vomiting and also a very characteristic sign of opiate administration, the constricted, or 'pin-point' pupil of the eye (miosis). The action of opiates on the muscles of the intestines causes constipation, accounting for their use in antidiarrhoeal preparations.

Tolerance

Tolerance develops to many, but not all, of the effects of opiates so that increasing doses have to be taken to obtain the desired effect (of analgesia or euphoria, for example). Ultimately a regular user may be consuming a daily dose of opiate many times greater than that which would kill an opiate naive individual. If drug administration is interrupted, by a period of imprisonment, for example, tolerance is lost and if the old dose is suddenly resumed, it leads to intoxication which may be fatal. Cross-tolerance occurs between different opiates; this means that theoretically it does not matter which opiate an addict takes. If he or she cannot obtain the preferred opiate (usually heroin), a more easily available one may be substituted.

Finally, it should be noted that tolerance does not usually develop to miosis (pupil constriction) so that regular opiate users retain the characteristic, pin-point pupils.

Physical dependence

Physical dependence on opiates develops if drug administration is regular and continuous, but becomes apparent only if regular administration of the drug ceases. While opiates are being taken there is no objective evidence of the existence or the severity of physical dependence. If drug administration is interrupted, or if other drugs that oppose the action of opiates (opiate antagonists) are given, the symptoms and signs of the abstinence syndrome develop (Table 3.1). Its severity is an indication of the degree of physical dependence that had developed.

The severity of physical dependence depends on the particular opiate being taken, the dose and the duration of chronic administration. As tolerance to opiates increases and the daily dose increases, so the severity of dependence increases, but it reaches a maximum or 'ceiling' for each drug. Beyond this, further increases of dose have little effect on the degree of physical dependence as measured by the severity of the abstinence syndrome. Each opiate has its own capacity to induce physical dependence;

Table 3.1 Opiate abstinence syndrome: symptoms and signs

Grade 0
Drug-craving
Anxiety
Drug-seeking behaviour

Grade 1
Yawning
Sweating
Running eyes and nose
Restless sleep

Grade 2
Dilated pupils
Gooseflesh ('cold turkey')
Muscle twitching
Hot and cold flushes; shivering
Aching bones and muscles
Loss of appetite
Irritability

Grade 3
Insomnia
Low-grade fever
Increased pulse rate
Inceased respiratory rate
Increased blood pressure
Restlessness
Abdominal cramps
Nausea and vomiting
Diarrhoea
Weakness
Weight loss

drugs such as codeine and dextropropoxyphene, even in very high dosage, do not cause physical dependence to match that caused by morphine or heroin.

Opiate abstinence syndrome

The signs and symptoms of opiate abstinence may be graded (Table 3.1) to indicate the different stages and the severity of the abstinence syndrome. This grading is clinically convenient, if somewhat arbitrary, as the symptoms and signs of any particular grade may not all be present simultaneously.

The severity and timing of the abstinence syndrome, its onset, peak and duration of symptoms, all depend on a variety of factors, including which opiate was being taken, its dose and for how long it had previously been taken. Generally, an opiate with a short duration of action, such as heroin, has an abstinence syndrome of earlier onset, shorter duration and greater intensity than a longer-acting drug such as methadone. Similarly, the larger the dose of opiate, the more intense the symptoms and signs of withdrawal. The personality of the addict, his or her expectations and the ability to tolerate the discomfort of withdrawal are also important.

The opiate abstinence syndrome, although extremely unpleasant, is rarely life endangering in an otherwise healthy person. It is, however, very distressing for the individual concerned who can think of nothing except an overwhelming and urgent need for opiates. Consciousness is unimpaired so that the addict is painfully aware of what is happening and feels generally so wretched that he or she may say anything, whether true or not, in an attempt to receive earlier attendance from a doctor and quicker relief of symptoms.

The abstinence syndrome can be immediately relieved by the administration of any opiate; not necessarily the one that has been taken previously. Other sedative drugs may provide partial symptomatic relief, but will not reverse the symptoms and signs of the abstinence syndrome in the way that opiates do.

Psychological dependence

Psychological dependence on opiates is severe and accounts for the desire and craving for drugs that eventually disrupts the addict's life, which may become wholly devoted to obtaining more drugs. Unfortunately, psychological dependence does not end when drug withdrawal has been achieved. It persists long after the pain and discomfort of the abstinence syndrome have abated and accounts for the high relapse rate of opiate addiction.

Opiate receptors

Although opiates, in one form or another, have been used by humans for centuries, it is only during the last 20 years that considerable progress has been made in understanding their mechanism of action. The first step was the discovery within the brain of opiate receptors. These are specialized sites on the cell membranes, with a very specific shape to which opiates bind. Drugs which fit the receptor and activate it are called agonists. Other drugs, which bind to the receptor but do not activate it, thereby preventing other opiates from binding to it, are called antagonists (see p. 80). There appear to be three major categories of opiate receptors, designated mu (μ), kappa (κ) and delta (Δ), with sub-types of each category. Each type of receptor is activated only by opiates conforming to its particular shape and therefore has different sensitivities to different opiates and develops selective tolerance to different opiates. They are distributed differently throughout the central and peripheral nervous systems, with the μ and Δ receptors concentrated in areas involved in the transmission and perception of pain and the control of respiration.

Opiate receptors have now been identified not only in humans but in all vertebrates examined so far, as well as in some invertebrates. An obvious implication is the existence of naturally occurring (endogenous) opiate(s) in these animals as it seems very unlikely that a receptor which is so widely distributed in the animal kingdom should have as its only ligand a substance of plant origin. To date, three distinct 'families' of endogenous opiate peptides have been identified:

1   the enkephalins (Met- and Leu-enkephalin) which are composed of five amino acids each, identical except for the fifth amino acid;
2   beta-endorphin with 30 amino acids;
3   dynorphin with 17 amino acids.

They are coded by separate genes, occur in different anatomical cell groups in the brain and may have distinct biological functions. All three known classes of opiate peptides are found in one or more sites that are known to be part of the body's intrinsic system for pain modulation under physiological conditions, and it appears that endogenous opiates activate the Δ receptors which modify transmission in pain pathways.

What then of dependence on opiates? Do changes occur in this system of opiate transmitters and receptors to account for certain individuals becoming (or remaining) opiate abusers? So far, progress in this field has been limited, although interesting: tolerance develops to endogenous opiates *in vitro* and *in vivo* and cross-tolerance develops between morphine and endogenous opiates. An abstinence syndrome can be precipitated by the opiate antagonist, naloxone, in rats dependent on endogenous opiates and even more interestingly, human beta-endorphin, administered intravenously to opiate-dependent individuals produces a marked improvement in the abstinence syndrome. Its beneficial effect on diarrhoea, vomiting, tremor and restlessness lasts for several days suggesting that endogenous opiates may well be deficient in the abstinence syndrome, their production perhaps having been suppressed by the administration of opiate drugs. Assays of endogenous opiates in dependent individuals have, however, produced inconclusive results. This might be because the assays were done on opiate peptides in blood, and it is unlikely that blood levels reflect levels in the central nervous system. Furthermore, blood levels may be less important than rates of biosynthesis and turnover.

Studies on opiate receptors have similarly been unhelpful as neither the number of receptors nor their properties (ability to bind opiates) seems to be altered in the dependent state. However it appears that chronic (agonist) action at μ or κ receptors can cause tolerance and physical dependence within the neural systems which are affected by these receptors. Thus withdrawal of the agonist drug – that is, one which binds to and activates the receptor – after a long period of administration, or its displacement by a drug with antagonist properties, precipitates a withdrawal syndrome which is quite specific for the receptor type. μ receptor physical dependence, for example, produces severe withdrawal manifestations with intense drug-seeking behaviour. There appears to be little cross-tolerance between the different receptors so that a drug with κ agonist properties cannot suppress the withdrawal syndrome caused by a μ agonist withdrawal.

Different opiate drugs

There have been many attempts to separate, by means of chemical modification, the desirable analgesic action of opiates from their dependence-producing property. Many new drugs have been synthesized either by changing the chemical structure of naturally occurring opiates, or by synthesizing completely new drugs. These are often introduced with extravagant claims that they do not cause dependence. As their use becomes more widespread, however, their dependence-producing potential usually becomes more obvious, and so far all of the clinically useful opiate analgesics share similar structural characteristics and possess a general similarity of action. Any differences between them tend to be differences of degree rather than of nature.

In particular, it has been found that morphine and all the closely related morphine-like opiate drugs have a high affinity for the μ receptor (which was, in fact named μ for the drug morphine). They have less affinity for κ and Δ receptors. Thus all of these drugs can be described as μ agonist opiates, or as prototype μ agonists. Their low affinity for σ receptors probably accounts for the fact that they rarely cause hallucinations or dysphoria.

Morphine

Morphine is a naturally occurring opiate alkaloid. It was first isolated in 1803 and was named after Morpheus, the Greek God of sleep and dreams, because of its sedative, sleep-inducing properties. Although it can be taken orally, the development of the hypodermic syringe facilitated its widespread clinical use. It is still frequently used in the management of severe pain, but suffers from the drawback that it often causes nausea and vomiting. Perhaps for this reason it is not particularly popular as an illicit drug of abuse or dependence.

Papaveretum (omnopon)

Papaveretum is a mixture of morphine and other opium alkaloids. It is often used for pre-operative medication, but is rarely abused, and then usually by members of the medical profession.

Diamorphine (heroin)

Diamorphine was first marketed as the 'heroic' (or powerful) cure for morphinism. It was claimed to be non-addictive, but this soon proved to be untrue. It is made from morphine by a chemical process known as acetylation, which though simple in theory, requires considerable equipment and the expertise of a competent chemist. Nevertheless, it is prepared in large quantities illicitly in fairly primitive 'laboratories' close to the source of opium. The resultant white powder is much easier to transport and smuggle than opium and is now available in most places in the world, its source varying according to local and international politics.

Heroin is a more potent analgesic than morphine, and is used medicinally in a dose of 5–10 mg 4 hourly. It is less likely to cause nausea or constipation and has a much greater euphoric effect. Perhaps for these reasons it is the drug of choice of most opiate-dependent individuals. It may be taken orally or administered by intramuscular, intravenous (mainlining) or subcutaneous (skin-popping) injection. A popular way of taking it is called 'chasing the dragon', in which the heroin is heated on a piece of foil and the resultant fumes are inhaled. This method, although just as likely to cause dependence, is safer than injecting, which is associated with a number of serious complications. Because 'chasing the dragon' is easier and safer than injecting, it may encourage those who would not have dared to inject to experiment with heroin and subsequently become addicted. In time, as the individual's habit becomes larger and therefore more expensive to maintain, or if the heroin is in short supply (and again more expensive), it is more likely to be taken by intravenous injection. This delivers all the available drug right into the bloodstream providing the addict with the best 'kick' ('high', 'rush') possible for that dose of heroin.

Methadone (Physeptone)

Methadone is a synthetic opiate analgesic with a long duration of action (about 24 hours) so that one daily administration to an opiate-dependent individual is sufficient to prevent the onset of the abstinence syndrome. For this reason it is the opiate most frequently prescribed in the treatment of opiate dependence. Although also available in tablet or injectable form, it is usually prescribed as methadone mixture which is unsuitable for injection and has little black market value. Most addicts receive between 30 and 80 mg methadone daily. Despite cross-tolerance between the different opiates, opiate-dependent individuals claim to be able to tell the difference between heroin (their drug of choice) and methadone, which does not give them the euphoric 'high' that they seek. In addition, methadone often causes increased sweating, a side effect which does not seem to occur with other opiates and for which there is no physiological explanation.

Although it is a potent analgesic, it is rarely prescribed for this purpose.

Pethidine (Pethilorfan, Pamergan; meperidine, Demerol in USA)

Pethidine is a synthetic opiate widely used clinically as an analgesic in childbirth and post-operatively. It is a frequent drug of abuse for opiate-dependent individuals in the medical or related professions.

Dipipanone (with cyclizine as Diconal); dextromoramide (Palfium)

These are two synthetic opiate drugs which, during the late 1970s and early 1980s, were very popular with opiate-dependent individuals in the UK. They were often prescribed by independent doctors whom the addicts consulted because the drug-dependence treatment units (DDTUs) were (and are) unwilling to prescribe the injectable opiates which the addicts sought.

Although intended for oral use, Diconal tablets were often crushed, dispersed in water and injected, resulting in the expected complications of self-injection. Tablets surplus to requirement were sold on the black market. Because of the increasing frequency of dependence on dipipanone, it was brought under the same control as heroin and cocaine, so that only doctors with a licence from the Home Office may now prescribe dipipanone to addicts. More recently, because illicit heroin is widely available on the black market, dextromoramide and dipipanone have become less attractive to addicts.

Dextropropoxyphene (Doloxene)

Dextropropoxyphene is a mild opiate analgesic derived from methadone, but with less addictive and analgesic potential. Although available in capsule form, it is much more popularly combined with paracetamol as Distalgesic. Abuse of Distalgesic is not uncommon and overdosage is particularly serious, because of the combination of hepatotoxicity due to paracetamol and respiratory depression due to dextropropoxyphene.

Codeine

Codeine is another alkaloid found in crude opium. It is a much less effective analgesic than morphine and is therefore used for the relief of mild to moderate pain only; it is often combined with aspirin or paracetamol. Its constipating effect is utilized in the treatment of diarrhoea and it is also used as a cough suppressant. It must not be forgotten, however, that codeine and its derivatives (pholcodine, dihydrocodeine) are opiates with a liability for abuse and dependence, albeit less than that of morphine or heroin. As some of these preparations (e.g., codeine phosphate and pholcodine syrups and linctuses) are available without prescription, 'over the counter', opiate addicts can buy them easily. They sometimes use them to supplement supplies from other sources or to prevent the onset of the opiate abstinence syndrome.

Opiate agonist–antagonists

During the search for effective opiate analgesics free from the dependence liability of morphine and heroin, new drugs have been identified which are devoid of analgesic properties, and which oppose or antagonize the respiratory depressant effects of opiates. These drugs (e.g., naloxone, naltrexone) are known as opiate antagonists.

It is now understood that their properties arise because they bind to opiate receptors but do not activate them. For example, naloxone is a μ receptor antagonist which also binds to a lesser degree to κ and Δ receptors. It antagonizes the effect of morphine and related drugs by displacing them from their receptor sites. However, binding to receptors and activating them is not an 'all or none' phenomenon. Some drugs, described as partial agonists, may bind to a receptor but not activate it fully. In so doing they may displace a full agonist, thus reducing or 'antagonizing' its effects. Thus partial agonists are commonly described as agonist–antagonists, and unlike the full agonists, their effects do not increase in proportion to the dose administered, but appear to have a 'ceiling'. It is also important to appreciate that as well as having different affinities for the different receptor sites, a particular drug may be a full agonist at one receptor and an antagonist or partial agonist at another.

Because classical opiate dependence appears to be so firmly linked to μ receptor activity, it seems likely that a partial μ agonist might have less abuse and dependence liability than the prototype μ agonists. Much recent research has therefore concentrated on the mode of action of different drugs at the different receptor sites and a number of agonist–antagonist opiates are now available. However, the abuse liability of a particular drug is more than the mathematical sum of its activity at several receptor sites. Other factors, such as its solubility, the ease with which it enters the nervous system and the firmness with which it binds to the receptor site may all be important. Unfortunately, there is no single animal species which can provide a completely reliable model for predicting the abuse and dependence liability of opiate drugs and these problems usually become apparent only when the drug has become widely available for use by humans outside the laboratory setting.

Pentazocine (fortral)

Pentazocine is a partial μ agonist with agonist activity at κ receptors. It may precipitate withdrawal symptoms in opiate-dependent individuals. When administered by injection it is a more potent analgesic than codeine or dihydrocodeine, but it sometimes causes hallucinations and thought disturbance. High doses may also cause respiratory depression, raised blood pressure and tachycardia. Although its dependence liability is less than that of morphine or heroin, cases of abuse and dependence have been reported and in certain places abuse has become widespread. In some places in the USA, for example, pentazocine abusers add crushed tablets of the antihistamine, tripelennamine, which is known to enhance the reinforcing and analgesic effects of pentazocine, to crushed tablets of pentazocine, and inject this mixture, known as 'T's and 'blues', subcutaneously or intravenously. The effect was said to be indistinguishable from the 'rush' or 'high' caused by heroin and lasted 5–10 minutes. Repeated injection of this mixture may cause convulsions. However, the non-μ actions of pentazocine at κ receptors, which cause progressive increases in dysphoria and other undesirable subjective effects, tend to limit its abuse potential.

Self-injection with pentazocine causes characteristic fibrotic changes in the skin and muscle.

Buprenorphine (temgesic)

Buprenorphine is a partial μ receptor agonist with a long duration of action because of tight receptor binding. It is an effective analgesic which is administered sublingually (under the tongue) or by injection. Oral administration is unsatisfactory because the drug is metabolized very rapidly by the liver.

An unusual property of buprenorphine is that, after chronic administration, the onset of the abstinence syndrome is delayed. There are few, if any, signs of withdrawal during the first 48 hours and only mild signs from the 3rd to the 10th day. In one study, more marked withdrawal effects were reported on the 14th day. Heroin addicts dependent on a small dose of opiate can be transferred on to buprenorphine which can be withdrawn fairly easily because of the delayed onset of the abstinence syndrome. While they are taking buprenorphine, the subjective effects of self-administered heroin are reduced, presumably because buprenorphine is acting as an antagonist on the μ receptors. Thus, theoretically, the rewarding properties of heroin are impaired and the likelihood of future administration should be reduced. However, if buprenorphine is given to individuals dependent on large doses of opiates, its antagonist properties precipitate the onset of withdrawal symptoms. Despite early optimism, the abuse potential of buprenorphine is causing concern. Opiate addicts are clearly able to identify buprenorphine as an opiate when it is administered in sufficient quantity (0.8–2.0 mg) and there are reports of abuse and dependence from several countries. Tablets intended for sublingual administration are being crushed and injected by addicts.

It is interesting that naloxone in doses of up to 4 mg does not precipitate the buprenorphine withdrawal syndrome, although higher doses can reverse the effects of buprenorphine and should theoretically precipitate withdrawal in dependent individuals.

Butorphanol

Butorphanol is an agonist–antagonist opiate with affinity to μ and κ receptors. Like other μ agonists it has analgesic and respiratory depressant properties; it can also cause psychotomimetic symptoms. It can also precipitate symptoms of withdrawal when administered to morphine-dependent individuals. Although butorphanol has positive reinforcing properties in animals, there have been only occasional reports of dependence upon it. This is probably because, like pentazocine, it tends to produce undesirable subjective effects, rather than the sought-after euphoria induced by morphine and other prototype μ agonists.

Nalbuphine (Nubain)

Nalbuphine is a partial μ agonist with a high affinity for κ receptors. Thus it produces analgesia, sedation and some respiratory depression and it does not cause psychotomimetic symptoms. It can reverse the respiratory depression caused by full μ agonists and precipitates the withdrawal syndrome if given to individuals dependent on these drugs. Experienced morphine-users usually recognize nalbuphine as morphine-like, and after a period of chronic administration of nalbuphine, naloxone precipitates a mild withdrawal syndrome. So far, however, there have been very few cases of abuse.

The drugs mentioned in this section do not form a comprehensive list of opiate analgesics. They were selected because they are common, or fairly common, drugs of abuse or dependence, or because they are used to treat opiate dependence. Other opiates are available and may more rarely be the subject of abuse; dependence upon them is similar to that described in this section.

Sedative hypnotics

Sedative hypnotic drugs can be conveniently classified into two groups:
1   the barbiturates, which dominated this area of therapeutics for half a century;
2   the more modern non-barbiturates which were developed because of all the disadvantages and dangers of the earlier drugs.
Since the 1960s the benzodiazepine non-barbiturates have been of overwhelming importance in terms of the number of prescriptions issued and the number of individuals receiving these drugs. However, both barbiturate and non-barbiturate sedative hypnotic drugs have many similar pharmacological properties.

Effects

Sedative hypnotic drugs have a depressant effect on the brain. In small doses they relieve anxiety, inducing a sense of relaxation. In a slightly larger dose they cause drowsiness and sleep, shortening the time until its onset and prolonging its duration. Even when taken in small, hypnotic doses, these drugs have a 'hang-over' effect the following day, often leaving the patient feeling 'drugged' and drowsy. Slowing of performance occurs, measurable under laboratory conditions and manifesting itself in daily life by an inability to concentrate, to make quick decisions or to carry out tasks as quickly and efficiently as usual. Driving a car or operating machinery after taking them the night before may therefore be hazardous.

In excessive doses, such as those taken in deliberate self-poisoning, sedative hypnotic drugs cause a prolonged deep coma with respiratory depression (slow, shallow breathing) and low blood pressure. Death, due to respiratory failure, may occur quite suddenly and unexpectedly with barbiturates, although an overdose of a benzodiazepine alone is unlikely to be fatal.

Tolerance

Tolerance develops rapidly to some of the effects of sedative hypnotics drugs. After taking them for a few days or weeks, the patient is again taking longer to go to sleep and the duration of sleep returns to normal. To achieve the original and desired improvement in sleep the dose has to be increased. After a while the habitual user may show little sign of sedation and may be sleeping for only an hour or two more than usual on a night-time dose that would be profoundly sedating for anyone not used to taking these drugs.

Tolerance also develops to the anxiolytic effect of these drugs, so that they rapidly become ineffective if prescribed in a normal, therapeutic dosage. It is dangerous to increase the dose, however, because this increases the risk and the severity of physical dependence.

Physical dependence

Physical dependence on sedative hypnotics drugs is characterized by the manifestations of the abstinence syndrome, and by a state of chronic intoxication which develops in those who habitually take very large doses.

It is difficult to be precise about the dose or the duration of consumption of these drugs necessary to cause physical dependence, because it varies according to the criteria of dependence that are adopted. For example, withdrawal of therapeutic doses of benzodiazepines given for only a few weeks may lead to anxiety, depression, tremor and somatic symptoms. Because these are often similar to the symptoms of the original illness, it used to be thought that they were evidence that treatment should be continued for longer. Now, however, it is appreciated that they are genuine symptoms of withdrawal (rebound) and that during this stage, anxiety may increase to an intensity above that in the pre-drug period. This type of rebound phenomenon is particularly marked in patients stopping medium-acting benzodiazepines, such as lorazepam, and the importance of prescribing these drugs for short periods only (2–4 weeks) is stressed. Another form of rebound anxiety occurs, particularly with shorter-acting compounds, when there may be interdose anxiety associated with falling blood levels as the time for the next dose approaches.

Similarly, withdrawal of the normal hypnotic dose of sedative hypnotics drugs may precipitate nightmares, broken sleep with vivid dreams and increased REM (rapid eye movements) which may persist for several weeks. This is known as rebound insomnia and its appearance following the abrupt withdrawal of benzodiazepine hypnotics suggests that even modest doses can cause mild physical dependence. Higher doses (say diazepam 60 mg daily) taken over a period of 1–2 months would be sufficient to cause noticeable physical dependence with many of the signs listed below, although there is considerable individual variability of response and some people may be vulnerable to severe consequences of withdrawal, having taken a much smaller dose.

Sedative hypnotic abstinence syndrome

The symptoms and signs of sedative hypnotic withdrawal develop progressively. They include weakness, anxiety, tremor, dizziness, insomnia, impaired concentration, loss of appetite, nausea and vomiting, dysphoria, headaches, incoordination, heightened sensory perception, lethargy, depersonalization, tiredness, blurred vision, facial burning sensation, hot and cold feelings with sweating and muscle aching. All of these symptoms may be experienced when patients are withdrawn from long-term treatment (3 months) with a benzodiazepine administered in normal dosage (30 mg/day or less). Perceptual symptoms vary considerably from patient to patient and can be very distressing. It should be emphasized that these symptoms are genuine manifestations of withdrawal and are not a resurgence of the condition for which the sedatives were originally prescribed; thus patients who were prescribed benzodiazepines for non-psychiatric reasons may experience perceptual symptoms, anxiety and insomnia when their medication is stopped. The abstinence syndrome usually begins within 2 days of drug withdrawal although it may be delayed for over a week; it may occur despite dose tapering, but usually subsides over a period of a few weeks.

If larger doses of sedative hypnotics have been taken, withdrawal will lead to an increased pulse rate (more than 100/min) with a further increase (of more than 15/min) on standing. Standing is also associated with a fall in blood pressure. There is muscle twitching and tremor, increased reflexes and dilated pupils. These unpleasant, but not particularly dangerous symptoms may, however, be followed by *grand mal* convulsions (fits) which may progress to life-threatening status epilepticus, in which the patient has fits continuously. A psychotic state, resembling alcoholic delirium tremens in which the patient is very agitated and confused and suffers auditory and visual hallucinations may also occur.

Although the sedative hypnotic withdrawal syndrome is the same in its broad outline regardless of which class of drug is responsible, there are differences between different drugs. Fits and delirium are more common after barbiturate withdrawal, while milder symptoms such as anorexia, agitation and insomnia are more common after benzodiazepine withdrawal.

Chronic intoxication

Because there is an upper limit to tolerance to sedative hypnotic drugs and because dependent individuals often increase their daily consumption beyond this point, chronic intoxication is a common feature of their condition. This resembles intoxication with alcohol and is characterized by difficulty in thinking, slow and slurred speech, poor comprehension and memory, and emotional lability. Irritability and moroseness are common. It is interesting that abusers seem less aware of their mood changes and behavioural impairment when taking high doses of benzodiazepines than with high doses of barbiturates.

Chronic intoxication with barbiturates, which is now less common than formerly, is accompanied by neurological symptoms and signs: nystagmus (jerky, involuntary movements of the eyes), double vision, squint, difficulty in visual accommodation, unsteadiness and falling. With larger doses the increasing sedation leads to the subject falling, sleep and eventually respiratory depression and death. In fact, one of the main risks of chronic barbiturate use and the consequent development of tolerance is that the gap between the intoxicating dose and the fatal dose is dangerously reduced.

Psychological dependence

Psychological dependence on sedative hypnotic drugs is manifested by craving for the drug and by drug-seeking behaviour. Animals will perform an action repeatedly to obtain these drugs, thereby demonstrating their reinforcing properties. However, sedative hypnotics are less powerful reinforcers of behaviour than are opiates or cocaine, and undoubtedly cause less severe psychological dependence.

Although psychological dependence on barbiturates has long been recognized, it was thought at first that benzodiazepines were free from this disadvantage. However, the considerable difficulty experienced by many benzodiazepine users in managing without their drugs, even when they were withdrawn gradually to prevent the onset of physical symptoms, has contradicted early beliefs and hopes. It is now recognized that benzodiazepines can and do cause psychological dependence and that this is closely related to the dose that is taken and the duration of administration. For this reason the indications for prescribing them are now defined very strictly, and it is recommended that they should be prescribed in the smallest effective dose for a period that does not usually exceed 4 weeks.

Barbiturates

Barbiturate drugs are all derived from a single chemical substance, barbituric acid. The first to be synthesized was barbitone (Veronal) which was introduced into clinical practice in 1903 when it was welcomed as the solution to one of man's oldest and most intractable problems – insomnia.

Over the years many different barbiturates have been synthesized. Some very short-acting barbiturates are administered intravenously for the induction of general anaesthesia (e.g., thiopentone, methohexitone). Other, long-acting compounds such as phenobarbitone and methylphenobarbitone are used to treat epilepsy. Neither of these two types of barbiturates has been involved in problems of abuse and dependence and concern has centred on barbiturates of medium duration of action which used to be prescribed for the treatment of anxiety or insomnia. These include amylobarbitone, butobarbitone, pentobarbitone and quinalbarbitone. The similarities between all of these drugs are more striking than their differences.

Non-barbiturate, non-benzodiazepine sedative hypnotics

Because of the disadvantages and dangers of barbiturates and particularly their dependence liability and their serious effects when taken in overdose, many attempts were made to synthesize safer sedative hypnotics. These included drugs such as meprobamate (Equanil), glutethimide (Doriden), dichloralphenazone (Welldorm) and methaqualone, which when they were introduced, were hailed like the barbiturates before them, as an answer to a prayer for a safe hypnotic. Clinical experience, however, revealed that their effects on the nervous system are similar to those of barbiturates, that tolerance develops together with physical and psychological dependence. When taken in overdose all of these drugs show features of poisoning similar to those of barbiturate overdose although some, such as glutethimide, which is no longer marketed in the UK, are particularly dangerous. Methaqualone used to be available in combination with an antihistamine (Mandrax) and became a very common drug of abuse. None of these drugs is important therapeutically now.

Benzodiazepines

Because the above drugs were no more satisfactory than barbiturates the search continued for safer and better alternatives. The benzodiazepines were introduced into clinical practice in the 1960s and an enormous number have now been synthesized. Like barbiturates they possess powerful anti-epileptic properties, although they are rarely used in the long-term treatment of epilepsy because their effectiveness wanes within a few months. However, a benzodiazepine (diazepam or clonazepam) is the drug of choice for the emergency treatment of the life-threatening condition of major status epilepticus. In addition, benzodiazepines have muscle relaxant properties permitting their use for the relief of muscle spasm or spasticity. They differ from earlier sedative hypnotics drugs in being much safer when taken in overdose. Indeed, very large doses of benzodiazepines rarely cause sufficient respiratory depression to kill the patient unless another drug or alcohol has been taken simultaneously. Their safety in overdose is a very important property in societies where deliberate self-poisoning with psychoactive drugs has become very common.

The main advantage of benzodiazepines over older drugs in this class is their ability, in low doses, to relieve anxiety without causing undue sedation. This was undoubtedly the basis for their early popularity, when their potential for producing dependence was not appreciated, and a vast range of benzodiazepines was synthesized. Their similarities are more striking than their differences which mostly depend on their duration of action. The early benzodiazepines (e.g., diazepam, chlordiazepoxide) are long-acting drugs, mainly because they are converted in the body to active metabolites such as desmethyldiazepam which itself has a half-life of 72 hours or more.

These drugs have the disadvantage that they often cause a prolonged hang-over, leaving the patient feeling 'drugged' for some time. For this reason, shorter acting benzodiazepines (e.g., lorazepam, oxazepam) were developed, which bypass desmethyldiazepam in their metabolic pathways and which are more suitable as day-time anxiolytics and as hypnotics with minimal hangover. However, these short-acting drugs cause rapid rises and falls in blood levels so that withdrawal phenomena are more common and patients may crave the next tablet to relieve their distressing symptoms. Dependence on them often seems more severe and more difficult to treat than dependence on benzodiazepines with a longer duration of action, although there is no scientific evidence that a particular benzodiazepine is any better or worse than any other, in terms of therapeutic effectiveness or dependence liability.

Cross-tolerance

It is not surprising that cross-tolerance develops between different barbiturates and that any barbiturate can be taken to prevent or treat the abstinence syndrome caused by withdrawal of another. It is perhaps less expected that a considerable degree of cross-tolerance also exists with other central nervous system depressants such as alcohol, benzodiazepines and other non-barbiturate hypnotics including chlormethiazole. The existence of this cross-tolerance emphasizes the intrinsic similarities of all of these drugs, whatever their differences in terms of chemical structure, etc. The discovery of separate benzodiazepine receptors in human brain tissues may go some way towards explaining the differences that do exist. These receptors are associated with the receptor sites for the neuroinhibitor γ-aminobutyric acid (GABA) and benzodiazepines appear to act by promoting the depressant effect of GABA on the brain, thus inducing sedation and sleep.

Stimulant drugs

Amphetamine

Amphetamine is the general name given to a class of synthetic drugs that are similar in effect to a substance produced by the body called adrenaline. Adrenaline acts as a transmitter in part of the nervous system known as the sympathetic nervous system which prepares the body for 'fight or flight', releasing sugars stored in the liver and increasing heart and respiration rates. Amphetamines, because they mimic many of the effects of adrenaline, are known as sympathomimetic amines. They appear to act by releasing the neurotransmitters noradrenaline and dopamine, by inhibiting their re-uptake and perhaps also by a direct agonist action on the receptor sites for these two chemicals.

The least potent of the amphetamines is amphetamine sulphate which was marketed in 1932 as a nasal decongestant in the form of an inhaler (Benzedrine). It was soon realized that one of the side effects of Benzedrine was sleeplessness and it was thus that the stimulant effect of amphetamine was revealed.

Amphetamine sulphate is in fact a mixture of two forms of amphetamine, chemically indistinguishable and differing only in the direction in which they rotate plane polarized light. Dextrorotatory amphetamine (D-amphetamine) is approximately twice as powerful a central stimulant as the racemic compound which contains both forms of amphetamine, and three to four times as potent as laevorotatory amphetamine (L-amphetamine).

Effects

Amphetamine is a powerful central stimulant producing an elevated mood and making the user feel energetic, alert and self-confident. Task performance that has been impaired by boredom or fatigue is improved, accounting for the popularity of amphetamine among students working for examinations. Feelings of hunger and fatigue are reduced and there is increased talkativeness, restlessness and sometimes agitation. Some individuals may, however, become anxious and irritable. Because it is a sympathomimetic drug, amphetamine causes increased heart rate and blood pressure, palpitations, dilated pupils, dry mouth and sweating; L-amphetamine has a greater effect on the cardiovascular system than D-amphetamine.

Acute intoxication with amphetamine is characterized by dizziness, sweating, chest pain, palpitations, hypertension and cardiac arrhythmias. Body temperature may be raised and convulsions often occur.

Tolerance

Tolerance develops to some but not all of the effects of amphetamine. Those taking it for its euphoric, mood-elevating effect find that they have to escalate the dose progressively to maintain this effect and may take 250–1000 mg daily. However, because they have also become tolerant to its cardiovascular effects they do not suffer from adverse side effects. Because tolerance also develops to the appetite-suppressant effect of amphetamine, it is not effective in the treatment of obesity. It is, however, useful in the treatment of narcolepsy, a rare condition in which the sufferer keeps falling asleep suddenly and inappropriately; tolerance does not develop to the awakening effect of amphetamine and narcolepsy remains one of the few therapeutic indications for amphetamine (10–60 mg daily). Amphetamine and its derivatives have a paradoxical effect on hyperkinetic children, reducing their antisocial behaviour and increasing their attention span. As tolerance does not develop to these effects, amphetamine (or methylphenidate) is sometimes used in the management of this condition, although the effect of long-term treatment is not clear.

In addition to the development of tolerance, amphetamine can also produce sensitisation, which is sometimes called 'reverse tolerance'. It has been observed in animals, when single daily doses of the drug that do not, at first, cause hyperactivity or stereotyped behaviour, can start to induce this behaviour if injections continue over a period of several weeks. This effect is believed to be mediated by the release of dopamine in the striatum (part of the mid-brain) and it has been suggested that this is the basis of the stereotyped behaviour that is sometimes observed in amphetamine and cocaine addicts.

Cross-tolerance develops between different amphetamines, but not between amphetamine and cocaine despite their many similarities.

Physical dependence

Although chronic amphetamine users may escalate their dose until they are taking large quantities, the existence of physical dependence is disputed. After long-term use, or after a binge of drug-taking lasting a few days, abrupt withdrawal is commonly followed by feelings of fatigue, depression and hunger, and a need for sleep (the 'crash'). Although these may be the manifestations of a withdrawal syndrome it has been suggested that they are the normal reaction to the lack of sleep and food that occurs with chronic amphetamine use. Depression at this time may be so severe that suicide is a real risk.

Psychological dependence

Psychological dependence on amphetamine undoubtedly develops and chronic users experience intense craving and exhibit drug-seeking behaviour. This craving may last, with varying intensity, for several weeks, responding to emotions and to drug-related stimuli. Laboratory experiments on animals confirm that amphetamine has powerful reinforcing properties.

Adverse effects

The most serious consequence of amphetamine abuse is a psychotic illness which may be difficult to distinguish from schizophrenia. It is characterized by paranoid delusions and by auditory and visual hallucinations. It usually develops if amphetamine has been taken for a long time and the dose has been escalated. It is particularly common if methylamphetamine is injected, but can occur with oral use and may even develop after a single, oral dose of amphetamine. The symptoms usually remit within 1 week of drug withdrawal.

Another complication of chronic amphetamine abuse is automatic, stereotyped behaviour in which some action such as tidying a handbag, fiddling with a radio or touching/picking at the skin on the face or extremities may continue for hours at a time. Scratching or picking at the skin is often associated with tactile hallucinations and with delusions of being infested with parasitic insects.

Derivatives

Since the introduction of amphetamine into medical practice many other drugs have been synthesized for their stimulant or appetite-suppressant effects. Methylamphetamine, an injectable amphetamine, was available in the 1960s, but was withdrawn from retail pharmacies when there was a veritable epidemic of intravenous methylamphetamine abuse with many cases of psychosis. Benzphetamine was used for the treatment of obesity because of its appetite-suppressant properties, but problems of dependence soon became apparent. Since then a range of drugs have been produced. Most are chemically similar to amphetamine, have rapidly become drugs of abuse and have been brought under strict control. They include methylphenidate (Ritalin), phenmetrazine (Preludin), diethylpropion (Apisate), phentermine (Duramin) and mazindol (Teronac). Slight modifications of chemical structure have produced drugs such as fenfluramine and chlorphentermine with less stimulant properties, but their role in the long-term management of obesity remains questionable.

Pemoline

Pemoline is an amphetamine-like drug which decreases appetite and has central stimulant effects. Its therapeutic usefulness is rated as low and in large doses it may produce hyperactivity, dyskinesia, seizures, insomnia and hallucinations.

The euphoric effects induced by pemoline are significantly less than those of amphetamine and its reinforcing properties appear very limited. In addition, it is not soluble in water so that there is less likelihood of it being injected. It is perhaps not surprising therefore that there have been few case reports of dependence on pemoline although large quantities are diverted illicitly, mainly to countries in West Africa. Abuse has been reported from several countries and pemoline has been suspected in some cases of drug abuse by athletes and in the doping of race horses.

Cocaine

Cocaine is an alkaloid prepared from the leaves of the coca bush, *Erythroxylum coca*, which grows in the mountainous regions of South America (Colombia, Bolivia, Peru). Traditionally, the leaves were (and are) chewed by the natives – apparently without ill effect – to alleviate fatigue, hunger and cold. They were used by the Incas in religious ceremonies as well as socially and for medicinal purposes.

Cocaine itself was first isolated in the 1880s and its oral consumption became widespread throughout the USA and Europe as it was included in tonics, patent medicines, soft drinks and even wine. Its pharmacological properties were investigated by Sigmund Freud who noted its local anaesthetic and psychic effects. He initially recommended it as a cure for morphine addiction, but later became aware of its dependence liability.

The process of extracting cocaine is carried out in illegal factories often situated in the jungle close to where the coca shrubs are grown. Cocaine hydrochloride of a high degree of purity is obtained. It is a white powder easy to transport and smuggle and is often diluted ('cut') with adulterants such as sugar, amphetamine or local anaesthetics.

Routes of administration

Cocaine may be administered by almost any route. Intravenous use has long been popular with 'serious' drug users because the drug reaches the brain rapidly and subjective effects, including an intense rush or high, are reported within 1 or 2 minutes. They also abate rapidly, over the next 30 minutes or so.

A common way of taking cocaine is by sniffing (snorting) it. A line of cocaine hydrochloride (20–30 mg) is laid out and inhaled through a straw and the drug is absorbed through the vascular mucous membranes lining the nose. Because cocaine causes vasoconstriction (narrowing of the blood vessels), drug absorption is slowed and there is no rush. However, a period of pleasurable stimulation and euphoria occurs, lasting for 20–40 minutes. Sniffing is simpler than injecting and carries no risk of infective complications, but repeated intranasal use of cocaine damages the nasal mucous membrane causing chronic inflammation (rhinitis) and sometimes a perforated nasal septum.

Smoking cocaine has recently become popular. This practice originated in South America in the 1970s when coca paste, a crude derivative of coca leaves, was mixed with tobacco or marijuana and smoked. Cocaine hydrochloride is unsuitable for smoking because it decomposes at high temperatures. However, when the cocaine alkaloid is freed from its hydrochloride base by a chemical reaction involving ether, it has a melting point of 98°C and is volatile at temperatures above 90°C. It therefore vaporizes very easily when heated, and the drug is rapidly and efficiently absorbed from the lungs.

Another form of cocaine freebase is crack which is prepared by a simple process of 'cooking' cocaine with baking powder and water. The baking powder precipitates out any impurities or adulterants, leaving pure, crystalline cocaine which is cracked into chips which are marketed in small phials. Because each phial contains only a very small quantity of cocaine, it is comparatively cheap, so that cocaine, once available only to the wealthy, has become accessible to many more people.

Purified cocaine base is usually smoked in a glass water pipe or it may be sprinkled on a tobacco or marijuana cigarette. It produces a sudden, intense high, (the 'rush' or 'flash') comparable to that produced by intravenous injection, because the cocaine is absorbed very rapidly by the large surface area of the lungs and reaches the brain within seconds. The euphoria abates equally quickly, leaving the user feeling restless and irritable and craving for another dose. The cocaine user often appears unable to titrate or adjust the dosage and the frequency of administration and the quantity inhaled escalates rapidly. Inhalations may be repeated as often as every 5 minutes during binges that may last from hours to days. Smoking continues until supplies are finished or the user falls asleep exhausted.

Effects

Cocaine is a powerful central nervous system stimulant producing increased energy, wakefulness, activity, confidence and facilitating social interchange. Most important of all it is a powerful euphoriant, giving the user a great feeling of well-being.

This euphoriant property is utilized when cocaine is included in elixirs (e.g., 'Brompton Cocktail') used for the treatment of pain in terminally ill patients. These elixirs also contain heroin or morphine, and cocaine counteracts what might otherwise be an undesirable degree of sedation.

The physical effects of cocaine include a raised pulse rate, blood pressure and temperature, and dilated pupils. In addition to its local anaesthetic properties, cocaine also causes local vasoconstriction (narrowing of blood vessels) so that it was once widely used in ear, nose and throat surgery because it reduced haemorrhage. Now, however, it has been replaced by less toxic synthetic local anaesthetics. It is still used in eye drops for ophthalmic surgery.

Very large doses taken by those who are not used to it cause hypertension, cardiac arrhythmias and convulsions. Death may occur due to cardiac or respiratory arrest.

Tolerance

It used to be believed that tolerance to cocaine did not occur and that large doses were taken only in a search for greater euphoria, rather than because small doses were no longer effective. These observations were based on cocaine users who snorted cocaine hydrochloride intermittently, in what was described as 'usual' recreational doses, which were probably insufficient to induce tolerance.

Now that pure cocaine freebase is available, a very different picture is emerging. Some users may take huge doses – 30 g in 24 hours has been reported – that would undoubtedly be toxic to a cocaine-naive individual, but which the regular user can take without serious complication because of the development of tolerance to the hyperthermic, convulsant and cardiovascular effects of cocaine. It is less clear whether tolerance develops to the euphorigenic properties of cocaine; if it does, this would contribute to dose escalation. However, as the dose and frequency of consumption increase, dysphoric effects of cocaine, such as irritability, suspiciousness and restlessness occur, suggesting that there is a ceiling to tolerance of cocaine's psychic effects.

Tolerance does not seem to develop to the reinforcing effect of cocaine.

Physical dependence

A variety of symptoms have been described following cocaine withdrawal by users who habitually consume very large doses. The symptoms include lethargy, depression, apathy, social withdrawal, tremor, muscle pain and disturbances of eating and sleeping (as well as EEG (electroencephalograph) changes). When severe, they form a syndrome known as the 'crash'.

Despite long-standing opinion to the contrary, it is difficult to believe that the crash could be anything but the cocaine abstinence syndrome, although it does not cause the major physiological disruption associated with the more familiar abstinence syndromes of opiates or sedative hypnotics.

Psychological dependence

Cocaine causes severe psychological dependence with craving and drug-seeking behaviour so intense that the normal pattern of life is disrupted and everything becomes subservient to the need to obtain cocaine. In the early stages, a weekend user, accustomed to having a good time if he or she takes cocaine, finds that nothing is quite as enjoyable without it, and eventually that he or she is incapable of enjoying anything if cocaine is not taken. Consumption extends gradually through the week and it is then often taken specifically to relieve stress, because of the learned experience of 'feeling better' after cocaine. Severe psychological dependence may develop quite rapidly, often without the user being aware that his or her drug use is problematical.

In animals, cocaine is a powerful primary reinforcer: laboratory animals exposed to cocaine will repeat an action more and more frequently in order to obtain more cocaine and, given free access to it, will take the drug to the exclusion of food so that they lose weight and die. Until recently there was little evidence that cocaine has such compelling effects in humans and it was thought to be a 'safe' recreational drug. The advent of pure cocaine freebase has dramatically changed this view. Not only has it become apparent that cocaine can cause tolerance and physical dependence, but new patterns of consumption of cocaine have developed, with freebasers smoking cocaine almost continuously until either they or the supply of drug are exhausted – a behaviour pattern remarkably similar to that observed in laboratory animals. It has been suggested that this pattern of drug use is caused by the high concentrations of cocaine in the brain that are achieved by smoking cocaine freebase, and that last for only a few minutes before a rapid decline in concentration occurs. It is possible, for example that it is the sharp contrast between the 'rush' and withdrawal that generates the drive to use more drug within a short period.

Cocaine toxicity/psychosis

As the dose and frequency of use of cocaine increase, adverse reactions may occur. These start with feelings of anxiety, restlessness and apprehension and progress to suspiciousness, hypervigilance and paranoid behaviour.

Stimulation of the nervous system occurs causing muscle twitching, nausea and vomiting, increases in pulse and blood pressure, irregular respiration and sometimes convulsions. In cases of severe toxicity, this is followed by depression of the nervous system with circulatory and respiratory failure, loss of reflexes, unconsciousness and death.

Cocaine psychosis has also been described with persecutory delusions and repetitive (stereotyped) behaviour such as compulsively taking a watch or radio apart and reassembling it or repeatedly tidying or rearranging a set of objects. There may be auditory hallucinations and sometimes tactile hallucinations, classically described as a sensation of insects crawling under the skin ('cocaine bugs') and causing incessant picking at the skin, or scratching. These symptoms are indistinguishable from the toxic symptoms caused by other stimulants such as amphetamine, but last for a shorter time and may come to medical attention less often.

Because of the adverse effects of cocaine when it is taken in high dosage, the cocaine user finds him or herself in a dilemma. The unpleasant symptoms of drug withdrawal and above all the intense craving for cocaine, make discontinuing it almost impossible, but continued consumption of large doses leads to the unpleasant symptoms outlined above. Other drugs, such as alcohol and other central nervous system depressants, may then be taken to counteract the unwanted effects of cocaine and the drug abuser may become (unwittingly) physically dependent on them too. Overdose and intoxication with these drugs is also common. It should also be noted that cocaine is often adulterated with synthetic local anaesthetics such as procaine or lignocaine which, when consumed in large doses, may cause convulsions.

Khat

Khat is a tree, *Catha edulis*, that grows at high altitude in East Africa, Yemen and Democratic Yemen where the leaves and young shoots have been used for their stimulant effect for hundreds of years. Modern methods of transport have made it easy to export khat and to bring regular supplies of fresh leaves to markets in towns and cities in Democratic Yemen, Ethiopia, Somalia, Yemen, Kenya and Tanzania. Recent reports suggest that it may be exported more widely for the benefit of expatriate communities.

Nowadays khat is usually chewed, although in the past an infusion of the leaves was prepared (Arabian or Ethiopian tea). The khat leaves are plucked from the twig and are chewed; the juicy extract is swallowed and the leafy residue is kept as a wad in one side of the mouth. In Yemen it is usually taken in a group setting at special parties, drinks are served and tobacco is smoked either as cigarettes or in a water pipe.

One alkaloid, cathine, was identified in khat a century ago. More recently, other substances, including cathinone, have also been isolated.

Effects

Khat affects the digestive system commonly causing anorexia and constipation. Stomatitis (inflammation of the mouth), gastritis and dyspepsia have also been reported. In the cardiovascular system there is a temporary increase in pulse rate and blood pressure, palpitations and flushing of the face.

Khat is chewed because of its ability to produce cerebral stimulation. Because of this it was traditionally consumed by tribal people when travelling, and nowadays is taken by long-distance lorry drivers and by students preparing for examinations. It produces a general sense of well-being and when taken in a group setting (as it traditionally is) it elevates the mood of the group and promotes social interaction. After a few hours however the mood of the group changes and some participants become restless and irritable. It may cause sleeplessness which in turn may lead to the abuse of alcohol or sedative hypnotics drugs. It has been reported that khat may (rarely) cause a toxic psychosis or schizophrenic reaction. Its use may sometimes precipitate a functional psychosis in predisposed individuals.

Dependence

There is no evidence of a clear cut abstinence syndrome and thus no evidence of physical dependence on khat. Psychological dependence does develop, and in cities in Somalia and Yemen it is estimated that a consumer may spend 25% of his daily earnings in khat, thus causing financial hardship to his family.

Although the problems associated with the use of khat may seem minor in comparison with those of other drugs of abuse, khat should not be ignored. Until recently it had been used only locally where it was grown, and even now because the leaves must be fresh when they are chewed, their area of distribution has remained fairly localized. However, the active ingredient of khat, cathinone, has now been isolated and in experiments on laboratory animals, has been shown to have primary reinforcing properties similar to those of cocaine. If pure cathinone were to become available on the street, it is possible that it would cause severe psychological dependence and that it would be extensively abused. Already, in countries where khat is not cultivated and has to be imported, its use raises major socioeconomic issues and these, together with the medical complications of its use, have been considered by some countries serious enough to warrant the introduction of preventive measures (prohibition).

There are clear similarities between the present state of khat abuse and the way in which cocaine abuse began. Already, khat is being cultivated for export. It would indeed be tragic if the rest of the world waited in ignorance while a new drug of dependence and abuse was systematically extracted, marketed and exported. The lessons learned from the history of cocaine should not be forgotten too quickly.

Hallucinogens

Lysergic acid diethylamide (LSD)

LSD was first synthesized in 1938 by Hofmann. It is derived from ergot, a fungus that grows on rye grains and is a white, crystalline powder soluble in water and effective in such minute quantities that doses are measured in micrograms (μg). It is taken orally and its effects can be felt with a dose of only 25 μg although a more usual dose would be 100 μg. It was originally sold on sugar cubes and on small, flat strips known as microdots, and is now available on squares of paper, rather like stamps.

The physical effects of LSD consumption are apparent within a few minutes. They include nausea, headache, dilated pupils, raised pulse rate, a small and variable alteration of blood pressure and perhaps an increase in body temperature.

The mechanism of action of LSD and related drugs is not clear. They act at multiple sites in the central nervous system, with an agonistic action at presynaptic receptors for 5-hydroxytryptamine (5-HT, serotonin) in the mid-brain, where the firing rate of neurones was sharply reduced following small systemic doses of LSD.

Effects

The psychological effects of LSD are very variable, depending on the expectations and mood of the subject and the setting in which the drug is taken. Their onset follows the somatic symptoms and they persist for several hours.

Characteristically there are changes in perception, especially in the more experienced user. These affect all senses, particularly vision and may take many different forms: stationary objects appear to move and change shape; some things become minute while previously ignored details loom large and assume importance; colours become more intense. There is often a 'cross-over' of perceptions (synaesthesia) so that sounds are 'seen' or 'felt' and colours are 'heard'. Distortions of body image are common: a limb may appear to shrink, or become enormous and may seem completely separate from the rest of the body. The perception of time is often distorted too, with 'clock' time passing very slowly.

Although LSD and similar drugs are often described or classified as hallucinogens, these perceptual changes are often illusions (the altered perception of an existing object) rather than true hallucinations (perception in the absence of stimulus). The latter do occur sometimes, although auditory hallucinations arise less frequently than in naturally occurring psychoses.

In addition to these striking perceptual changes, LSD also affects thinking processes and mood, and induces feelings that are rarely, if ever, experienced at other times. The user may feel that he or she has achieved union with and a unique understanding of mankind, God and the universe, but often lacks the language to describe what has obviously been a profound experience. Sometimes the experiences are wonderful and exalting although they may be overwhelmingly frightening. It is thus not surprising that the mood of the LSD user is labile, moving through anxiety, apprehension, gaiety and depression in a way that may be incomprehensible to an observer. The subject may be withdrawn and introspective, preoccupied with these experiences and, because LSD also affects thought processes, may show impaired concentration, distractibility and illogical thinking and be totally out of touch with others and unable to explain what is happening.

It should now be apparent why LSD and other similar drugs are often described as psychedelic or mind-expanding; it enables the user to experience a mental state which he or she would otherwise be unlikely to achieve. There is no evidence, however, that these apparently profound and, at the time, very meaningful experiences affect the personality or subsequent behaviour in a beneficial way. However, at one stage, LSD was used as an aid to psychotherapy, because it was believed that it would enable events of psychodynamic importance to be re-lived.

Tolerance and dependence

Tolerance to the effects of LSD develops so rapidly that a second dose of the drug taken within 24 hours has less effect than the first, and after three or four daily doses, subsequent administration has little or no psychological effect. Because of this there is no incentive to take it regularly on a daily basis, psychological and physical dependence do not develop and withdrawal phenomena are not observed. Tolerance is lost equally rapidly and after 3 or 4 days of abstinence, full sensitivity to the effects of LSD is regained. Chronic users usually take LSD once or more a week, often in large doses. Tolerance to the cardiovascular effects of LSD is less pronounced.

Adverse effects

The most common adverse effect of LSD is a 'bad trip' – an unpleasant, often terrifying drug experience that leads to a temporary episode of over-whelming anxiety and panic which may last for up to 24 hours. A bad trip cannot be predicted or prevented and may occur to any user, even after a number of previously pleasurable experiences. Its occurrence is presumably related in some way to the mental state of the user and the setting in which drug consumption occurred.

Serious, even fatal, accidents may occur during a period of LSD intoxication. They may be due to the individual's belief in supernatural powers or in an ability to perform the impossible – such as flying, walking on water, etc. Such events receive much publicity but occur only rarely.

Spontaneous, involuntary recurrences of the drug-induced experience (flashbacks) are fairly common after LSD use and may be troublesome if they occur frequently. They may also be precipitated by the use of another drug such as cannabis.

It is not clear whether LSD can cause prolonged psychotic illness. When such an illness does occur after LSD use, it is generally believed that it would have occurred anyway and that its onset was merely precipitated by LSD. Nevertheless, given the psychotomimetic properties of LSD, it is possible that it plays a more causal role in vulnerable individuals.

Other hallucinogenic drugs

There are several drugs whose psychological effects are similar to those of LSD and which are also described as hallucinogenic, psychedelic or psychotomimetic. Many are derived from plants which have been used for a long time in religious rituals. Indeed it has been suggested that there are hundreds of thousands of species of hallucinogenic plants in the world. Mescalin, for example, is obtained from the peyote cactus which is traditionally chewed by Indians in Mexico, while psilocin and psilocybin come from a particular ('magic') mushroom in Mexico; lysergic acid monoethylamide, which has mild hallucinogenic properties, is found in the seeds of the morning glory plant; and there are hallucinogens in plants such as nutmeg, mace and deadly nightshade. Cross-tolerance occurs between LSD, mescaline and psilocybin.

In addition to naturally occurring drugs, a whole range of synthetic compounds are available, including DMT (dimethyltryptamine), DMA (dimethoxyamphetamine) and DOM (dimethoxymethylamphetamine) which are similar in their effects to LSD, but also have some amphetamine-like properties. DOM is also known as STP (standing for serenity, tranquillity and peace) and has a longer duration of action than LSD.

Other drugs, such as MDA (methylenedioxyamphetamine) and MMDA (methoxymethylenedioxyamphetamine) are probably LSD-like but have other properties as well.

The particular problems posed by these new drug analogues are discussed in the section on 'designer' drugs (see p. 111).

Phencyclidine (PCP)

PCP also produces changes in mood and perception, but is quite distinct from the psychedelic drugs described above. It is related to pethidine and induces a marked sensory blockade. First introduced as a veterinary anaesthetic, its property of causing patients to feel detached from bodily sensations and therefore unaware of pain, suggested a revolutionary approach to anaesthesia for humans. However, this was soon abandoned because it so often made patients agitated and deluded. It became, however, a drug of abuse particularly in the USA where it is known as 'angel dust'. It is relatively easy to synthesize illicitly and is often passed off as LSD. It is usually smoked or snorted.

Effects of PCP vary according to the dose consumed but as there is great individual variation of response, even small doses may cause profound effects in some people. The desired effect is a euphoric sensation of floating, usually accompanied by mild numbness of the extremities, but the cerebellar effects of PCP simultaneously cause staggering gait, slurred speech and nystagmus. Slight increases in dose may precipitate severe muscular rigidity, hypertension and a non-communicative state. The risk of convulsions and coma becomes greater if more than 20 mg is consumed.

The psychological effects of PCP are very unpredictable; there may be perceptual disturbances, hallucinations, elevation of mood, restlessness, anxiety or paranoia. Sometimes the patient is frankly psychotic and there may be aggressive and bizarre behaviour. The acute effects of PCP last for 4–6 hours, which is followed by a long period of 'coming down'.

Tolerance and dependence

Tolerance to the effects of PCP develops in animals and humans. Most of those who abuse it probably take it about once a week, although some people have 'runs' of using it for 2 or 3 days at a time. Craving for the drug occurs in some people and the depression and disorientation that occurs after a run of drug use may represent a mild abstinence syndrome. The fact that monkeys will self-administer PCP (but not LSD) also suggests that it may have some dependence potential. However, it is rarely abused in Europe (yet).

Cannabis

Cannabis is obtained from the Indian hemp plant, *Cannabis sativa*, which is grown in many countries as a source of rope fibre. When the plant is fully grown, its flowers and upper leaves are covered with a sticky resin which contains psychoactive substances collectively known as cannabinoids. There are probably more than 50 of these, of which the most important is Δ-9-tetrahydcannabinol (THC). The potency of a particular preparation of cannabis is related to its THC content which in turn depends on the part of the plant that is gathered and the environmental conditions, particularly the climate, where it is grown. Special varieties of *Cannabis sativa* are cultivated specifically for their resin in some tropical countries in the Caribbean, South America, South East Asia, Indian Subcontinent, etc.

Preparations

Various preparations of cannabis are available, often known by different names in different countries.

1   *Bhang*: the dried leaves and flowering tops of uncultivated plants, which are infused and drunk.

2   *Marijuana*: the dried leaves and flowering tops of uncultivated plants, which are smoked.

3   *Ganja*: small upper leaves and flowering tops of cultivated female plants, which are smoked. It is about three times as potent as marijuana.

The THC content of these three herbals preparations is between 1 and 10%.

4   *Hashish/charas/cannabis resin*: the pure resin from the flowering tops and leaves of female plants. It is in the form of a sticky brown cake which is usually smoked. The THC content varies between 8 and 15%.

5   *Liquid cannabis/Hashish oil*: this is obtained by subjecting cannabis resin to extraction with a non-aqueous solvent. After filtration and evaporation, a brown syrupy liquid is obtained into which tobacco is dipped before smoking. It may contain up to 60% THC.

An average marijuana cigarette in the UK usually contains 300–500 mg of herbal material with a THC content of perhaps 1–2%. Even if smoked by an experienced user, only 50% of the available THC is absorbed and so the estimated dose of THC from one cigarette is in the region of 2.5–5.0 mg. However, the dose may also vary because heat converts some inactive compounds into THC and can inactivate psychoactive cannabinoids.

Absorption and fate of THC

THC is absorbed very quickly across the large surface area of the lungs and plasma concentrations peak very quickly (10–30 minutes). THC binds tightly to blood proteins but because it is so fat soluble it is readily absorbed by organs such as the brain which have a high fat content and is released only slowly back into the bloodstream. It is metabolized (broken down), mostly in the liver, to 11-hydroxy THC, which is 20% more potent than THC itself, and to other products with unknown or relatively little psychoactive effect. The effects of a single marijuana cigarette are apparent within minutes and last for 2–3 hours. When cannabis is consumed orally, the onset of action is slower than if it is smoked and a larger dose is required to obtain the same effects, which then last longer.

Because of their fat solubility, THC and its metabolites remain for long periods of time in the fatty tissues of the body. Thus, 5 days after a single injection of THC, 20% remains stored and 20% of its metabolites remain in the blood; complete elimination of a single dose may take 30 days. Given this slow rate of clearance, it is likely that repeated administration may lead to accumulation of THC and its metabolites in the body. An awareness of these pharmacokinetics is relevant to any discussion about the long-term effects of cannabis.

Effects

The physical effects commonly associated with cannabis use include dryness of the mouth, hunger, reddening of the eyes and reduced pressure in the ocular fluid of the eyes. There may be increased blood pressure (together with postural hypotension) and a dose-related increase in heart rate. Chronic, high dosage effects of cannabis are reported to include reduced testosterone level and sperm count, as well as reduced fertility in women and reduced fetal birth weight. Gynaecomastia may occur.

The psychological effects of smoking a marijuana cigarette are well known. The desired and sought after effects are euphoria, self-confidence, relaxation and a general sense of well-being. There is often an altered perception of time, which may appear to be passing more slowly than usual, and the perception of hearing, taste, touch and smell may seem to the subject to be enhanced, although there is no objective evidence of this on formal testing. It may be difficult for the subject to concentrate and memory may be impaired. Sometimes these experiences are not pleasurable and the subject becomes anxious, agitated and suspicious, occasionally experiencing a severe panic reaction. Although there is no conclusive evidence, it is likely that the ability to drive a car safely is adversely affected by cannabis consumption.

The mental set of the subject and the setting in which cannabis is taken may both influence the drug-induced experience, although laboratory experiments have provided conclusive evidence that the psychological effects of cannabis are due to its THC content. In small doses, equivalent to smoking one marijuana cigarette, THC causes changes in mood (usually euphoria) and altered perception. With bigger doses ($200–250 \mu g/kg$; approximately 15 mg THC for an average, 70 kg man), there is marked distortion in visual and auditory perception, and hallucinations occur in most subjects together with sensations of depersonalization and derealization. Thinking becomes confused and disorganized and paranoid feelings are common. With even higher doses, a frank toxic psychosis develops.

It appears, therefore, that THC, the main constituent of cannabis, is a psychotomimetic drug; in other words it can produce a state similar to that of a psychotic illness and this effect depends on the dose that is administered. In the laboratory the reaction of the same individual to the same dose is reproducible on different occasions and some individuals are unusually sensitive to THC, experiencing psychosis even at low doses.

Tolerance

The development of tolerance to the effects of cannabis has long been a controversial issue. In Western countries it is often claimed that cannabis does not cause tolerance, on the grounds that experienced users continue to obtain a 'high' from their first cigarette of the day. Indeed, the phenomenon of reverse tolerance has been described, when experienced users may report more subjective experiences than novices. These observations and opinions are contradicted by the experience of countries where heavy, regular consumption of cannabis is common. In these countries, very large doses may be consumed (hundreds of milligrams of THC) that would undoubtedly be toxic to a drug-naive individual, suggesting that tolerance to the effects of THC has indeed developed.

Laboratory experiments too confirm the existence of tolerance to cannabis-induced changes in mood, tachycardia (increased heart rate), decreased intra-ocular pressure and impairment of performance in psychomotor tests. Tolerance develops rapidly, within a few days of regular drug use, and decays rapidly when drug use ceases. It is generally much less obvious than tolerance to heroin or cocaine, and the irregular small doses of cannabis that are usually consumed in Western countries may not be sufficient to cause a noticeable degree of tolerance. Furthermore, there appears to be an upper limit to tolerance to cannabis, which may vary from individual to individual, and once this is reached further increases in dose may precipitate the onset of psychotic symptoms.

Dependence

Similar controversy surrounds the question of dependence on cannabis. Again, it is not surprising that dependence is reported most frequently in those countries where cannabis is consumed regularly and in large quantities. In this situation, cannabis withdrawal is followed by some discomfort and an abstinence syndrome, the hallmark of physical dependence, has been described. It is characterized by irritability, restlessness, decreased appetite, weight loss and insomnia. These clinical observations are supported by the observation under laboratory conditions of a withdrawal syndrome in volunteers who had taken high doses of THC for several weeks. This experiment confirmed that the syndrome is relatively mild, starting a few hours after the cessation of drug administration and lasting for 4–5 days.

On the other hand, there is no evidence in terms of craving or drug-seeking behaviour that psychological dependence occurs, and animal studies suggest that cannabis has only weak primary reinforcing properties.

Cannabis psychosis

Worldwide, millions of people smoke marijuana and consume cannabis in different forms, and there have been many reports, from all over the world, of 'cannabis psychosis' – a psychotic illness arising after the consumption of a large quantity of cannabis. It is characterized by the sudden onset of confusion, generally associated with delusions, hallucinations and emotional lability. Temporary amnesia, disorientation, depersonalisation and paranoid symptoms are also common. This toxic mental state may persist for a few hours or a few days.

This syndrome is well recognized and frequently reported in those countries, such as India, West Indies and South East Asia, where heavy consumption of cannabis is common, but its existence is often questioned in the UK and other Western countries. Here, the THC content of the cannabis that is available is often low and even 'experienced' users usually smoke only one or two cigarettes, perhaps two or three times a week – a far cry from Jamaican heavy users whose consumption of THC is estimated to be 420 mg daily. As toxic psychosis is a dose-related effect of cannabis, it is only to be expected that there would be a smaller incidence of the syndrome in the UK, although it seems likely that there is a general lack of awareness of its existence and consequent under-diagnosis. Furthermore, it seems likely that many users are familiar with the effects of cannabis and are able to titrate their intake to avoid unpleasant effects. Mild intoxication is undoubtedly dealt with, without recourse to medical advice.

It has also been suggested, although there is little firm evidence, that cannabis can cause a functional psychosis – a paranoid schizophrenia-like illness in a setting of clear consciousness. There are many alternative explanations for any apparent relationship between cannabis and psychosis: that the patient was psychotic anyway and cannabis use was incidental or merely aggravated the existing condition; that the patient was potentially psychotic and this was precipitated by cannabis which cannot cause psychosis in a 'normal' individual; that the illness preceded and indirectly caused cannabis use. Although these and other explanations may be true, they do not preclude the existence of a cannabis-induced functional psychosis, and those who are experienced in the sequelae of prolonged and heavy cannabis abuse have observed subtle differences between true paranoid schizophrenia and the psychotic illness that sometimes develops in cannabis abusers. For example, the latter are more likely to have hypomanic symptoms, but less likely to have 'schizophrenic-type' thought disorder. Their illness responds very swiftly to antipsychotic medication, but tends to relapse if cannabis use is resumed.

There is, however, no evidence that cannabis causes a chronic psychosis that persists after drug use is discontinued, although some patients may effectively 'maintain' themselves in a psychotic condition by continuing to consume large quantities of cannabis.

Flashbacks

Flashbacks are spontaneous, involuntary recurrences of drug-induced experiences after the effects of the drug have worn off. They have been described following cannabis use, but the generally accepted wisdom is that they only occur if the patient has previously used other psychotomimetic drugs such as LSD – although the flashback may then be of a cannabis-induced experience. In some cases flashbacks have occurred within hours of using cannabis; given the prolonged presence of THC in the body, these symptoms can hardly be said to be occurring in the absence of the drug.

Amotivational syndrome

Amotivational syndrome is a phrase coined to describe a condition of chronic apathy attributed to long-term, heavy cannabis use. It is characterized by the asocial, non-directional behaviour of a 'drop-out' who appears to have none of the usual goals of life. There is controversy about whether the amotivational syndrome actually exists and if it does, whether it is causally related to cannabis use or whether both conditions (cannabis use and amotivational syndrome) are manifestations of underlying psychopathology.

Chronic brain damage

It has also been suggested that prolonged use of cannabis eventually leads to brain damage or atrophy. Again, there is no conclusive evidence to support this hypothesis.

Volatile solvents

The inhalation or 'sniffing' of volatile solvents became a focus of attention in the UK during the 1970s and early 1980s when it was closely related to the punk sub-culture. It was, however, like most forms of drug abuse not a new phenomenon but a 'variation on a theme' – an epidemic of a condition that previously had warranted only occasional anecdotal case reports of health professionals inhaling anaesthetic gases, of industrial solvent workers who abused solvents and so on. When it became widespread among young teenagers it provoked lurid reports in the popular press, but little in the way of systematic research so that comparatively little is known about this form of drug abuse. Specifically, and partly because of the large number of chemicals involved, there is scant information about the development of tolerance and dependence. Although the panic of the 1970s has subsided, solvent abuse persists, especially among teenagers, and there are sporadic reports of 'outbreaks' of this form of drug abuse in different countries.

Typically, in the UK, if glue sniffing occurs in a particular locality, it is a group activity, more popular among boys than girls. The majority will experiment with it for a short time and then stop, with about one-tenth continuing to sniff in groups for a few months. A small number will continue solvent sniffing for many years, usually in a more solitary fashion.

The substances that have been abused include a wide range of commercial and domestic products, such as glues (containing toluene and related hexanes), nail varnish and removers, (amyl acetate and acetone), gas lighter fuel (butane) and cleaning fluids (trichloroethylene). The active constituents are volatile hydrocarbons which evaporate at room temperature, giving off fumes that can be inhaled. Aerosol products are also abused for the sake of the propellants they contain – substances such as butane or chlorinated fluorocarbons. It is obvious that all of these products are widely available and fairly cheap so that any youngster who wants to abuse them can obtain them easily.

Methods of administration

The usual method of sniffing is to put some of the chosen product on to a piece of material, or into a paper or plastic bag (often a potato crisp bag), which is then held over the mouth and nose while deep breaths are taken. If air is exhaled into the bag, the carbon dioxide content of the air–vapour mixture increases, enhancing the drug experience. Where sniffing is a group activity, the same bag may be passed around the group. A very dangerous practice, with a high risk of death by suffocation, is to pour some of the solvent into a large plastic bag which is put right over the head so that air is excluded completely and the vapour is more concentrated. Aerosols may be sprayed directly into the mouth.

As the subject breathes in and out, the solvents are rapidly absorbed through the large surface area of the lung and enter the bloodstream. Most are highly lipid soluble and are rapidly distributed throughout the nervous system where they depress many vital functions and produce the desired 'high' within a few minutes. Many are excreted, unchanged, through the lungs producing a characteristic odour on the breath, but others are metabolized and excreted in the urine. It is difficult to test urine for solvent abuse because of the wide variety of substances involved.

Effects

The desired effect of solvent abuse is euphoria – which may be achieved within a few minutes after just a few breaths. It is similar to being intoxicated with alcohol, but the intoxicated condition can be attained much more rapidly by using solvents. Like alcohol, most solvents act as central nervous system depressants, but because the higher centres of the brain that control behaviour are depressed first, the apparent initial effect of solvent abuse is of stimulation and of disinhibition. There may be feelings of omnipotence and recklessness so that dangerous behaviour of an impulsive or destructive nature may ensue.

Other effects vary according to the solvent being inhaled, the amount being taken and the method and duration of inhalation, as well as the previous habits of the individual. They include giddiness, ataxia (unsteadiness), slurred speech and impaired judgement. Some subjects experience hallucinations which are usually visual and often frightening. Other physical symptoms include nausea and vomiting, sneezing, coughing and diarrhoea. These effects wear off quite quickly, usually in less than an hour, leaving the user feeling drowsy. Repeated inhalation, which is a common practice, may result in disorientation, fits and eventual unconsciousness with depression of respiration and heart rate.

A glue-sniffer's rash, although uncommon, has been described, believed to be due to the repeated application of a plastic bag containing solvent over the mouth and nose. The rash is symmetrical in distribution and consists of red papules and pustules extending from each nostril up the nasal fold and across the bridge of the nose.

As well as the dangerous consequence of suffocation if a plastic bag is placed right over the head, asphyxia may also occur due to inhalation of vomit during unconsciousness. Deaths have also been reported due to cardiac arrhythmias, which seem to occur most frequently if aerosol propellant gases are sprayed directly into the mouth. It has been suggested that many solvents sensitize the heart muscle, so that it reacts abnormally to stress by beating irregularly. It may, therefore, be important not to startle an individual who is intoxicated with solvents. Fatal accidents sometimes occur during solvent intoxication; they may be the consequence of bizarre behaviour due to disorientation and hallucination, and are particularly likely if inhalation takes place in a dangerous situation – near a canal, for example, or on a roof top.

Over the last decade there has been a steady upward trend in the number of deaths attributable to solvent abuse. Lighter fuel now accounts for 40–50% of these deaths because, when sprayed directly into the mouth, rapid cooling causes mucosal tissue in the airways to swell, leading to obstruction and suffocation.

The toxic effects of many solvents are well known, particularly from experience in industrial medicine, and there is no doubt that some substances are very toxic and can cause severe tissue damage. However, the relevance of findings from chronic, low-dose exposure of factory workers to the repeated, acute, high-dose exposure of the adolescent solvent abuser is not clear. The chronic effects reported include liver and kidney damage, bone marrow depression, anaemia, encephalopathy and neuropathy. Many long-term effects are reversible if solvent abuse is stopped. Permanent brain damage seems to be rare although it can occur particularly after long-term abuse of solvents. Chromosome damage has also been reported as well as blood abnormalities, but these effects of solvent abuse have not been conclusively proven.

Tolerance

It appears that tolerance to the effects of a particular solvent can develop if abuse persists over a long period – say of 6–12 months. Some individuals may then be abusing several pints of solvent each week.

Dependence

There is no doubt that psychological dependence on solvents develops in many young abusers who find it very difficult to reduce their consumption or stop altogether. True physical dependence with a defined withdrawal syndrome probably does not occur although 'hangover' effects (headaches, nausea, drowsiness, etc.) may be prominent in heavy abusers. It is not clear whether these are the residual effects of the abused solvents or a 'withdrawal' syndrome due to absence of drugs from the body.

Designer drugs

The term 'designer drugs' is used to describe clandestinely produced substances pharmacologically similar to drugs of abuse that are already strictly controlled by national and international law; so-called designer drugs are subtly different in chemical structure so that they remain out of reach of the law. They are in fact drug analogues deliberately synthesized to produce the euphoria or 'high' of controlled drugs, but able to be manufactured, sold and abused without risk of penalty.

The idea of producing analogues of a parent drug is neither new nor rare. Indeed, pharmaceutical companies perpetually try to produce analogues and have synthesized many. However, it was first done for the purpose of avoiding the law in the 1960s when hallucinogenic amphetamine analogues of mescaline were synthesized. Since then analogues of phencyclidine and methaqualone have been produced and, more recently, analogues of opiates have been identified. These are usually derivatives of either fentanyl or pethidine and are substituted for heroin. They are easy to produce and inexpensive, yet very potent and so are a source of considerable profit to the producer. Because of their potency they are taken only in very small doses and are therefore very difficult to detect by routine chemical analysis.

Fentanyl itself is a very potent synthetic opiate analgesic widely used during operative anaesthesia. A number of clandestinely produced analogues have been identified, some of which are 250 times as potent as heroin. This means that 1 g of the analogue can produce 500 000 doses to be traded on the street as 'heroin' or 'China white'. Because of their potency these analogues carry a high risk of fatal overdose.

Analogues of pethidine are also more potent than the parent drug, but the clandestine production of one such analogue, MPPP, yields a number of impurities including a neurotoxic by-product, MPTP. This damages dopamine-containing neurones in the nervous system, causing a severe, irreversible neurological condition resembling Parkinson's syndrome and characterized by tremor, muscular rigidity, slowness of movement and speech, and a mask-like, expressionless face. This occurred, tragically, in several young people who had self-administered intravenously MPPP/MPTP that had been purchased as heroin. Another pethidine analogue, PEPAP, may contain a similarly neurotoxic by-product and it is possible that more intravenous drug abusers who have been exposed to these substances in the past, may develop Parkinson's syndrome at a later stage.

Ecstasy

Another important group of designer drugs derive from the hallucinogenic amphetamines. MDMA (3,4, methylene-dioxymethamphetamine) known as 'Ecstasy', 'E', 'XTC' or 'Adam', and MDE ('Eve') are analogues of the controlled drug MDA (see p. 102). Like the parent compound, these new drugs induce a state of altered consciousness, enhance visual, auditory and tactile perceptions and produce mild intoxication. They are also thought to damage serotonin-containing neurones in the nervous system.

In the UK, the use of Ecstasy is intrinsically linked to a particular music scene, that involves energetic dancing at large parties ('raves') held in venues such as disused warehouses. Many hundreds of young people attend, often travelling long distances to do so. Drugs like MDMA are sold at these parties, although it may be mixed with LSD, amphetamines, etc.

MDMA has been widely abused in the USA and has been openly promoted as a legal euphoriant, thus illustrating the problem posed by designer drugs. Because drug control laws usually define drugs in terms of their chemical structure, it is easy to side-step these laws by slightly changing the chemical structure of the drug. If the cumbersome process of changing the law is initiated so that the new drug is included, it is very easy to redesign the drug so that the new analogue remains out of reach. The difficulty of controlling these dangerous substances is compounded by the problems of identifying them in very low concentrations and then of describing them, ensuring that legislation cannot keep up with the constantly changing drug scene. This problem has been countered in the USA where designer drugs have caused most trouble, by new legislation which makes it an offence to manufacture and distribute designer drugs (defined as a substance, other than a controlled substance, with a structure substantially similar to controlled drugs or designed to produce an effect substantially similar to that of a controlled drug). This law, which shifts the emphasis away from the actual substance of abuse and towards the process of manufacture and distribution, will obviate the need for new legislation to be passed to cope with the ever-changing chemical repertoire.

In the UK, action has been taken against designer drugs in anticipation of future problems. Carfentanil and lofentanil which are analogues of fentanyl are now included in Class A of the Misuse of Drugs Act, as are any analogues of fentanyl and pethidine which may appear in future as drugs of abuse. This means that they are subject to the strictest controls and that the penalties for their misuse are severe (see Chapter 11).

Steroids

Anabolic steroids are drugs or hormonal substances, chemically and pharmacologically related to testosterone, that promote muscle growth. They occur naturally in the body, playing an important role in the development and functioning of the reproductive organs. They are 'anabolic' because they increase the retention of nitrogen in the body, a basic constituent of protein, thus promoting the growth and development of muscle tissue. They have limited medical use but are taken inappropriately by individuals for whom increased body size or increased muscle power is perceived as important – individuals such as body-builders, bouncers, doormen and even policemen, as well as weight-lifters and athletes. Others may use steroids to increase their self-esteem, or to improve their appearance when stripped for the beach, etc.

There is no accurate information about the extent of non-medical steroid use in the UK but it appears that the majority of users are males aged 17–35, while there is some evidence of its growing popularity among younger teenagers too (mostly boys). In the US, it has been estimated that there are 2–3 million people abusing these drugs, including half a million teenagers. Attention has focused on their use by sportsmen and women

who believe that these drugs will make them stronger, faster, more competitive and more aggressive.

Not surprisingly, accurate data relating to the effects of steroids relates
to their medical use for patients rather than their unsupervised use by athletes. However, it is generally accepted that they can increase muscle
strength if they are used during periods of intense training and in conjunction with a carefully controlled high protein diet. Used in isolation they
may increase muscle mass but not strength.

A wide variety of anabolic steroids is available for non-medical use.
Most are manufactured in underground laboratories, but some intended for
veterinary use have been diverted for human consumption. They are available in both oral and injectable forms and different steroids may be used
simultaneously ('stacking'). It appears that they are often taken in a cycli-
cal fashion with rest periods in between. During a cycle, the dose of steroids
may be gradually increased during the first part of the cycle, and then
tapered down near the end of the cycle; this pattern of dose management is
called a 'pyramid'.

Adverse effects

Anabolic steroids may cause abnormalities of liver function tests although
these usually return to normal when drug-taking ceases. They can cause
facial acne and, if taken by children, may stunt growth.

More serious complications may also occur; these include a rare form of
hepatitis and liver tumours. Steroids may also cause hypertension and have
been implicated in coronary heart disease. They affect sexual function and
when taken by women can cause virilization. Adverse psychiatric effects,
including confusion, sleep disorder, depression, hallucinations and paranoid
delusions, can also occur, albeit rarely. A corollary of the desired effects of
increased competitiveness and aggression is that users may become
irritable, short-tempered and potentially violent – the so-called 'roid rage'.

Where steroids are taken by injection there is the possibility of syringes
and needles being shared and a consequent risk of HIV infection. Indeed at
some needle exchange schemes, steroid users account for a significant proportion of attenders; this appears to reflect the popularity of bodybuilding
and the difficulty of obtaining suitable injection equipment for oil-based
steroids.

Unlike most of the other substances that are frequently misused, steroids
do not have an immediate psychoactive effect and they do not have reinforcing properties. In the UK, they are Prescription Only Medicines that
can only be sold by a pharmacist working in a registered pharmacy, but it

is not illegal to possess or import them for personal use. Non-medical steroid use is therefore different in many ways to other forms of substance misuse: it is not illegal (although non-medical use is banned by the various sports authorities); most steroid-users are health conscious, welcoming health checks and the opportunity to obtain sterile injection equipment; and they rarely misuse other drugs although there are some reports of amphetamine use. Nevertheless, it *is* a form of substance misuse; it is carried out secretively; and it is easy to understand that an athlete who achieves success while taking steroids, may develop great faith in their effects and become psychologically dependent upon them. The relationship between steroid misuse and other forms of substance misuse is highlighted by experience in the US, where anabolic steroids were made controlled drugs in 1991. Since then, 185 investigations of major dealers have been reported and 6 million dosage units and $2.5 million have been seized. Most cases have involved international trafficking with steroids originating from all over the world. It has also been found that many traffickers are involved in drugs other than steroids, most notably cocaine.

Over-the-counter medicines

Most drugs of abuse or those with dependence liability are controlled under the Misuse of Drugs Act 1971 and come within the scope of the Misuse of Drugs Regulations 1985 (see Chapter 11), requiring a doctor's prescription before they are dispensed. However there are many other medications with a potential for misuse, which are available from a pharmacist, 'over the counter', without the need for a doctor's prescription. For example, there is a range of cough mixtures and treatments for diarrhoea that contain codeine or similar drugs with opiate-like effects while the familiar remedy of kaolin and morphine mixture contains a dilute tincture of morphine itself. Similarly, there are nasal decongestants containing stimulant-like drugs, and a range of antihistamines which are predominantly sedative in their effects.

These drugs are a cause for concern for a variety of reasons. Firstly, drug-dependent individuals are well-informed about them and may use them deliberately to supplement other sources of supply. While most are formulated in such a way that they are not suitable for injection, there have been reports of users trying to extract active ingredients for this purpose. Secondly, many are compound preparations, containing more than one active ingredient. If the drug that the user wants is present only in low concentration, large quantities of the compound will be taken, perhaps resulting in toxicity from the other constituents.

Another important area of concern is that some individuals may take these drugs regularly over many years in an inappropriate fashion. Uninformed self-medication, however well intentioned, can lead to dependence upon the drugs with attendant risks to personal health. The extent of this type of use is, of course, unknown. However, it has been estimated that there are more than a quarter of a million analgesic abusers in the UK. They buy, over the counter, from pharmacists, supermarkets, newsagents and even slot machines, compounds containing aspirin and other 'minor' analgesics. Taken in excess for a prolonged period these may cause serious renal damage and have been implicated as a cause of renal tumours.

Herbal preparations and 'natural' medicines

In recent years there has been burgeoning interest in so-called 'natural' remedies and foods because of a belief that herbal preparations, vitamins and minerals can only be beneficial and lack the side effects of modern, synthetic drugs. In fact, many modern drugs are derived originally from plants and are carefully formulated, under very strict controls, to ensure consistency of ingredients and dose. In contrast, natural preparations are not subject to the same controls and, despite an often blind trust in their safety, may cause serious side effects if taken in excess. Some may have mood-altering effects: for example in the USA, some herbal tea bags, popular because they were caffeine-free, in fact contained about 5 mg cocaine per bag. Similarly, so-called 'Asthma cigarettes' contain stramonium leaves with hyoscine as an active ingredient, that may cause hallucinations.

Self-medication with herbal laxatives, such as preparations of senna or ipecac, may cause serious complications if doses are excessive. This may occur in association with eating disorders such as bulimia and anorexia, when there may be profound and life-threatening electrolyte disturbances. Another group of natural remedies with a long history of self-medication are the aphrodisiacs. Prolonged use of ginseng, for example, is said to cause a 'ginseng abuse syndrome', with hypertension, oedema, diarrhoea, skin rashes, insomnia and depression.

The combined use of drugs and alcohol

Despite considerable evidence that alcohol and drugs are used and misused concurrently, services for substance misusers and research into substance misuse usually focus either on drugs or on alcohol with little interaction between the two areas. With the behaviours overlapping, and the substances themselves interacting, it seems appropriate to consider, albeit briefly, the particular problems associated with the combined use of drugs and alcohol.

For example, epidemiological research shows that in the UK, cigarettes and alcohol are the first and second drug tried by schoolchildren. Thus it is not surprising that patients seeking treatment for drug abuse commonly give a history of alcohol use too. Indeed, recent evidence suggests that the prevalence of combined use in a population of alcoholics and/or drug addicts ranges from 29 to 95%. For example, one study in the USA reported that, out of 298 drug abusers seeking treatment for cocaine abuse, 29% could be described as dependent on alcohol while about 62% met the criteria for having been dependent on alcohol at some previous time. Similarly, in another study, this time of clients in alcohol treatment agencies, the percentage using alcohol with drugs ranged from 57% for methadone to 95% for speed and amphetamines, while other drugs reported to have been used included crack, cocaine, heroin, sedatives and hallucinogens as well as codeine and other opiates. Similar findings have been reported from other countries; in Australia, for example, there was a 45% prevalence of combined drug and alcohol use in a sample of 313 heroin users, while in Canada 20–45% of a sample of 427 patients meeting DSM-III criteria for alcohol abuse or dependence reported combined use of benzodiazepines and alcohol.

The reasons for combining different substances vary from person to person. Sometimes they may be combined in a search for enhanced effect, as for example when cocaine abusers also use alcohol to potentiate cocaine euphoria. Interestingly the same drug combination has been reported to have been used so that alcohol would counteract the negative acute effects of cocaine. Among alcoholics, the use of benzodiazepines is associated with a tendency to self-medicate for anxiety, while there is evidence that some injecting drug users uses alcohol to enhance sexual activities and pleasure.

When different substances are taken simultaneously, they can interact in a number of different ways. Firstly, of course, they may act independently of one another so that the observed effects are no more and no less than if they were taken separately. Alternatively they may have a summative or additive effect, or work synergistically or, indeed, have an antagonistic effect. The underlying mechanisms for such interactions are usually not clear although a possible mechanism for drug–alcohol interaction has now been described: at low blood alcohol concentrations, alcohol is mainly metabolized by alcohol dehydrogenase, leaving the microsomal ethanol-oxidizing system free to metabolize other drugs. At high blood alcohol concentrations, the latter system is utilized for alcohol metabolism so that the metabolism of other drugs is slowed and their effects are prolonged. This would explain why alcohol can enhance the psychomotor deficits associated with psychoactive drugs such as benzodiazepines, and perhaps why drug abusers who are involved in the combined use of drugs and alcohol, report more severe drug dependence. However, it must be remembered that many other factors, such as the dose–time response may also be important.

In practice, although antagonistic effects are possible, the behavioural effects of combined use are similar to those commonly associated with either alcohol or illicit drugs but are elevated. Thus the combined use of alcohol and cerebral depressants usually produces impaired performance on driving and similar skills. Impairment of reaction time, attention and alertness have all been reported and it seems likely that they contribute to the causation of incidents such as traffic accidents, fires, falls, etc.

The combined use of drugs and alcohol has several implications for treatment. Firstly, a longer course of treatment may be needed as a result of the need to avoid possible harm arising from the interaction between drugs administered in treatment and the drug combination taken by the patient. More specifically, alcohol detoxification may be necessary before treatment for the drug problem can be initiated. In more general terms and in view of the prevalence of combined drug and alcohol use, the second major implication for treatment services is that there is a clear argument for combining the services offered to drug and alcohol dependent individuals.

References and further reading

Allen D (ed.) (1987). *The Cocaine Crisis*. Plenum Press, New York.

Ashton H (1984). Benzodiazepine withdrawal: an unfinished story. *British Medical Journal*, **288**, 1135–1140.

Cami J, Bigelow GE, Griffiths RR & Drummond DC (eds) (1991). Clinical testing of drug abuse liability (Special issue). *British Journal of Addiction*, **86**, 1525–1652.

Drake PH (1988). Khat chewing in the Near East. *Lancet*, **1**, 532–533.

Fehr KO & Kalant HA (eds) (1983). *Cannabis and Health Hazards. Proceedings of an ARF/WHO Scientific Meeting on Adverse Health and Behavioural Consequences of Cannabis Use*. Toronto Addiction Research Foundation, Toronto.

Freeman H & Rue Y (eds) (1987). *The Benzodiazepines in Current Clinical Practice*. Royal Society of Medicine, London.

Ghodse AH (1994). Combined use of drugs and alcohol. *Current Opinion in Psychiatry*, **7**, No. 3, 249–251.

Ghodse AH (1986). Cannabis psychosis. *British Journal of Addiction*, **81**, 473–478.

Goldstein A (1983). Some thoughts about endogenous opioids and addiction. *Drug and Alcohol Dependence*, **11**, 11–14.

Grabowski J (ed.) (1984). *Cocaine: Pharmacology, Effects and Treatment Abuse*. NIDA Research Monograph. Department of Health & Human Services, Rockville.

Ives R (ed.) (1986). *Solvent Misuse in Context*. National Children's Bureau, London.

Jaffe JH (1991). Drug addiction and drug abuse. In Goodman HG, Goodman LS, Rall TW *et al.* (eds). *Goodman and Gilman's: The Pharmacological Basis of Therapeutics,* 522–574. Pergamon Press, New York.

Johanson CE & Yanagita T (eds) (1987). Benefit-risk ratio assessment of agonist-antagonist analgesics (Special Issue). *Drug and Alcohol Dependence,* **20**, 289–409.

Lader M (1983). Dependence on benzodiazepines. *Journal of Clinical Psychiatry,* **44**, 121–127.

Madden S (1990). Identifying the problem. In: Ghodse AH & Maxwell D (eds). *Substance Abuse and Dependence,* 30–52. Macmillan Press, London.

National Research Council Institute of Medicine (1982). *Marijuana and Health.* Report of a study by a committee of the Institute of Medicine, Division of Health Sciences Policy. National Academy Press, Washington DC.

Pelicier Y (ed.) (1993). *Benzodiazepines.* Report of the World Psychiatric Association Presidential Educational Task Force.

Petursson H & Lader M (1984). *Dependence on Tranquillisers.* Oxford University Press, New York.

Watson JM (1980). Solvent abuse by children and young adults. *British Journal of Addiction,* **75**, 27–36.

Wesson DR & Smith DE (1977). *Barbiturates: Their Use, Misuse and Abuse.* Human Sciences Press, New York.

World Health Organization (1985). *WHO Expert Committee on Drug Dependence. Twenty-Second Report.* WHO Technical Report Series 729. WHO, Geneva.

World Health Organization (1987). *WHO Expert Committee on Drug Dependence. Twenty-Third Report.* WHO Technical Report Series 741. WHO, Geneva.

World Health Organization (1988). *WHO Expert Committee on Drug Dependence. Twenty-Fourth Report.* WHO Technical Report Series 761. WHO, Geneva.

World Health Organization (1991). *WHO Expert Committee on Drug Dependence. Twenty-Seventh Report.* WHO Technical Report Series 808. WHO, Geneva.

4

Assessment

Introduction

Careful, detailed and thorough assessment of individuals presenting with drug-related problems is essential if they are to receive effective help. The purpose of the assessment is to identify the nature and severity of the drug-related problem; to understand why it arose, to assess its consequences and to establish the strengths and weakness of the patient and his/her situation. Armed with this information, it is possible to formulate and develop a treatment programme to help that particular individual to live a full life, integrated into society without the need for drugs.

The need for a very thorough assessment is crystallized by that last phrase, 'without the need for drugs'. While it is comparatively easy, in the sense of it being a straightforward procedure, to achieve drug withdrawal, continued abstinence ('staying off' – relapse prevention) presents much more long-term and challenging problems. After all, having achieved abstinence, the drug-abusing individual usually finds him/herself in the same situation, with the same personal problems and the same personal resources – and with the same drugs readily available on demand. Nothing will have changed except a temporary interruption of drug administration and it is perhaps only to be expected that the same behaviour should be resumed and often immediately. The key to staying off is change – in the individual, his/her life situation or the availability of drugs – and the whole point of the assessment procedure is to identify areas where change can be effected so that the need for drugs is reduced or, better still, eliminated.

It is not surprising that full assessment of the individual and all the antecedent and consequent problems is necessarily a lengthy procedure, and if the patient is referred to a specialist drug-dependence treatment unit (DDTU) it usually takes a couple of weeks. During this time the patient attends the DDTU on several occasions and sees different members of the multidisciplinary team. Their enquiries may overlap to a certain extent, but gradually a picture is built up of the patient's drug problem and how it has developed over the years, the family background, present social and financial circumstances and so on. These findings, together with the results of laboratory tests on blood and urine, are presented at a meeting of the multidisciplinary team and an individual treatment plan can be worked out.

A particular reason why assessment takes such a long time is that many patients attending DDTUs are, or claim to be, dependent on opiates and/or other drugs, and one of their reasons for attending the unit may be to obtain a prescription for drugs. Although this prescription may be the only way of retaining a patient in treatment, it is very important that it should not be handed out indiscriminately to everyone who claims to need it; a regular prescription for methadone, for example, could convert an occasional user of opiates into an opiate-dependent individual or it could be sold on the black market. Accurate diagnosis of dependence status is therefore very important.

The full assessment procedure is described below. It is intended only as a guide, to be modified according to the patient's needs, the presenting problem and the resources available to the professional being consulted.

Drug history

The purpose of this part of the history is to find out specifically and accurately about the patient's drug-taking behaviour, both at the present time and in the past, and to establish its importance in the patient's life as a whole. It must be appreciated from the beginning that the history given by the patient may be inaccurate and sometimes deliberately untruthful. The amount of drug taken may be understated, so that the apparent problem is minimized; alternatively it may be exaggerated in an attempt to get a larger dose prescribed. Illicit activity may be concealed. Truthful accounts are more likely to be obtained in a non-judgemental situation and when confidentiality is assured.

It is first of all very important to establish why the patient is seeking help at this time and whether any specific event has precipitated their attendance. Information should be obtained about the first exposure to drug taking and subsequent drug taking should be similarly explored, ending up with recent patterns of abuse, including the methods and routes of drug administration. This part of the history taking may be very complicated if the patient is or has been a polydrug abuser, and it is usually simplest to take each drug in turn, in chronological order of first use and to elicit all the relevant information for each drug separately. Specific enquiries should be made about amphetamines, methylphenidate (Ritalin), cocaine, cannabis, LSD, methadone, heroin, dipipanone (Diconal), barbiturates, methaqualone (Mandrax), benzodiazepines (diazepam, lorazepam, etc.) or other sedatives. A similar history should also be obtained about the use of tobacco or alcohol. The physical, psychological, social and legal consequences of drug use should be established and information elicited about previous attempts at help seeking and the other agencies with which the patient may have been in contact.

A format for obtaining all this information is outlined in Table 4.1. It

Table 4.1 Outline of drug history scheme

---

1 Reason for referral
Type of help sought

2 First exposure
Age
Which drug
Mode of administration
Circumstances
  where
  who/how initiated
  source of drug
Reaction to drug

3 Subsequent use
Which drug(s)
  dose
  frequency of administration
  route
  date and age of becoming a regular user
  periods of heavy use
  maximum regular amount taken
  effects of drug
Reasons for continuation
Circumstances of drug taking: solitary/with friends
Preferred drug(s)
Periods of abstinence
  voluntary
  enforced
  reasons for relapse

4 Recent use (last 4–6 weeks)
Drug(s):
  dose
  frequency
  route

Continued

Table 4.1 *Continued*

Any withdrawal symptoms
Evidence of increasing tolerance; escalating dose
Source of supply
Price paid
Continued use despite evidence of harm

5 *History of self-injecting*
Age first injected
Duration of injecting
Frequency
Route: subcutaneous/intramuscular/intravenous
Site

6 *HIV risk behaviour*
Source of injection equipment
Sharing of injection equipment
 last time shared
 number of others shared with
Knowledge about sterilization procedures
Knowledge about sources of clean equipment
Heterosexual/homosexual risk behaviour
Use of condoms
Sexual behaviour when intoxicated
Knowledge of HIV issues and transmission

7 *Consequences and complications of drug use*
Physical illness: malnutrition; hepatitis; jaundice; abscesses; septicaemia; deep vein
 thrombosis; overdose; road traffic and other accidents; symptoms of abstinence
 syndrome
Mental illness: episodes of drug-induced psychosis; intoxication leading to drowsiness
 and confusion; dementia
Social problems: associated with drug use; amount spent weekly on drugs; source of
 that money; time spent on drug taking, neglect of other activities.
Occupational problems: difficulties at work; suspensions; jobs lost.
Legal problems: drug-related criminal record; any pending court cases

8 *Contact with other treatment agencies or sources of help*
e.g., DDTUs; doctors; probation services; local authorities; voluntary agencies, religious
organisations, self help groups, etc.

suggests the most fruitful lines of questioning to elicit the maximum information, so that a full picture of the patient's drug taking is built up. It is then possible to identify the main drug problem(s) for each patient, to find out if they are physically and/or psychologically dependent on drugs and to gain some idea of the severity of the drug dependence. The severity of drug dependence may be manifest in several ways, including duration of drug abuse, the quantity of drugs taken, the amount of drug-related activity compared to other activities in their life, the route of administration and the degree and extent of risk-taking behaviour.

A systematic assessment questionnaire, incorporating a scoring system for the severity of drug-related problems and the needs of the patient is included in Appendix 2. This is useful both for research purposes and for treatment planning.

Life history

Even a young drug abuser has a life behind him or her – a life history of many years, of which drug taking forms only a part. Having explored, defined and understood the drug taking, it is necessary to find out about all the other parts of the life history that provide the essential background to the foremost problem of drug abuse. It is said that to know all is to understand all; finding out about the life history of the drug abuser, about his/her environment, experiences and personality, aids the helper in understanding the whys and wherefores of the drug taking. Reaching this understanding creates an empathy between the drug abuser and the professional helper that is the basis of any future therapeutic relationship.

The areas of the life history to be covered include the family history, which should specifically explore drug use by other members of the patient's family and their knowledge of and attitude towards the patient's drug taking. Other important information should be obtained about the patient's early history and academic record and, if there is any doubt, a specific enquiry should be made about the patient's ability to read and write. Their employment record should also be ascertained, but if it is impossible to enumerate all jobs or the number of jobs then the longest job held and the 'average duration' of jobs should be recorded. The marital and psychosexual history are of importance, as is the menstrual history if a female patient is dependent on opiates; these drugs sometimes cause amenorrhoea and the early stages of pregnancy may not be diagnosed. It is also necessary to gain some idea of the patient's home circumstances, although a more detailed account will be elicited in the course of the social-work assessment. An up-to-date account of the patient's legal history should be obtained and, perhaps most important of all, the patient's personality before drug taking started should be explored. Here, information from parents, friends or other relatives may be very helpful, if the patient agrees to their participation in the enquiry.

A suggested format for establishing the patient's life history is provided in Table 4.2.

Table 4.2 Outline of life-history scheme

1 Family history
Age and occupation of parents and siblings (if deceased: date and cause of death,
    together with patient's age at the time)
Description of parents' personality and their past and present attitudes towards patient
History of illness or delinquency in family members
Drug use (including alcohol, tobacco) by other family members
Knowledge of patient's drug use by other family members, and their attitude towards it
Relationship between various members of family

2 Early history
Birth history
Early development including time of milestones
Childhood neurotic traits (bed-wetting, sleep walking, tantrums, etc) and periods of
    separation from parents
Childhood illnesses
Home life and atmosphere

3 School
Schools attended
Educational attainments
Relationships with staff and peers
Truancy
Further education
Vocational training

4 Employment
Age of starting work
Jobs held:
    dates
    duration
    wage
    job satisfaction
    reason for change

5 Marital and psychosexual history
Date of marriage; spouse's name, age and occupation
Children; names and ages
General marital adjustment; any periods of permanent or temporary separation
The same information should be collected for any further marriages or cohabitations
Partner's drug taking and knowledge of, and attitude to, patient's drug taking
Sexual inclinations and practices: masturbation; sexual fantasies; homosexuality;
    heterosexual experiences; contraception; sterilization

6 Menstrual history
Age when periods started

Continued p. 126

Table 4.2 *Continued*

Length of cycle
Dysmenorrhoea
Premenstrual tension
Periods of amenorrhoea
Date of last menstrual period
Climacteric symptoms

7 Previous illnesses
Physical:
   major illnesses and accidents
   dates of admission to hospital
   accidental overdoses
Psychiatric:
   all psychiatric admissions and treatments
   attendance at psychiatric clinics
   suicidal attempts; deliberate self-poisoning

8 Home circumstances
Address; whom is patient living with
Present income; its source
Financial or domestic problems

9 Legal history
Number of arrests, court appearances, convictions
Periods in detention centre, approved school, Borstal, prison
Periods of probation
Nature of offences
Outstanding court cases
Disqualification from driving

10 Previous personality–before drug use
Interests, hobbies
Social relations–family, friends
Mood; mood swings
Character: obsessionality, ambitions, future plans
Religious beliefs and observances
Evidence of personality disorder (ICD-10 F60)

Social-work assessment

The patient (or client, when seen by a social worker) may be interviewed initially in the social worker's office or in a community venue, but a home visit, if the patient agrees, is often very helpful in permitting a first-hand appraisal of living conditions and lifestyle. In addition, information may be gathered from partners, relatives or a probation officer – but, of course, only with the consent of the patient.

It must be remembered throughout the assessment that many drug abusers have been in conflict with the law and that they may have felt rejected by the caring professions in the past. They may still be involved in illicit activities which they fear may come to light in the course of a social enquiry. Thus, some abusers may be deceitful, devious and manipulative, and although they may have sought help voluntarily, they often remain suspicious of those who try to help them. To establish some degree of empathy with them, it is necessary to understand the motivation behind this behaviour, much of which is a learned response to pressures from peers, families and professionals. Only in an atmosphere of trust and confidentiality can the need – or otherwise – for social intervention be identified and the balance of positive and negative factors in the patient's environment and social networks be accurately assessed. The particular points to be addressed in more detail in the social work assessment are shown in Table 4.3.

Once the information in Table 4.3 has been elicited, a much clearer picture will have emerged about the patient's needs. Some patients, for

Table 4.3 Outline of social work history scheme

1 Accommodation
Locality
Tenure
Condition
Whom the patient is living with

2 Employment
Work experience and capabilities
Need for vocational guidance and training
Attitude towards work

3 Finances
Income
Benefits
Debts

4 Social functioning
How the day is spent

5 Social networks
Friends and family
Agencies
Involvement with drug sub-culture
Extent of loneliness and isolation

example, may require assistance with problems relating to their material conditions. Practical advice and sometimes active intervention in difficulties related to housing, welfare benefits and debts may be welcomed, and some patients may benefit substantially from help in seeking training or in finding a job. Other patients require intervention on the grounds that there is a risk of neglect or abuse to children living in the household (see p. 272), and sometimes there are particular family factors which warrant including one or more of the patient's family in the treatment plan. For example, it may be helpful to arrange for a pre-school child to attend a day nursery or to refer a relative to a self-help support group. Sometimes a decision is made to involve the whole family in family therapy. Finally, because many patients are already involved with other helping agencies, there may already be a professional worker taking an interest in their case, so that liaison is appropriate.

Perhaps the most important question to be addressed in the social-work assessment is what sort of long-term help the patient will require. Because rehabilitation, the reintegration of the individual into society, is the statutory responsibility of the social services, the social worker is the key health-care professional involved in this very long-term project and needs to assess what sort of therapeutic environment will be best for each patient. For example, for some patients complete removal to a drug-free therapeutic community may be the best way of achieving a permanently drug-free lifestyle. For others, this may be impractical or undesirable and placement in a hostel or day hospital may be more appropriate. Some, while remaining at home, may benefit from practical help and advice about changing their pattern of living in relation to work, leisure and social life, and some may benefit from individual or group psychotherapy.

These choices are made largely, but not solely, on the basis of the social-work assessment, and the social worker is involved in their initiation if the patient is to be placed elsewhere, but more often their work involves seeing the patient on a regular basis for help, advice and counselling.

Family assessment

A more complete picture of the patient's drug-taking, lifestyle and background can be obtained if other members of the family are also interviewed. They may, for example, be able to confirm important details in the history and to elaborate upon them. However, a family assessment goes far beyond factual information-gathering and seeks to explore the extent to which the drug-taking behaviour of the patient may have been, and still is being, affected by family attitudes and dynamics, and the effect of the drug taking on the family. The fuller understanding of the patient's problem gained by such an assessment is of crucial importance in planning a treatment programme which is tailored to the individual's needs and is therefore more likely to succeed. In particular, it may indicate a need for family therapy and/or support for other family members.

The proportion of patients for whom a family assessment is considered appropriate and who give their consent for it is likely to be small, as the confidentiality of their consultation is often of paramount importance to drug abusers. Those who do give their consent can be divided into three groups:

1   patients in their late teens or early twenties, attending with their parents;
2   patients who attend with their non-drug-using partner;
3   patients who attend with their drug-using partner.

If the patient lives at home and attends with his/her parent(s), their knowledge of their child's drug taking is assessed; whether, for example, they suspected the drug taking themselves or were told by their child or by someone else. Their attitude towards the drug taking is explored and, in particular, how they perceive their child's drug taking in relation to their own use of drugs (tobacco, alcohol, prescribed drugs, etc.). It is important to establish the nature of drug-related family behaviour; whether, for example, family members collude to some degree with the patient's use, whether the patient splits the family, or if family members try to shield each other from the full knowledge of the patient's drug taking. If, for example, there are secondary gains for the patient, vis-à-vis family dynamics, achieved by virtue of drug-taking, it may be extremely difficult, if not impossible, to eliminate this behaviour without some kind of family therapy. The assessment should also estimate the strength of the family unit and, in particular, of the parents' marriage, to see how much support they will be able to offer the patient during the very stressful situation of drug withdrawal; whether indeed the family wish to be involved in the treatment plan; and how much support they themselves may need too.

The assessment, if the patient attends with a non-using partner, is in some ways similar to that outlined above. Again, it is necessary to gauge his/her knowledge and attitude towards the patient's drug taking, and to assess the contribution of the dynamics of the relationship to maintaining drug-taking behaviour. The stability and strengths of the marriage/partnership must be explored, as must the partner's strengths and weaknesses, so that his/her need for support is fully understood. It may be helpful to find out if the partner was instrumental in bringing the patient to treatment, how this came about, and if there are any conditions attached to this situation.

When a patient attends with a drug-using partner, the assessment must address quite different problems, as it is necessary to establish the nature and severity of the partner's drug problem too, and his/her motivation to attend for treatment. The problems of uncoordinated drug withdrawal in couples should be discussed, together with the possibility of coordinated treatment. An important issue to be assessed is whether the using partner is likely to sabotage treatment or to encourage the abuse of prescriptions. Once again, the relative strengths of both individuals should be examined and any supports that they share should be identified.

Physical examination

Physical examination is an important part of the assessment procedure, permitting confirmation of details supplied in the history and sometimes providing new information. Objective signs of intoxication or withdrawal may contribute to the assessment of the severity of physical dependence, and sequelae of drug abuse that require medical intervention can be identified. The findings on physical examination vary according to the drug(s) of abuse and the method of their administration. No attempt is made in this brief account to cover all possible physical manifestations and complications of drug abuse, nor to deal with the differential diagnosis of unconsciousness due to drug overdose (see Chapter 7). Rather, it is intended as a guide to physical signs that may be recorded during the routine examination of a patient presenting with a drug problem, and offers some explanation as to how they have arisen.

General appearance

An appearance of *general neglect* coupled with poor nutritional state suggests a lifestyle that has become totally concerned with drugs, ignoring personal hygiene, food, clothes, etc. Marked *weight loss* is particularly seen with chronic use of stimulants such as amphetamines. Scars on the head may indicate injuries sustained during convulsions (usually in the course of sedative hypnotic withdrawal).

Gait

An *unsteady gait* (ataxia), often in association with *slurred speech* (an appearance similar to drunkenness), suggests intoxication with sedatives.

Eyes

Watering eyes occur during opiate withdrawal. *Nystagmus* is indicative of intoxication with sedative hypnotics. *Pin-point pupils* suggest the recent administration of opiates, while *dilated pupils* occur in the opiate abstinence syndrome. Dilated pupils may also occur following the use of amphetamine, cocaine, hallucinogens and anticholinergic drugs. *Jaundice* of the scleral conjunctivae suggests hepatitis, probably secondary to non-sterile injection or to the abuse of volatile solvents. Dilatation of conjunctival blood vessels results in *red eye*, usually due to cannabis abuse but sometimes to solvents. Jerky nystagmus may be seen in chronic barbiturate intoxication.

Nose

Congestion of the nasal mucosa (lining of the nose) occurs if drugs have been snorted. Ulceration or perforation of the nasal septum may occur, traditionally due to cocaine, but it also occurs if heroin is snorted. A *runny nose* (rhinorrhoea) is due to opiate withdrawal and leads to constant *sniffing*. A *red, spotty rash* around the nose and mouth may be due to solvent sniffing.

Mouth

There is a high incidence of *dental caries* in those who are dependent on opiates; this is attributable to poor dental hygiene and a predilection for sweet food. A particular type of carious lesion has been described which is larger than usual and found only on the labial and buccal surfaces of the teeth. Several teeth may have been lost in this way, or in the course of convulsions during the sedative hypnotic abstinence syndrome. Breath odour may indicate abuse of solvents or alcohol.

Skin

Because many people with a serious drug problem inject their drugs and do so repeatedly, the skin bears many marks *(stigmata)* of their drug-taking behaviour. Often these are due to the introduction of infection because of dirty injection techniques. Thus *abscesses* are common and there may also be the *scars* of healed abscesses.

Many drugs that are injected were manufactured and intended only for oral consumption; they have physical properties that render them totally unsuitable for injection and which can cause serious complications if they are administered in this way. Oral barbiturates, for example, when dispersed in water, are very acidic and highly irritant to the body's tissues. If injected subcutaneously (skin-popping), skin necrosis may occur, leading to *shallow, sterile abscesses* which heal leaving *shallow, punched-out scars* These are frequently multiple and may be found anywhere on the body, but usually on the extremities.

Intravenous injection is, however, the preferred route of administration by most long-term, drug-dependent individuals, mainly because it provides maximum effect from the minimum amount of drug (and therefore gives best value for money). The veins of the arms are most accessible and stigmata of injection should be sought on the front of the elbows. *Needle puncture marks* may be seen in the skin overlying the veins which may be *red* and *inflamed* due to *thrombophlebitis*; there may be *peripheral swelling (oedema)* of the extremities due to the venous obstruction. This is particularly common if barbiturates are injected. Repeated injection leads to *pigmentation of the skin* over the veins (*tracking*) which may feel *hard* and *stringy* due to fibrosis after repeated thrombosis. When the veins of the arm can no longer be used for injection, others are used instead – in the foot, groin, neck – anywhere into which the frantic drug abuser can get a needle. Any of these sites may become thrombosed and infected, often by skin bacteria, because the skin is rarely cleaned before injection. Evidence of the use of neck veins, or of others even more extraordinary, indicates very severe dependence and this behaviour, repugnant even to other drug-dependent individuals, suggests a serious underlying personality disorder. *Decorative tattoos* may be placed to conceal evidence of drug injection.

Because of the progressive difficulty of intravenous injection, accidental injection into an adjacent artery sometimes occurs. If barbiturates are administered in this way they may cause acute arterial spasm which, if severe and prolonged, may lead to *gangrene* necessitating subsequent *amputation*. This is most frequently seen in the hand, where attempts to inject barbiturates into the small blood vessels have led to amputation of one or more fingers (or parts of fingers).

Gooseflesh (pilo-erection) is a wellknown cutaneous sign of the opiate abstinence syndrome, while patients withdrawing from sedatives and alcohol may *sweat* profusely.

Cardiovascular system

Raised pulse rate (tachycardia) may be due to drug withdrawal (opiates, sedatives) or to intoxication with stimulant drugs, which may also cause irregularities of the heart (arrhythmias). *High blood pressure* may occur following the administration of amphetamine and similar drugs, while *low blood pressure* may occur following the administration of opiates and sedatives (although tolerance develops to this effect in chronic users). If the barbiturate abstinence syndrome is suspected, pulse and blood pressure should be measured with the patient supine and then standing; a fall in blood pressure (*orthostatic hypotension*) and an *increase in heart rate of more than 15* is suggestive of barbiturate withdrawal.

A diagnosis of endocarditis should be considered in any drug abuser with a *fever* and a *heart murmur* and, as prompt treatment may be life saving, a high index of suspicion should be maintained (see p. 233).

Respiratory system

Examination of the chest may be quite normal, although there may be signs of *pulmonary embolism, infarction* and of increased pulmonary blood pressure (*pulmonary hypertension*). Chest infections are common and there is a reported association between heroin use and asthma.

Abdomen

Enlargement of the liver (hepatomegaly) is common in those who inject drugs and is strongly suggestive of hepatitis. Because tolerance does not develop to the constipating effect of opiates, the colon (lower bowel) may be *distended with faeces* and easily palpable. In a female patient, the possibility of pregnancy should not be forgotten; it is not unknown for amenorrhoea to be attributed to drug abuse (opiates) and for pregnancy to be far advanced before it is diagnosed.

Neuromuscular system

Tremor and muscle twitching are signs of the opiate abstinence syndrome. Repeated intramuscular injection of some drugs, particularly pentazocine and pethidine produces severe *wasting of the muscle(s)* into which the drug is injected; there may be *fibrosis* that entraps peripheral nerves and sometimes calcification. Peripheral nerves may also be damaged by accidental, intraneural injection of a drug.

Lymphatic system

Enlarged lymph nodes in axillae and groins are common if drugs are injected because of the repeated introduction of infection; they are usually bilateral, and if unilateral this indicates preferential injection on that side.

Lymphadenopathy may carry a more sinister implication now as it also occurs in AIDS. Lymphatic obstruction due to repeated episodes of infection and inflammation may contribute to the development of chronically *'puffy'* hands, with a characteristic, *brawny oedema* – typical of those who inject barbiturates into their hands and forearms.

Test of physical dependence on opiates (naloxone hydrochloride)

Physical dependence on opiates can be assessed using the opiate antagonist naloxone hydrochloride. Naloxone 0.4–0.8 mg (1–2 ml) is administered intramuscularly; this has no effect if the patient is not physically dependent on opiates. If the patient is physically dependent, the signs and symptoms of the opiate abstinence syndrome will become apparent within minutes of injection. If unduly distressing, they can be relieved to some extent by giving morphine 15–30 mg; the patient should then be kept under observation for a couple of hours for signs of opiate intoxication because naloxone has a shorter duration of action than morphine. The patient's consent must always be obtained and the naloxone test should not be done if the patient is pregnant, as it may induce abortion.

Testing with naloxone is a procedure used more frequently by some treatment centres than others and is rarely used in the UK. It can only assess pharmacological need and should never be the sole component of the assessment procedure. Recent research at St George's Drug Dependence Treatment and Research Centre suggests that naloxone eye drops may be a useful development of the naloxone test (Ghodse Opiate Addiction Test). When administered to one eye of an opiate-dependent individual they produce pupil dilatation of that eye only, with no systemic effects of opiate withdrawal. They have no effect if the individual is not physically dependent on opiates. Unfortunately, there is no similar test for the assessment of physical dependence on non-opiate drugs.

Mental state examination

Examination of the mental state is an essential component of the assessment procedure. Firstly, it may identify a coexistent psychiatric illness, such as depression, schizophrenia or agoraphobia, that requires treatment and which may be (or may have been) a contributory factor in the initiation and/or continuation of drug abuse. In addition, because most drugs of abuse have psychoactive properties, it is logical to seek the psychological consequences of their consumption. They may cause hallucinations or delusions, for example, or they may affect cognitive state, mood and thought. However, these symptoms and signs are not drug specific and cannot be diagnostic. Similar symptoms may arise during intoxication with one drug and in the abstinence syndrome of another. Their incidence and severity vary according to the dose consumed, individual sensitivity to the effect of the drug and the development of tolerance and physical dependence.

Nevertheless, the skilled interpretation of psychological signs and symptoms can make a significant contribution to the assessment of a drug-abuse problem, particularly when these observations are considered in conjunction with the history of drug taking and the results of laboratory investigation. It should be stressed, however, that many patients – probably the majority – present with a perfectly normal and appropriate mental state. In addition, many of the drug effects outlined below are very subtle and are not easily discernible even by experienced observers.

As part of the examination of the patient's mental state, it is important to ascertain the degree of understanding and awareness of the extent to which his/her drug abuse is problematic and to establish whether the patient is able to attribute any abnormal psychic experiences, such as abnormal visual perceptions, to their use of psychoactive drugs.

Enquiries should also be made as to their motivation for seeking treatment at the current time, including external motivators such as forensic, employment or social factors, and intrinsic factors such as the psychological or medical sequelae of drug use. The patient's use of commonly employed defence mechanisms such as denial, minimization, rationalization and projection should also be explored and the interviewer should be alert to evasiveness and manipulative behaviour.

Finally, it is important to establish whether the patient is agreeable to treatment and the kind of treatment that they are requesting, which may, at times, differ from what the clinician feels is most appropriate.

General behaviour

Restlessness, anxiety and *irritability* may be caused either by intoxication with stimulants or hallucinogens, or by the withdrawal of opiates and sedatives. The latter may also be associated with muscle twitching and tremulousness. When due to stimulants, restlessness may be accompanied by repetitive behaviour patterns, incessant *fiddling* and *picking at the skin*. Restlessness and anxiety due to opiate withdrawal may be so severe that the patient cannot tolerate or endure the interview; there may also be repeated *yawning*. In contrast, *quiet, withdrawn behaviour* may follow consumption of sedatives or opiates which in higher doses cause drowsiness. General *apathy* follows stimulant withdrawal, and preoccupation with inner psychic phenomena after use of cannabis or hallucinogens may also lead to withdrawn behaviour. Hostile, aggressive behaviour, and sometimes violence, may occur with stimulant intoxication and also occurs as a paradoxical reaction in chronic intoxication with sedative hypnotics.

Talk

General *talkativeness* and pressure of speech is common in patients intoxicated with stimulants, who may flit from one topic to another. Cannabis too may induce chattiness. *Lack of spontaneous speech* and *monosyllabic answers* are common in those who have recently taken opiates and sedatives, but can also occur if the patient is preoccupied with the wretchedness of the abstinence syndrome of these drugs. Formal thought disorder occurs much less frequently in drug-induced psychosis than in other psychotic conditions (e.g., schizophrenia).

Mood

Changes in mood, which are often frequent and rapid (labile mood) are commonly associated with drug abuse. For example, elated mood with excessive cheerfulness, energy and confidence can follow stimulant abuse and may mimic mild hypomania. Abrupt withdrawal from stimulants in heavy users can precipitate sudden intense feelings of depression and anxiety ('the crash'), often with suicidal ideation; hypersomnolence may also be a feature. This is followed by a period of milder depressive symptoms characterized by apathy, anhedonia and anergia. Alcohol and sedative misuse may be associated with depression of mood which usually improves after a period of abstinence. Feelings of guilt, worthlessness and hopelessness are commonly expressed by chronically dependent individuals and it should be remembered that they have an increased risk of suicide; the possibility of this should always be explored during mental state examination.

A feeling of mental detachment, well-being and quiet euphoria is described by opiate users, while marked anxiety and depression are associated with withdrawal in dependent individuals. 'Bad trips', undesired and unpleasant drug experiences, associated especially with hallucinogens and stimulants, may result in marked panic attacks, depersonalization and feelings of extreme terror.

Thought content

A general *suspiciousness* of other people is a common consequence of regular consumption of stimulants and *ideas of reference* and *paranoid delusions* may be apparent. These may also occur after the administration of hallucinogens and cannabis.

Abnormal experiences and beliefs

Hallucinations are common after stimulants, hallucinogens and cannabis. Auditory and tactile hallucinations are typical of stimulant administration, and if the patient also suffers from *delusions* these are likely to be paranoid in nature. Paranoid delusions may also occur following cannabis consumption. The hallucinogens give rise to a wide variety of illusions and hallucinations; frank psychosis may ensue and flashbacks are common. Hallucinations and delusions may also occur in the course of sedative withdrawal. Abnormal beliefs in supernatural powers (e.g., the ability to fly) have been described during LSD use, sometimes with fatal consequences.

Cognitive state

A wide range of psychoactive drugs may *impair the patient's general awareness and his/her ability to concentrate and attend to the interview. Disorientation* and *confusion* may arise with stimulant or sedative intoxication. Withdrawal in heavy sedative abusers often produces a *delirious state* similar to alcoholic delirium tremens. *Impairment of short-term memory* and *amnesic periods* (memory blackouts) occur during periods of sedative and alcoholic intoxication.

Psychological assessment

Psychological assessment of the patient involves personality testing using standardized inventories to measure the patient's cognitive state, personality and social functioning and to identify specific deficits. In particular, the patient's suitability for different treatment options is assessed. For example, patients suffering from overwhelming anxiety may benefit from instruction in relaxation techniques; some patients may require social skills and assertiveness training; others, suffering from phobias, might benefit from desensitization. There is a wealth of psychological intervention which may be employed to reduce or eliminate the patient's need for psychoactive drugs, and psychological assessment aims to identify those patients to whom this may usefully be applied. In addition, psychological assessment may help to identify an individual's particular skills and aptitudes, facilitating more appropriate vocational guidance and rehabilitation.

Special investigations

Laboratory investigations may be helpful in assessing the general health status of the patient and in detecting adverse consequences of drug abuse – due either to the drug itself or to the methods of its administration, or to the lifestyle of the patient.

Haemoglobin

Venepuncture may be very difficult in chronic injectors because easily accessible veins are likely to be thrombosed. Haemoglobin and full blood count may provide evidence of nutritional deficiencies (iron, vitamins) that have led to anaemia. Anaemia can also occur if the bone marrow is depressed by solvent abuse and in the presence of chronic infection – in which case the ESR (erythrocyte sedimentation rate) will probably be raised too. A raised white cell count is common in drug abusers due to the frequency of infective complications of self-injection.

Urea

A raised blood urea suggests damage to the kidneys. This may occur in the course of solvent abuse, and may also be due to intravenous heroin use which can cause a nephrotic syndrome with protein in the urine. Renal damage is common and severe in those who abuse analgesics such as aspirin.

Liver function tests

These are often abnormal in those who inject drugs due to a high incidence of hepatitis. Typically, the liver enzymes serum glutamic oxalo-acetic transaminase (SGOT), serum glutamic pyruvic transaminase (SGPT) and alkaline phosphatase (AP) are raised; bilirubin may be raised even if jaundice is not apparent clinically. Liver damage can also be caused by solvent abuse and by the adulterants of illicit drugs.

Wasserman reaction

In the midst of current concern about AIDS, the risk of syphilis in drug abusers who inject their drugs is rarely mentioned. However, syphilis is transmitted in exactly the same way as AIDS, so that those at risk of one are equally at risk from the other, and the Wasserman reaction (WR) test for syphilis should not be omitted.

Hepatitis B

The variety of hepatitis most common in injecting drug abusers is hepatitis B, which is detected in the body by various markers or antigens. Most tests for hepatitis B seek to identify an antigen on the surface of the viral particle, named hepatitis B surface antigen (HBsAg), formerly known as Australia antigen. This can be detected in the blood, not instantly after infection, but after a variable incubation period (2–6 months). The body responds to the viral antigens by producing antibodies (hepatitis B antibodies) and their presence denotes prior infection with hepatitis B virus. Any patient who has injected drugs should be tested for the presence of HBsAg and for its antibodies. Tests for other types of hepatitis – hepatitis A, hepatitis C and delta virus – are not done routinely, but are reserved for the investigation of a patient with a clinical diagnosis of hepatitis.

Test for HIV antibody

The test for HIV antibodies is available at most DDTUs and some patients may ask to have it done. Others, such as those who continue to share needles, patients with unexplained symptoms, and women who are pregnant or planning pregnancy, should be advised to be tested. The patient's consent must always be obtained and the test should never be carried out until the full implications of the result – whatever it may turn out to be – have been discussed with the patient at a special counselling session (p. 238).

Precautions for taking specimens from drug abusers

Because drug abusers who inject drugs are a high-risk group for HIV and AIDS, the clinical and laboratory workers who deal directly with them and/or their specimens (of blood/urine, etc.), have a potential occupational risk of becoming infected. In fact, there have been very few such cases, but if this good record is to be maintained, high standards of operational practice are essential to avoid inadvertent infection. As no cases of AIDS have been attributable to air-borne droplet infection, precaution is concentrated on preventing accidental parenteral infection. These precautions apply when dealing with any drug abuser who self-injects, and not just to those known at the time to be HIV-positive.

Particular care must be taken when needles, etc. are used for invasive procedures, which should be carried out by experienced staff wearing suitable protective clothing (e.g., gown/gloves/apron, as appropriate). Needles should be removed from syringes with the utmost care and should be placed in the correct puncture-proof bin for final disposal. Accidental puncture wounds should be treated promptly by thorough washing and encouraging bleeding, and should be reported. Pre-existing skin wounds or abrasions should be kept covered.

Specimens of blood or urine should be placed in secure containers and then sealed in individual plastic bags before sending them to the laboratory. The accompanying request forms should be kept separate from the specimen containers and should indicate clearly that there is a risk (or suspicion of risk) that the specimens may be infected with HIV. Any spillage of potentially infected body fluids must be dealt with straightaway, ensuring disinfection.

These procedures have received special emphasis since the advent of AIDS, although they are no more rigorous than those that should be employed to prevent contamination with hepatitis B virus, which is much more infective and easier to transmit than HIV. They apply to all specimens obtained from high-risk patients, not just blood, and must be observed irrespective of the investigation for which the sample was taken.

Chest X-ray

Chest X-rays should be carried out routinely. They may be completely normal, but following a period of unconsciousness (e.g., after an overdose) there may be evidence of aspiration pneumonia. In those who inject drugs, the signs of pulmonary embolism, infarction or hypertension may be apparent.

Bacteriological investigation

Swabs from all infected lesions should be sent to the laboratory for culture and sensitivity testing. Infection is often due to 'unusual' microorganisms, that rarely cause problems in those who do not inject drugs, but which gain access to the body by means of non-sterile injection techniques. It is important that they should be identified so that anti-infective treatment can be prompt and appropriate.

Laboratory investigation for drugs

The laboratory plays an important role in the diagnosis and management of many cases of drug abuse and dependence, often because the individuals concerned are not always truthful about their drug consumption and an independent, objective source of information is particularly useful. However, all laboratory investigations, including tests for drugs, have their limitations, and the significance of the results can only be fully appreciated if these limitations are understood, and if the results are interpreted in the context of information gained from the history and examination of the patient.

The choice of body fluid for drug analysis depends on a number of factors that are different for each drug, but the principal consideration is the distribution of the drug between the body fluids, notably blood and urine. This varies according to the length of time the drug has been in the body and the dose.

Once the drug has entered the body, whether by the respiratory system, the alimentary canal or by injection, it circulates in the blood, either as the free drug or bound to a protein. However, to produce its action on the body, the drug must pass from the bloodstream to the body cells and it is only the free, non-protein-bound drug that can enter the body cells. The drug is rendered inactive and/or removed from the body by a variety of processes.

It may be combined (conjugated) in the liver with other chemical substances and the inactive conjugate subsequently excreted in the urine. Alternatively, it may be chemically altered (often in the liver) to produce pharmacologically active metabolites which, like the parent drug, may then undergo conjugation in the liver and excretion by the kidney. Damage to the liver (in hepatitis, for example) may reduce its ability to metabolize drugs.

The concentration of the drug in the blood at a particular time represents the amount of drug available to the body cells at the time the blood sample was taken and depends on the dose and on the rates of absorption and elimination. The time taken for the blood concentration to decline by 50% is known as the drug's half-life. Drugs with a short half-life (e.g., heroin, cocaine) have blood levels that decrease rapidly with time, and that cannot easily be correlated with dose unless additional information is available.

Usually, urine samples are preferred for the analysis of drugs of abuse. Specimens are readily obtainable and, because the concentration of a drug in urine is much higher than in blood, it can be detected more easily and for longer after drug administration. A disadvantage of using urine is that some drugs are present only as metabolites which are common to a number of parent drugs; thus the detection of a particular metabolite may not identify exactly which drug was consumed. Blood has the advantage that the parent drug can be measured, but only if the sample is collected soon after the drug was taken. Another advantage is that tampering with a blood sample is more difficult than with a urine sample.

Testing for drugs, therefore, usually takes place on urine samples (hair and saliva may also be used), and it is, of course, essential to be absolutely sure that the urine specimen being tested has actually come from the patient being assessed – substitution of specimens is not unknown. Clearly, a single urine specimen cannot provide all the answers about an individual's drug taking, but repeated tests can help to build up a more complete picture of drug taking over a period of time.

An additional benefit of urine testing is that it may have a significant deterrent effect on illicit drug taking. If those attending for the treatment of a drug problem know that they may be asked for a urine sample, and know that a positive result will have adverse consequences, they may be less willing to risk illicit drug misuse. Random urine testing may thus help to prevent relapse.

Table 4.4 shows how different drugs are distributed in blood and urine. The figures in the table are only average values and will vary from patient to patient, as well as with the frequency of dosing and the dose of the drug.

Hair analysis

Techniques have now been developed to use hair samples to investigate an individual's consumption of drugs. It has been suggested that, because hair grows at a relatively constant rate of about 1cm per month, the concentration of drugs at different points on the hair shaft can be used to measure the time that has elapsed since the drug was taken. Although there may be factors that limit interpretation, there is a theoretical potential for hair samples to be used for detailing an individual's recent drug history, and this has been used both in the clinical setting and in forensic casework. Nevertheless, this is a technique in its infancy and there cannot yet be complete confidence in the reliability of results obtained from hair analysis.

Laboratory methods

Chromatography is a method for separating chemical substances that depends on differences between their rates of transfer between a moving stream of liquid or gas and a stationary material, usually a finely divided solid or film of liquid on the surface of such a solid. With *thin-layer chromatography (TLC)*, the finely divided, solid stationary material is spread as a thin layer on a sheet of glass. In *high-performance liquid chromatography (HPLC)* the stationary material is packed into a steel tube and the moving

Table 4.4 Drug distribution in blood and urine. (Source: Bucknell & Ghodse, 1991)

	Blood		Urine	
	Half-life* (hours)	Blood level (μg per ml)†	90% excretion (days)‡	Unchanged drug (%)§
CNS depressants				
Barbiturates				
Phenobarbitone	100	10–40	16	25
Butobarbitone	40	0.3–5.0	7	5
Amylobarbitone	24	0.3–5.0	6	1
Chlormethiazole	5	0.27–2.0		5
Benzodiazepines				
Diazepam	48	1.15–3.0	7	
CNS stimulants				
Amphetamine	12	1.01–0.1	3	3
Methylamphetamine	9	0.02–0.8	1.5	43
Cocaine	1	0.1–0.5	2	4
Narcotic analgesics				
Heroin	0.5			nil
Morphine	3	0.05	1	5
Codeine	3	0.01–0.1	1	
Methadone	15	0.05–0.07	2	4
LSD	3	0.004		1
Cannabis	30	0.007	12	

*Half-life: time in hours for the blood level to decrease by 50%.
†Blood level: the lower value is the likely blood level after a single, therapeutic (or usual) dose; the upper value is the likely value during chronic administration.
‡90% excretion: time in days for 90% of the drug to be excreted in the urine
§Unchanged drug: percentage of the unchanged drug excreted in the urine.

stream of liquid is pumped through at high pressure, while in *gas–liquid chromatography (GLC)*, a moving stream of gas is pumped through at high pressure.

Immunoassay depends on the interaction between the substance being measured and a specific antibody to that substance. The antibody is produced in animals (in the same way that antibodies are produced in humans during vaccination procedures) by previously injecting the chemical substance of interest, or a derivative, into an animal which responds by synthesizing the antibody. This is then isolated from the blood of the animal and can be used to detect the original chemical substance in other samples. The measurement of drugs using *radioimmunoassay* (RIA) or *enzyme immunoassay* (EMIT) relies on the use of reagents labelled with a radioactive marker or enzyme respectively.

Mass spectrometry, by accurate analysis of molecular weight can determine molecular structure and hence identify specific drugs.

The two screening methods that are used most commonly are TLC and EMIT. These methods can detect a wide variety of drugs including barbiturates, morphine, methadone and amphetamine. Confirmation of positive results is usually achieved by specific GLC or HPLC. In addition, specific immunoassay methods are available for some drugs and their metabolites. The most sensitive and specific method, available in some specialized laboratories, is GLC linked to a mass spectrometer.

Sophisticated equipment is needed to carry out these tests. As it is expensive to install and run, it is available only in specialized centres that provide a drug-screening service with a high level of expertise for surrounding hospitals, thus achieving economy of scale. This means, however, that there may be a delay of several days between sending a urine specimen to the laboratory and receiving a report on the drugs it contains.

Interpretation of results

The interpretation of the results of analyses depends on the sensitivity and specificity of the analytical method used. Most laboratories use screening procedures for the common drugs that will only detect a single, minimum therapeutic dose for about 24 hours after administration. There are, however, large variations in drug metabolism and excretion between individuals so that the drug may be detected for less than 24 hours in some patients, but may persist for much longer in others. A negative result of a drug screen by these methods means only that the urine specimen contains less than the lowest amount detectable by the method. It does not necessarily mean the complete absence of the drug from the urine, nor that the drug has not been taken. Nevertheless, negative urine results may be very informative; for example, the repeated absence of opiates from the urine of an individual claiming to be dependent and seeking a prescription gives more precise information than a positive result which could mean either that the individual is dependent or that he/she is an occasional user.

Positive results must be interpreted in relation to the specificity of the method used. Identification of a drug solely by screening methods is fraught with difficulties and confirmation by a more specific method is essential for forensic work. However, due to constraints imposed by the pressure of work, time and money, many laboratories report results on the basis of screening procedures only. Thus, false positive results (a drug reported present when in fact it is absent) are not unknown. Awareness of this is very important because in attempting to assess the patient's drug consumption, excessive and misplaced reliance on the laboratory tests may be as misleading as unquestioning acceptance or automatic disbelief of the patient's account of his/her drug taking.

Drug-screening programmes

Following the lead of companies and corporations in the USA, there have been calls for drug-screening programmes in the UK for certain groups of individuals, and particularly for those whose mental impairment by drugs might put others at risk. Drug screening might involve either random testing or routine, regular testing, although neither is a foolproof method of detecting or preventing drug abuse. Leaving aside the important question of whether compulsory testing is an unacceptable infringement of individual rights, the usefulness of such a programme requires careful scrutiny. It has been claimed, for example, that drug testing may be beneficial because of its potential deterrent effect.

It has already been explained that negative results of urine testing for drugs do not necessarily mean that the individual concerned has not taken drugs. It might mean only that the dose was so small or had been taken so much earlier that the concentration of drug in the urine was too low to be detected by screening methods. Positive results too can be misleading. The available methods of screening urine are insufficiently accurate to be relied on and false positive results occur regularly. This problem could be overcome by the use of specific tests, but these are time consuming and expensive and therefore inappropriate for mass screening. Because of the limitations of drug-screening methods, the interpretation of the results is very important and this requires expert assessment of the history of drug use and the findings on clinical examination, which should be considered in conjunction with the result of the urine test.

Given the very loose association between safety in the workplace and the use of drug screening, and the problems associated with the latter, introduction of such programmes is likely to remain controversial. However, in some countries screening for drugs has already become quite fashionable, generating an inappropriate demand for the service and increasing the likelihood of screening being imposed. An alternative to screening is performance appraisal, carried out using computer/video technology to simulate real tasks for those whose impairment puts many others at significant risk. This approach seems preferable, because it emphasizes 'fitness to work', rather than querying drug abuse.

Summary

This chapter has been primarily concerned with the content of the assessment – what information to gather and, specifically, which questions to ask. The procedure that is outlined is not applicable to every situation in which a drug abuser seeks help: someone dropping in to an advice centre does not expect and is likely to feel resentful about detailed enquiries into their private life; a busy general practitioner may not have the time to explore the patient's background in the way that has been described. Clearly, it is up to the professional concerned to select appropriate areas and details of the assessment procedure, depending on the nature of the help that is required and the skills and resources available.

Although many of the questions and procedures described here may not be relevant to all professionals, the detailed nature of the elicited information emphasizes the complexity of drug abuse. It is not an isolated event in the person's life; many factors contributed to its developing in the past and many are contributing to its maintenance at the time that the individual asks for help. Undoubtedly, his/her drug taking has had adverse consequences and these are probably continuing. In this complex situation it is not helpful, at any level of intervention, to jump to hasty conclusions about the nature of the problem or to offer ill thought-out solutions. If drug abuse and drug dependence are perceived as ongoing interactions between the drug, the individual and society, then the purpose of the assessment is to tease out these interwoven threads, each of which is itself multistranded, to see how they are woven together.

For those with a long history of severe dependence, this teasing out is difficult and takes a long time, requiring all the approaches to assessment described in this chapter. Assessment comprises much more than information gathering, however. It is, after all, the time when the individual engages in, or is engaged in, treatment. Any such approach to any professional is difficult. Most patients, whatever their problem, are anxious in this situation, and when the problem is one of drug abuse or dependence the patient is likely to be very anxious indeed. It takes great courage to admit to a drug problem and to ask for help, especially if there have been previous attempts at dealing with it and previous failures. Anxiety may be disguised by hostile or aggressive behaviour; some patients, having taken drugs to give them courage to attend, may be intoxicated. Nevertheless, their seeking help is the all-important first step which they alone can take and which should be (must be) rewarded by positive responses from all involved in the assessment procedure. A snappy telephonist, an off-putting receptionist, a doctor or nurse riled by an uncooperative patient can precipitate that patient's walking out, not to return or to try again – at least not for some time. Positive, friendly, non-judgemental attitudes are essential – exactly the responses, in fact, that any patient, regardless of ailment, is entitled to expect, but even more important for drug abusers who may have had many previous experiences of rejection. As their behaviour often elicits adverse responses in those whom they encounter, a high degree of professionalism is necessary on the part of all involved staff, who may require special training and support.

For many drug abusers and especially those with long and complex drug problems, the assessment procedure itself may be a therapeutic process. The telling of the 'life history' – some of it spontaneously, some in answer to direct questions – helps the patient, perhaps for the first time, to see his/her drug taking in some sort of perspective. The account of the present social circumstances clearly identifies current problems and needs. This clarification to an outsider is, or can be, a clarification to the drug abuser too and what needs to be done, the way forward, can become apparent to both.

Assessment is not an end in itself. There is no point in defining the problem, understanding the antecedent circumstances and merely observing and recording the adverse consequences. The aim of assessment is to offer the patient an appropriate treatment programme. This will involve the drug of abuse certainly, but many other areas of the patient's life are likely to be affected too. Assessment should make apparent to both parties what changes are necessary, in which areas of the patient's life, and what the realistic expectations of such change are (although drug abuser and helping professional may not always agree). The skill of the helping professional lies in the accurate assessment of the problem and the accurate matching of the patient to treatment option.

Classification of substance-use disorders

There have been many approaches to classifying mental and behavioural disorders. The two most widely used systems are the World Health Organization's International Classification of Diseases and Related Health Problems, now in its tenth revision (ICD-10), and the American Psychiatric Association's Diagnostic and Statistical Manual of Mental Disorders, third edition, revised (DSM-III-R).

ICD-10

ICD-10 uses an alphanumeric coding scheme, based on codes with a single letter, followed by two numbers at the three-character level. Further detail is then provided by means of decimal numeric subdivisions at the four-character level. As it is designed to be a central ('core') classification for a family of disease- and health-related classifications, some members of the family of classifications are derived by using a fifth or even sixth character to specify more detail.

Within ICD-10, mental and behavioural disorders due to psychoactive substance use are classified within the block F10–F19. At this point it should be noted that the term 'disorder' is used throughout the classification, so as to avoid even greater problems inherent in the use of terms such as 'disease' and 'illness'. 'Disorder' is not an exact term, but in this context implies the existence of a clinically recognizable set of symptoms or behaviour associated, in most cases, with distress and with interference with personal functions. Social deviance or conflict alone, without personal dysfunction, is not included within this definition of mental disorder. Block F10–F19 contains a wide range of disorders of varying severity (from uncomplicated intoxication and harmful use to obvious psychotic disorders and dementia), that are all attributable to the use of one or more psychoactive substances (which may or may not have been medically prescribed).

The substance involved is indicated by means of the second and third characters (i.e., the first two digits after the letter F):

F10   mental and behavioural disorders due to use of *alcohol*;
F11   mental and behavioural disorders due to use of *opioids*;
F12   mental and behavioural disorders due to use of *cannabinoids*;
F13   mental and behavioural disorders due to use of *sedatives* or *hypnotics*;
F14   mental and behavioural disorders due to use of *cocaine*;
F15   mental and behavioural disorders due to use of other *stimulants* including *caffeine*;
F16   mental and behavioural disorders due to use of *hallucinogens*;
F17   mental and behavioural disorders due to use of *tobacco*;
F18   mental and behavioural disorders due to use of *volatile solvents*;
F19   mental and behavioural disorders due to *multiple drug use and use of other psychoactive substances*.

The identification of the psychoactive substance used may be made on the basis of self-report data, objective analysis of specimens of urine, blood, etc., or other evidence (presence of drug samples in the patient's possession, clinical signs and symptoms, or reports from informed third parties, as described earlier). Objective analysis provides the most compelling evidence of present or recent use, although this information is of limited value in relation to past use. Whenever possible, it is always advisable to seek corroboration from more than one source of evidence.

Although many drug users take more than one type of drug, the diagnosis of the disorder should be classified, whenever possible, according to the most important single substance (or class of substance) used. This may usually be done with regard to the particular drug, or type of drug, causing the presenting disorder. When in doubt, the code should be selected to identify the drug or type of drug most frequently misused, particularly in those cases involving continuous or daily use. Only in cases in which patterns of psychoactive substance taking are chaotic and indiscriminate, or in which the contributions of different drugs are inextricably mixed, should code F19 (disorders resulting from multiple drug use) be used.

Other points to be noted are as follows.

1   The misuse of non-psychoactive substances, such as laxatives or aspirin, should be coded by means of F55 (abuse of non-dependence-producing substances), with a fourth character to specify the type of substance involved.

2   Cases in which mental disorders (particularly delirium in the elderly) are due to psychoactive substances, but without the presence of one of the disorders in this block (e.g., harmful use of dependence syndrome), should be coded in F00–F09. Where a state of delirium is superimposed upon a disorder in this block, it should be coded by means of F1x.3 or F1x.4.

3   The level of alcohol involvement can be indicated by means of a supplementary code (from Chapter XX of ICD-10): Y90 (evidence of alcohol involvement determined by blood alcohol content) or Y91 (evidence of alcohol involvement determined by level of intoxication).

4   The fourth character (after the decimal point) specifies the clinical condition arising as a consequence of the use of a psychoactive substance. These are listed below and should be used, as required, for each substance specified, although it should be noted that not all four-character codes are applicable to all substances:

F1x.0   acute intoxication;
F1x.1   harmful use;
F1x.2   dependence syndrome;
F1x.3   withdrawal state;
F1x.4   withdrawal state with delirium;
F1x.5   psychotic disorder;
F1x.6   amnesic syndrome;
F1x.7   residual and late-onset psychotic disorder;

F1*x*.8   other mental and behavioural disorders;
F1*x*.9   unspecified mental and behavioural disorder.

F1*x*.0 Acute intoxication

Acute intoxication is defined as a transient condition following the administration of alcohol or other psychoactive substance, resulting in disturbances in level of consciousness, cognition, perception, affect or behaviour, or other psychophysiological functions and responses. This should be a main diagnosis only in cases where intoxication occurs without more persistent alcohol or drug-related problems being concomitantly present. Where there are such problems, precedence should be given to diagnoses of harmful use (F1*x*.1), dependence syndrome (F1*x*.2), or psychotic disorder (F1*x*.5).

The following diagnostic guidelines are important.

1   Acute intoxication is usually closely related to dose levels. Exceptions to this may occur in individuals with certain underlying organic conditions (e.g., renal or hepatic insufficiency) in whom small doses of a substance may produce a disproportionately severe intoxicating effect. Disinhibition due to social context should also be taken into account (e.g., behavioural disinhibition at parties or carnivals). Acute intoxication is a transient phenomenon and its intensity reduces as time passes. In the absence of further use of the substance, the effects will eventually disappear and recovery is therefore complete, except where tissue damage or another complication has arisen.

2   It should be noted that the symptoms of intoxication need not always reflect the primary actions of the substance: for instance, depressant drugs may led to symptoms of agitation or hyperactivity, and stimulant drugs may lead to socially withdrawn and introverted behaviour. The effects of substances such as cannabis and hallucinogens may be particularly unpredictable. Moreover, many psychoactive substances are capable of producing different types of effect at different dose levels. For example, alcohol may have apparent stimulant effects on behaviour at lower dose levels, may lead to agitation and aggression with increasing dose levels, and produce clear sedation at very high levels.

3   This diagnostic coding includes acute drunkenness in alcoholism, and 'bad trips' (due to hallucinogenic drugs).

The fifth character is used to indicate whether the acute intoxication is associated with any complications:

F1*x*.00   uncomplicated, this means that the intoxication is uncomplicated although the symptoms may be of varying severity, depending on the dose;
F1*x*.01   with trauma or other bodily injury;

F1*x*.02 with other medical complications, such as haematemesis or inhalation of vomit;

F1*x*.03 with delirium;

F1*x*.04 with perceptual distortions;

F1*x*.05 with coma;

F1*x*.06 with convulsions;

F1*x*.07 pathological intoxication. This grouping applies only to alcohol. It describes the sudden onset of aggression and often violent behaviour that is not typical of the individual when sober, very soon after drinking amounts of alcohol that would not produce intoxication in most people.

F1*x*.1 Harmful use

This is a pattern of psychoactive substance use that is causing damage to health. The damage may be physical (as in cases of hepatitis from the self-administration of injected drugs) or mental (e.g., episodes of depressive disorder secondary to heavy consumption of alcohol). The following diagnostic guidelines should be followed.

1   The diagnosis requires that actual damage should have been caused to the mental or physical health of the user.

2   Harmful patterns of use are often criticised by others and frequently associated with adverse social consequences of various kinds. The fact that a pattern of use or a particular substance is disapproved of by another person or by the culture, or may have led to socially negative consequences such as arrest or marital arguments is not in itself evidence of harmful use.

3   Acute intoxication (see F1*x*.0), or 'hangover' is not in itself sufficient evidence of the damage to health required for coding harmful use.

4   Harmful use should not be diagnosed if dependence syndrome (F1*x*.2), a psychotic disorder (F1*x*.5), or another specific form of drug- or alcohol-related disorder is present.

F1*x*.2 Dependence syndrome

This is defined as a cluster of physiological, behavioural and cognitive phenomena in which the use of a substance or class of substances takes on a much higher priority for a given individual than other behaviours that once had greater value. A central descriptive characteristic of the dependence syndrome is the desire (often strong, sometimes overpowering) to take psychoactive drugs (which may or may not have been medically prescribed), alcohol, or tobacco. There may be evidence that return to substance use after a period of abstinence leads to a more rapid reappearance of other features of the syndrome than occurs with non-dependent individuals.

A definite diagnosis of dependence should usually be made only if three or more of the following have been experienced or exhibited at some time during the previous year.

1   A strong desire or sense of compulsion to take the substance.

2   Difficulties in controlling substance-taking behaviour in terms of its onset, termination, or levels of use.

3   A physiological withdrawal state (see F1*x*.3 and F1*x*.4) when substance use has ceased or been reduced, as evidenced by the characteristic withdrawal syndrome for the substance, or use of the same (or a closely related) substance with the intention of relieving or avoiding withdrawal symptoms.

4   Evidence of tolerance, such that increased doses of the psychoactive substance are required in order to achieve effects originally produced by lower doses (clear examples of this are found in alcohol- and opiate-dependent individuals who may take daily doses sufficient to incapacitate or kill non-tolerant users).

5   Progressive neglect of alternative pleasure or interests because of psychoactive substance abuse; increased amount of time necessary to obtain or take the substance or to recover from its effects.

6   Persisting with substance abuse despite clear evidence of overtly harmful consequences, such as harm to the liver through excessive drinking, depressive mood states consequent to periods of heavy substance use, or drug-related impairment of cognitive functioning; efforts should be made to determine that the user was actually, or could be expected to be, aware of the nature and extent of the harm.

Narrowing of the personal repertoire of patterns of psychoactive substance use has also been described as a characteristic feature (e.g., a tendency to drink alcoholic drinks in the same way on weekdays and weekends, regardless of social constraints that determine appropriate drinking behaviour).

It is an essential characteristic of the dependence syndrome that either psychoactive substance taking or a desire to take a particular substance should be present; the subjective awareness of compulsion to use drugs is most commonly seen during attempts to stop or control substance use. This diagnostic requirement would exclude, for instance, surgical patients given opioid drugs for the relief of pain, who may show signs of an opioid withdrawal state when drugs are not given but who have no desire to continue taking drugs.

The dependence syndrome may be present for a specific substance (e.g., tobacco or diazepam), for a class of substance (e.g., opioid drugs), or for a wider range of different substances (as for those individuals who feel a sense of compulsion regularly to use whatever drugs are available and who show distress, agitation, and/or physical signs of a withdrawal state upon abstinence).

F1x.2 (dependence syndrome) includes chronic alcoholism, dipsomania and drug addiction. The diagnosis of the dependence syndrome may be further specified by the following five-character codes:

F1x.20   currently abstinent;

F1x.21   currently abstinent, but in a protected environment (e.g., in hospital, in a therapeutic community, in prison, etc.);

F1x.22   currently on a clinically supervised maintenance or replacement regime (controlled dependence) (e.g., with methadone, nicotine gum or nicotine patch);

F1x.23   currently abstinent, but receiving treatment with aversive or blocking drugs (e.g., naltrexone or disulfiram);

F1x.24   currently using the substance (active dependence);

F1x.25   continuous use;

F1x.26   episodic use (dipsomania).

F1x.3 Withdrawal state

This describes a group of symptoms of variable clustering and severity occurring on absolute or relative withdrawal of a substance after repeated, and usually prolonged and/or high dose, use of that substance. The onset and course of the withdrawal state are time-limited and are related to the type of substance and the dose being used immediately before abstinence. The withdrawal state may be complicated by convulsions. The following diagnostic guidelines are important:

1   a withdrawal state is one of the indicators of dependence syndrome (see F1x.2) and this diagnosis should also be considered;

2   withdrawal state should be coded as the main diagnosis if it is the reason for referral and sufficiently severe to require medical attention in its own right;

3   physical symptoms vary according to the substance being used. Psychological disturbances (e.g., anxiety, depression, and sleep disorders) are also common features of withdrawal. Typically, the patient is likely to report that withdrawal symptoms are relieved by further substance use.

It should be remembered that withdrawal symptoms can be induced by conditioned/learned stimuli in the absence of immediately preceding substance use. In such cases, a diagnosis of withdrawal state should be made only if it is warranted in terms of severity. It should also be noted that simple 'hangover' or tremor due to other conditions should not be confused with the symptoms of a withdrawal state.

The diagnosis of withdrawal state may be further specified by using the following five-character codes:

F1x.30 uncomplicated;

F1x.31 with convulsions.

F1x.4 Withdrawal state with delirium

A condition in which the withdrawal state (see F1x.3) is complicated by delirium.

Alcohol-induced delirium tremens should be coded here. Delirium tremens is a short-lived, but occasionally life-threatening, toxic-confusional state with accompanying somatic disturbances. It is usually a consequence of absolute or relative withdrawal of alcohol in severely dependent users with a long history of use. The onset usually occurs after withdrawal of alcohol but may, in some cases, appear during an episode of heavy drinking, in which case it should be coded here.

Prodromal symptoms typically include insomnia, tremulousness and fear, but the onset may also be preceded by withdrawal convulsions. The classical triad of symptoms includes clouding of consciousness and confusion, vivid hallucinations and illusions affecting any sensory modality, and marked tremor. Delusions, agitation, insomnia or sleep-cycle reversal, and autonomic overactivity are usually also present.

The diagnosis of withdrawal state with delirium may be further specified by using the following five-character codes:

F1x.40 without convulsions;

F1x.41 with convulsions.

F1x.5 Psychotic disorder

A cluster of psychotic phenomena that occur during or immediately after psychoactive substance use and are characterized by vivid hallucinations (typically auditory, but often in more than one sensory modality), misidentifications, delusions and/or ideas of reference (often of a paranoid or persecutory nature), psychomotor disturbances (excitement or stupor), and an abnormal effect, which may range from intense fear to ecstasy. The sensorium is usually clear but some degree of clouding of consciousness, though not severe confusion, may be present. The disorder typically resolves at least partially within 1 month and fully within 6 months.

The following diagnostic guidelines are relevant.

1   A psychotic disorder occurring during or immediately after drug use (usually within 48 hours) should be recorded here, provided that it is not a manifestation of drug withdrawal state with delirium (see F1*x*.4) or of late onset. Late-onset psychotic disorders (with onset more than 2 weeks after substance use) may occur, but should be coded as F1*x*.75.

2   Psychoactive substance-induced psychotic disorders may present with varying patterns of symptoms. These variations will be influenced by the type of substance involved and the personality of the user. For stimulant drugs such as cocaine and amphetamines, drug-induced psychotic disorders are generally closely related to high dose levels and/or prolonged use of the substance. A diagnosis of a psychotic disorder should not be made merely on the basis of perceptual distortions or hallucinatory experiences when substances having primary hallucinogenic effects (e.g., lysergide (LSD), mescaline, cannabis at high doses) have been taken. In such cases, and also for confusional states, a possible diagnosis of acute intoxication (F1*x*.0) should be considered.

3   Particular care should also be taken to avoid mistakenly diagnosing a more serious condition (e.g., schizophrenia) when a diagnosis of psychoactive substance-induced psychosis is appropriate. Many psychoactive substance-induced psychotic states are of short duration, provided that no further amounts of the drug are taken (as in the case of amphetamine and cocaine psychoses). False diagnosis in such cases may have distressing and costly implications for the patient and for the health services.

F1*x*.5 includes alcoholic hallucinosis, alcoholic jealousy and alcoholic paranoia.

The diagnosis of psychotic state may be further specified by the following five-character codes:

F1*x*.50   schizophrenia-like;
F1*x*.51   predominantly delusional;
F1*x*.52   predominantly hallucinatory (includes alcoholic hallucinosis);
F1*x*.53   predominantly polymorphic;
F1*x*.54   predominantly depressive symptoms;
F1*x*.55   predominantly manic symptoms;
F1*x*.56   mixed.

F1*x*.6 Amnesic syndrome

A syndrome associated with chronic prominent impairment of recent memory; remote memory is sometimes impaired, while immediate recall is preserved. Disturbances of time sense and ordering of events are usually evident, as are difficulties in learning new material.

Confabulation may be marked, but is not invariably present. Other cognitive functions are usually relatively well preserved and amnesic defects are out of proportion to other disturbances. The following diagnostic guidelines are important.

1 Amnesic syndrome induced by alcohol or other psychoactive substances coded should meet the general criteria for organic amnesic syndrome:

(a) memory impairment, as shown in impairment of recent memory (learning of new material), disturbances of time sense (rearrangements of chronological sequence, telescoping of repeated events into one, etc.);

(b) absence of defect in immediate recall, of impairment of consciousness, and of generalized cognitive impairment;

(c) history of objective evidence of chronic (and particularly high dose) use of alcohol or drugs.

2 Personality changes, often with apparent apathy and loss of initiative, and a tendency towards self-neglect may also be present, but should not be regarded as necessary conditions for diagnosis.

3 Although confabulation may be marked it should not be regarded as a necessary prerequisite for diagnosis.

F1x.6 includes Korsakov's psychosis or syndrome, induced by alcohol or other psychoactive substances.

F1x.7 Residual and late-onset psychotic disorder

A disorder in which changes of cognition, effect, personality, or behaviour, induced by alcohol or another psychoactive substances, persist beyond the period during which a direct, substance-related effect might reasonably be assumed to be operating. The following diagnostic guidelines may be helpful.

1 The onset of the disorder should be directly related to the abuse of alcohol or a psychoactive substance. Cases in which the initial onset occurs later than episode(s) of substance abuse should be coded here only where clear and strong evidence is available to attribute the state to the residual effect of the substance. The disorder should represent a change from or a marked exaggeration of the prior and normal state of functioning.

2 The disorder should persist beyond any period of time during which direct effects of the psychoactive substance might be assumed to be operative (see F1x.0, acute intoxication). Alcohol- or psychoactive substance-induced dementia is not always irreversible; after an extended period of total abstinence, intellectual functions and memory may improve.

3 The disorder should be carefully distinguished from withdrawal-related conditions (see F1x.3 and F1x.4). It should be remembered that, under

certain conditions and for certain substances, withdrawal-state phenomena may be present for a period of many days or weeks after discontinuation of the substance.

4 Conditions induced by a psychoactive substance, persisting after its use, and meeting the criteria for diagnosis of psychotic disorder should not be diagnosed here (use F1x.5, psychotic disorder). Patients who show the chronic end-state of Korsakov's syndrome should be coded under F1x.6.

Further specification of F1x.7 may be achieved by using the following five-character codes:

F1x.70 flashbacks, these may be distinguished from psychotic disorders partly by their episodic nature, frequently of very short duration (seconds or minutes), and by their duplication (sometimes exact) of previous drug-related experiences;

F1x.71 personality or behaviour disorder (meeting the criteria for organic personality disorder;

F1x.72 residual affective disorder (meeting the criteria for organic mood (affective) disorders;

F1x.73 dementia (meeting the general criteria for dementia);

F1x.74 other persisting cognitive impairment – his is a residual category for disorders with persisting cognitive impairment, which do not meet the criteria for psychoactive substance-induced amnesic syndrome (F1x.6) or dementia (F1x.73);

F1x.75 late-onset psychotic disorder.

F1x.8 Other mental and behaviour disorders

This diagnostic category is for any other disorder in which the use of a substance can be identified as contributing directly to the condition, but which does not meet the criteria for inclusion in any of the above disorders.

F1x.9 Unspecified mental and behavioural disorder

Unspecified mental and behavioural disorder induced by alcohol and drugs.

DSM-III-R

DSM-III-R, like ICD-10, acknowledges that no definition adequately specifies precise boundaries for the concept of mental disorder. However, each of the mental disorders is conceptualized as 'a clinically significant behavioural or psychological syndrome or pattern that occurs in a person and that is associated with present distress (a painful symptom) or disability (impairment in one or more important areas of functioning) or with a significantly increased risk of suffering death, pain, disability, or an important loss of freedom' Whatever the original cause, a mental disorder is a manifestation of behavioural, psychological or biological dysfunction. It should also be appreciated that there is no assumption that each mental disorder is a discrete entity with sharp boundaries between the different disorders.

A major difference between the ICD-10 and DSM-III-R is that the latter is a multiaxial system, requiring cases to be evaluated on several 'axes', each of which refers to a different class of information. The entire classification of mental disorders is contained within Axes 1 (Clinical Syndromes) and 2 (Developmental Disorders and Personality Disorders) and multiple diagnoses are made when necessary to describe the current condition.

Diagnostic guidelines are provided indicating the number and balance of symptoms usually required before a confident diagnosis can be made. Statements about the duration of symptoms are intended as general guidelines rather than strict requirements so that clinicians should use their own judgement about the appropriateness of choosing diagnoses when the duration of particular symptoms varies slightly from that specified.

Mental disorders related to substance use are classified in two areas of DSM-III-R – Psychoactive Substance Use Disorders and Psychoactive Substance-Induced Organic Mental Disorders.

Psychoactive substance use disorders

This diagnostic class covers the symptoms and maladaptive behavioural changes associated with more or less regular use of psychoactive substances. These changes are perceived as undesirable in most cultures and the underlying conditions are described as mental disorders, distinguishing them from non-pathological psychoactive substance use (e.g., drinking a moderate amount of alcohol).

There are two main categories of substance use disorder and their diagnostic criteria are summarized below.

Criteria for psychoactive substance dependence

Dependence can be diagnosed if at least three of the following symptoms have occurred, some of which have persisted for at least 1 month, or have occurred repeatedly over a longer period of time:

1   substance often taken in larger amounts or over a longer period than the person intended;

2 persistent desire or one or more unsuccessful efforts to cut down or control substance use;

3 a great deal of time spent in activities necessary to get the substance (e.g., theft), taking the substance (e.g., chain smoking), or recovering from its effects;

4 frequent intoxication or withdrawal symptoms when expected to fulfil major role obligations at work, school or home (e.g., not going to work because of a hangover; going to work or school while 'high'; intoxication while taking care of children), or when substance use is physically hazardous (e.g., driving while intoxicated);

5 Important social, occupational, or recreational activities given up or reduced because of substance use;

6 continued substance use despite knowledge of having a persistent or recurrent social, psychological or physical problem that is caused or exacerbated by the use of the substance;

7 marked tolerance; need for markedly increased amounts of the substance (i.e., at least a 50% increase) in order to achieve intoxication or desired effect, or markedly diminished effect with continued use of the same amount;

(NB The final two items listed (8 and 9) may not apply to cannabis, hallucinogens or phencyclidine.)

8 characteristic withdrawal symptoms;

9 substance often taken to relieve or avoid withdrawal symptoms.

Criteria for severity of psychoactive substance dependence

1 *Mild.* Few, if any, symptoms in excess of those required to make the diagnosis, and the symptoms result in no more than mild impairment in occupational functioning or in usual social activities or relationships with others.

2 *Moderate.* Symptoms or functional impairment between 'mild' and 'severe'.

3 *Severe.* Many symptoms in excess of those required to make the diagnosis, and the symptoms markedly interfere with occupational functioning or with usual social activities or relationships with others.

4 *In partial remission.* During the past 6 months, some use of the substance and some symptoms of dependence.

5 *In full remission.* During the past 6 months, either no use of the substance, or use of the substance and no symptoms of dependence.

Criteria for psychoactive substance abuse

Substance abuse can be diagnosed if all of the following criteria are fulfilled.

1   A maladaptive pattern of substance use indicated by at least one of the following:

   (a) recurrent use in situations in which use is physically hazardous (e.g., driving while intoxicated);

   (b) continued use despite knowledge of having a persistent or recurrent social, occupational, psychological, or physical problem caused or exacerbated by use of the substance.

2   Some symptoms persisting for at least 1 month or having occurred repeatedly over a longer period of time.

3   The patient has never met the criteria for Psychoactive Substance Dependence for this substance.

DSM-IV

Significant changes have recently been made in the diagnostic systems of the American Psychiatric Association, resulting in the development of DSM-IV, which has several important changes from the earlier DSM-III-R. For example, the stipulation in DSM-III that symptoms must 'have persisted for at least 1 month' is replaced with symptoms 'occurring at any time in the same 12-month period'. Broadening the dependence criteria will result in greater sensitivity of the dependence category, perhaps resulting in an increase in the breadth of individuals who are diagnosed with a disorder because it will no longer include only individuals who meet a significant number of criteria in a relatively short period of time. Another important change is grouping the criteria 'characteristic withdrawal symptoms' and 'substance taken to relieve or avoid withdrawal symptoms' into one category in DSM-IV, thus reducing the importance of physiological aspects of substance dependence by reducing the number of possible criteria. The criteria for substance dependence 'frequent intoxication or withdrawal when expected to fulfill major obligations at work, school or home or when substance use is physically hazardous' has been removed from DSM-IV, perhaps compromising the professional's ability to acknowledge the presence of impaired function in these locations; this may impair the diagnostic efficacy of the instrument.

   It is acknowledged in DSM-IV that it is often difficult to determine whether presenting symptoms are indeed substance induced – i.e., that they are the direct physiological consequence of substance intoxication or withdrawal, medication use or toxin exposure. Two additional criteria have therefore been added to each of the substance-induced disorders, with the intention of providing general guidelines and of allowing for clinical judgement in determining whether symptoms are substance-induced.

1   There is evidence from the history, physical examination, or laboratory findings of either:

(a) the symptoms developing during or within a month of substance intoxication or withdrawal:

(b) medication use is aetiologically related to the disturbance.

2   The disturbance is not better accounted for by a disorder that is not substance-induced. Thus, if the symptoms precede substance use, or persist for more than a month after its cessation, or are substantially in excess of what might be expected, given the type, duration, or amount of substance used, this would suggest the existence of an independent non-substance-induced disorder.

The DSM-IV criteria for substance dependence and abuse, as well as those for substance intoxication and withdrawal are listed below.

Criteria for substance dependence

The essential features of substance dependence are a cluster of cognitive, behavioural and physiological symptoms indicating that the individual continues use of the substance despite significant substance-related problems. There is a pattern of repeated self-administration that usually results in tolerance, withdrawal and compulsive drug-taking behaviour.

Diagnosis of dependence should be made if three or more of the following have been experienced or exhibited at any time during the last year.

1   Tolerance defined by either:

(a) the need for markedly increased amounts of substance to achieve intoxication or desired effect:

(b) a markedly diminished effect with continued use of the same amount of the substance.

2   Withdrawal, as evidenced by either of the following:

(a) the charactcristic withdrawal syndrome for the substance, or

(b) the same (or closely related) substance is taken to relieve or avoid withdrawal symptoms.

3   The substance is often taken in larger amounts over a longer period of time than was intended.

4   Persistent desire or repeated, unsuccessful efforts to cut down or control substance use.

5   A great deal of time is spent in activities necessary to obtain the substance, use the substance, or recover from its effects.

6   Important social, occupational, or recreational activities are given up or reduced because of substance use.

7   There is continued substance use despite knowledge of having had a persistent or recurrent physical or psychological problem that was likely to have been caused or exacerbated by the substance.

It should be specified whether physiological dependence is present or absent (i.e., either 1 or 2, above, is present).

The course of the dependence should also be described using one of six defined specifiers.

1   *Early full remission.* No criteria for dependence/abuse for at least 1 month, but for less than 12 months.

2   *Early partial remission.* One or more criteria for dependence/abuse have been met for at least 1 month but for less than 12 months (but the full criteria for dependence have not been met).

3   *Sustained full remission.* No criteria for dependence/abuse have been met at any time during a period of 12 months or longer.

4   *Sustained partial remission.* One or more criteria for dependence/abuse have been met, but not the full criteria, for a period of 12 months or longer.

5   *On agonist therapy.* This term should be used if the individual is on a pre-scribed agonist medication, and criteria for dependence/abuse have been met for that class of medication for at least the past month (except tolerance to, or withdrawal from, the agonist). This specifier may also be used for those being treated for dependence using a partial agonist or agonist/antagonist.

6   *In a controlled environment.* This specifier is used if the individual is in an environment where access to alcohol and controlled substances is restricted and no criteria for dependence/abuse have been met for the previous month (e.g., in prison, therapeutic community, locked hospital ward).

Criteria for substance abuse

The essential feature of substance abuse is a maladaptive pattern of substance use manifested by recurrent and significant adverse consequences related to the repeated use of substances, with clinically significant impairment or distress. This is manifested by one or more of the following occurring at any time during the same 12-month period:

1   recurrent substance abuse resulting in a failure to fulfil major role oblig-ations at work, school, or home (e.g., repeated absences, poor performance, expulsion or suspension from school, child neglect etc.);

2   recurrent substance abuse in situations that are physically hazardous (e.g., driving, operation machinery);

3   recurrent substance abuse-related legal problems;

4   continued substance abuse despite having persistent or recurrent social or interpersonal problems caused or exacerbated by the effects of the sub-stance (e.g., arguments and fights).

In addition, the symptoms should not have met the criteria for dependence on this class of substance.

Criteria for substance intoxication

1   The development of a reversible substance-specific syndrome due to the recent ingestion of (or exposure to) a substance.
2   Clinically significant maladaptive behavioural or psychological changes that are due to the effect of the substance on the central nervous system (e.g., belligerence, mood lability, cognitive impairment) developing during or shortly after use of the substance.

Criteria for substance withdrawal

1   The development of a substance-specific syndrome due to the cessation of (or reduction in) substance use that has been heavy and prolonged.
2   The substance-specific syndrome causes clinically significant distress or impairment in social, occupational or other important areas of functioning.
3   The symptoms are not due to a general medical condition and are not better accounted for by another mental disorder.

DSM-IV classification

In addition to the specifiers for substance dependence that have already been described, the following specifiers may also be utilized for substance-induced disorders:
with onset during intoxication (I)
with onset during withdrawal (W).

Within DSM-IV classification, the following substance-related disorders are separately enumerated and coded using the official coding system of the International Classification of Diseases, Ninth Revision, Clinical Modification (ICD-9-CM).

Alcohol-related disorders

Alcohol use disorders
   Alcohol dependence   303.90
   Alcohol abuse   305.00
Alcohol-induced disorders
   Alcohol intoxication   303.00
   Uncomplicated alcohol withdrawal   291.80
   Alcohol intoxication delirium   291.0

Alcohol withdrawal delirium   291.00
Alcohol-induced persisting dementia   291.20
Alcohol-induced persisting amnesic disorder   291.10
Alcohol-induced psychotic disorder   291.x
  with delusions   291.5
  with hallucinations   291.3
Alcohol-induced mood disorder   291.8
Alcohol-induced anxiety disorder   291.8
Alcohol-induced sexual dysfunction   291.8
Alcohol-induced sleep disorder   291.8
Alcohol-related disorder NOS   291.9

Amphetamine (or amphetamin-like)-related disorders

Amphetamine use disorders
  Amphetamine dependence   304.40
  Amphetamine abuse   305.70
Amphetamine-induced disorders
  Amphetamine intoxication   292.89
  Amphetamine withdrawal   292.0
  Amphetamine intoxication delirium   292.81
  Amphetamine-induced psychotic disorder   292.xx
    with delusions   292.11
    with hallucinations   292.12
  Amphetamine-induced mood disorder   292.89
  Amphetamine-induced anxiety disorder   292.89
  Amphetamine-induced sexual dysfunction   292.89
  Amphetamine-induced sleep disorder   292.89
  Amphetamine-related disorder NOS   292.9

Caffeine-related disorders

Caffeine-induced disorders
  Caffeine intoxication   305.90
  Caffeine-induced anxiety disorder   292.89
  Caffeine-related sleep disorder   292.89
  Caffeine-related disorder NOS   292.9

Cannabis-related disorders

Cannabis use disorders

Cannabis dependence   304.30
Cannabis abuse   305.20
Cannabis-induced disorders
  Cannabis intoxication   292.89
  Cannabis intoxication delirium   292.81
  Cannabis-induced psychotic disorder   292.xx
    with delusions   292.11
    with hallucinations   292.12
  Cannabis-induced anxiety disorder   292.89
  Cannabis-related disorder NOS   292.9

Cocaine-related disorders

Cocaine use disorders
  Cocaine dependence   304.20
  Cocaine abuse   305.60
Cocaine-induced disorders
  Cocaine intoxication   292.89
  Cocaine withdrawal   292.00
  Cocaine intoxication delirium   292.81
  Cocaine-induced psychotic disorder
    with delusions   292.11
    with hallucinations   292.11
  Cocaine-induced mood disorder   292.84
  Cocaine-induced anxiety disorder   292.89
  Cocaine-induced sexual dysfunction   292.89
  Cocaine-induced sleep disorder   292.89
  Cocaine-related disorder NOS   292.9

Hallucinogen-related disorders

Hallucinogen use disorders
  Hallucinogen dependence   304.50
  Hallucinogen abuse   305.30
Hallucinogen-induced disorders
  Hallucinogen intoxication   292.89
  Hallucinogen persisting perception disorder (flashbacks)   292.89
  Hallucinogen intoxication delirium   292.81
  Hallucinogen-induced psychotic disorder   292.xx
    with delusions   292.11
    with hallucinations   292.12

Hallucinogen-induced mood disorder   292.84
Hallucinogen-induced anxiety disorder   292.89
Hallucinogen-related disorder NOS   292.9

Inhalant-related disorders

Inhalant use disorders
  Inhalant dependence   304.60
  Inhalant abuse   305.90
Inhalant-induced disorders
  Inhalant intoxication   292.89
  Inhalant intoxication delirium   292.81
  Inhalant-induced persisting dementia   292.82
  Inhalant-induced psychotic disorder   292.xx
   with delusions   292.11
   with hallucinations   292.12
  Inhalant-induced mood disorder   292.84
  Inhalant-induced anxiety disorder   292.89
  Inhalant-related disorder NOS   292.9

Nicotine-related disorders

Nicotine use disorder
  Nicotine dependence   305.10
Nicotine-induced disorder
  Nicotine withdrawal   292.0
  Nicotine-related disorder NOS   292.9

Opioid-related disorders

Opioid use disorders
  Opioid dependence   304.00
  Opioid abuse   305.50
Opioid- induced disorders
  Opioid intoxication   305.50
  Opioid withdrawal   292.00
  Opioid intoxication delirium   292.81
  Opioid-induced psychotic disorder   292.xx
   with delusions   292.11
   with hallucinations   292.12

Opioid-induced mood disorder   292.84
Opioid-induced sexual dysfunction   292.89
Opioid-induced sleep disorder   292.89
Opioid-related disorder NOS   292.9

Phencyclidine (or phencyclidine-like)-related disorders

Phencyclidine use disorders
  Phencyclidine dependence   304.90
  Phencyclidine abuse   305.90
Phencyclidine-induced disorders
  Phencyclidine intoxication   292.89
  Phencyclidine intoxication delirium   292.81
  Phencyclidine-induced psychotic disorder   292.xx
  with delusions   292.11
  with hallucinations   292.12
  Phencyclidine-induced mood disorder   292.84
  Phencyclidine-induced anxiety disorder   292.89
  Phencyclidine-related disorder NOS   292.9

Sedative-, hypnotic-, or anxiolytic-related disorders

Sedative, hypnotic, or anxiolytic use disorders
  Sedative, hypnotic or anxiolytic dependence   304.10
  Sedative, hypnotic or anxiolytic abuse   305.40
Sedative-, hypnotic-, or anxiolytic-induced disorders
Sedative, hypnotic or anxiolytic intoxication   292.89
Sedative, hypnotic or anxiolytic withdrawal   292.0
Sedative, hypnotic or anxiolytic intoxication delirium   292.81
Sedative, hypnotic or anxiolytic withdrawal delirium   292.81
Sedative, hypnotic or anxiolytic persisting dementia   292.82
Sedative, hypnotic or anxiolytic persisting amnesic disorder   292.83
Sedative-, hypnotic- or anxiolytic-induced psychotic disorder   292.xx
  with delusions   292.11
  with hallucinations   292.12
  Sedative-, hypnotic- or anxiolytic-induced mood disorder   292.84
  Sedative-, hypnotic- or anxiolytic-induced anxiety disorder   292.89
  Sedative-, hypnotic- or anxiolytic-induced sexual dysfunction   292.89
  Sedative-, hypnotic- or anxiolytic-induced sleep disorder   292.89
  Sedative-, hypnotic- or anxiolytic-related disorder NOS   292.9

Polysubstance-related disorder

Polysubstance dependence   304.80

Other (or unknown) substance-related disorders

Other (or unknown) substance use disorders
  Other (or unknown) substance dependence   304.90
  Other (or unknown) substance abuse   305.90
Other (or unknown) substance-induced disorders
  Other (or unknown) substance intoxication   292.89
  Other (or unknown) substance withdrawal   292.0
  Other (or unknown) substance intoxication delirium   292.81
  Other (or unknown) substance persisting dementia   292.82
  Other (or unknown) substance persisting amnesic disorder   292.83
  Other (or unknown) substance-induced psychotic disorder   292.xx
  with delusions   292.11
  with hallucinations   292.12
  Other (or unknown) substance-induced mood disorder   292.84
  Other (or unknown) substance-induced anxiety disorder   292.89
  Other (or unknown) substance-induced sexual dysfunction   292.89
  Other (or unknown) substance-induced sleep disorder   292.89
  Other (or unknown) substance-related NOS   292.9

References and further reading

American Psychiatric Association (1987). *Diagnostic and Statistical Manual of Mental Disorders*, 3rd edn. (DSM-III-R). APA, Washington DC.

American Psychiatric Association (1994). *Diagnostic and Statistical Manual of Mental Disorders*, 4th edn. (DSM-IV). APA, Washington DC.

Donovan DM & Marlatt GA (eds) (1988). *Assessment of Addictive Behaviours: Behavioural, Cognitive and Physiological Procedures*. Guildford Press, Guildford.

Ferrara SD & Fernandez JCG (1987). Psychotropic drugs: organisation and role of the laboratory. In: Idanpaan-Heikkila J, Ghodse AH & Khan I (eds) *Psychoactive Drugs and Health Problems*. National Board of Health, Helsinki.

Ghodse AH, Bewley TH, Kearney MK & Smith SE (1986). Mydriatic response to topical naloxone in opiate abusers. *British Journal of Psychiatry*, **148**, 44–46.

Haertzen CA & Meketon MJ (1968). Opiate withdrawal as measured by the Addiction Research Centre inventory (ARCI). *Diseases of the Nervous System*, **29**, 450–455.

Hammersley R (1994). A digest of memory phenomena for addiction research. *Addiction*, **89**, 283–293.

McLellan AT, Luborsky L & Erdlen F (1980). The addiction severity index. In: Golthers E, McLellan AT & Druley KA (eds) *Substance Abuse and Psychiatric Illness*. Pergamon Press, New York.

Peachey JE & Loh E (1994). Validity of alcohol and drug assessment. *Current Opinion in Psychiatry*, **7, No. 3**, 252–258.

Steer RA & Schut J (1979). Types of psychopathology displayed by heroin addicts. *American Journal of Psychiatry*, **136**, 1463–1465.

Widiger TA & Smith GT (1994). Substance use disorder: abuse, dependence and dyscontrol. *Addiction*, **89**, 267–282.

World Health Organization (1974). *Detection of Dependence-Producing Drugs in Body Fluids. WHO Technical Report Series 556. WHO, Geneva.*

World Health Organization (1992). *The ICD-10 Classification of Mental and Behavioural Disorders. Clinical Descriptions and Diagnostic Guidelines.* WHO, Geneva.

World Health Organization (1993). *Health Promotion in the Work Place: Alcohol and Drug Abuse.* WHO Expert Committee. Technical Report Series 833. WHO, Geneva.

5

General measures of intervention

Introduction

Once assessment is completed, the crucial question of how to help a particular individual with their drug problem has to be answered. For some, the immediate response is pharmacological (see Chapter 6), although this is usually only a short-term measure and can only be one component of the total treatment response. But many who seek help have a drug problem with little or no physical dependence and for them there is no drug-specific treatment. For all drug abusers, therefore, it is essential to work out a long-term plan aimed at bringing about change in them and their lifestyle, so that they do not need to take drugs and can cope without them, even if they continue to be freely available.

A person's level of motivation for change is an important factor in determining the likely success of any intervention (and measurement of this will form part of the assessment interview). Of course, not every person presenting with a drug problem will be fully motivated to benefit from treatment, and a person's motivation for change will fluctuate depending on many factors. Most people have a degree of ambivalence, and a number of reasons for and against giving up or changing a habit, and the salience given to each of these can fluctuate even in a short time period. It may be helpful to think of motivation for change as a circle which the drug abuser may go round many times before achieving long-lasting change. The circle of motivation starts with the person not contemplating a change in their behaviour, either because of denial that a problem exists or because of a belief that the problem is unchangeable ('precontemplative' stage). The next stage is an awareness of the need and ability to change ('contemplative' stage) whilst nevertheless continuing with the behaviour. This is followed by a stage of active change, where the person's determination produces change-directed behaviour. The next part of the motivational circle is a 'maintenance of change' stage. One person may remain for several years at each stage, whilst someone else might experience all four on a daily basis.

The intervention offered will, to some extent, depend on the assessment of motivation for change, and it should not be assumed that everyone is at the active change state, nor that everyone will necessarily benefit from help directed at changing their behaviour. For most patients, however, some form of active-change treatment will be considered and a variety of treatment options are available. In virtually every case, if the treatment is to be of any value, it has to be on a voluntary basis and it is important that the patient participates in the choice of treatment option. Some treatments are directed at the underlying causes which may have initiated drug taking and/or are contributing to its continuation. Some help to resolve the problems associated with or consequent upon drug taking, and some deal more directly with the drug-taking behaviour itself, aiming to reduce or stop drug taking, regardless of other problems or circumstances. Some treatments may be directed at helping the client's motivation for change, rather than directly changing the behaviour, while others are aimed at helping to prevent relapse in those who have achieved change. The setting for these treatment options is likewise varied, from a residential programme through to self-help groups in the community. In recent years there have been considerable improvements in the provision of community treatments, often given by a multidisciplinary team seeing the patient at home or in another community venue.

Not all interventions are suitable for every patient, nor are they mutually exclusive. A patient, for example, may attend for drug counselling, undergo vocational rehabilitation and go to a local self-help group while, at the same time, his or her daily dose of opiates is being gradually reduced according to a treatment contract drawn up on a contingency-management basis. It is perhaps unlikely that a single individual would be on the receiving end of so many interventions, but the important point is that treatment plans must be drawn up thoughtfully, according to the needs of the individual, utilizing, as appropriate, a single intervention or a 'mix' of interventions, or components of different interventions. There is no one approach that is 'right' or 'best'. If there were, the problems of drug abuse and dependence would be rapidly overcome and petty controversies between the advocates of different treatment modalities would disappear.

Because there are no hard and fast rules about management, much depends on the skills of professional health-care workers in developing a treatment plan that meets the needs of the patient, and this in turn relies heavily on the findings of the assessment procedure. The key to successful intervention is to bring about change, and before that can be done, it is essential to know as much as possible about the existing situation.

The general measures of intervention that are briefly described in this chapter are mostly long-term measures, aimed at bringing about long term and fundamental changes. They are often collectively described as 'rehabilitation', and the fact that in this book rehabilitative interventions are described before 'treatment' (i.e., detoxification, maintenance, etc.) emphasizes the fact that for most drug abusers, long-term change is more important than short-term intervention and that the two stages of response should be considered and often initiated concurrently.

Psychotherapy

It has been apparent for many years that classical, analytically orientated psychotherapy is not suitable for drug-dependent patients. Early therapists emphasized the extreme difficulties encountered in trying to treat addicts, not least because it can be very difficult to engage them effectively in treatment and, if they do attend, their mental state may be adversely affected by drug use. In addition, such treatment is too time consuming and expensive to be a cost-effective option for treating the majority of problem drug users.

However, the term 'psychotherapy' embraces far more than Freudian or Jungian techniques of psychoanalysis. In its broadest sense it is a treatment involving communication between patient and therapist aimed at modifying or alleviating the patient's 'illness', and any encounter between the patient and a health-care worker thus offers an opportunity for psychotherapy. Awareness of the potential therapeutic value of this relationship and an appropriate structuring of the communication means that psychotherapy can become a component of an integrated approach to the treatment of drug dependence, rather than an alternative treatment strategy that is selected only occasionally.

Because many opiate-dependent individuals attend specialist treatment units regularly for long periods (months to years), possibly for opiate maintenance or for slow detoxification, long-term relationships can develop with clinic staff, which can be utilized to promote positive personality growth and psychological development. Similar opportunities arise with those who are dependent on sedative hypnotic drugs. It has been suggested that the supportive relationship that develops between patient and therapist becomes a substitute for drug use, just as drug dependency may be a substitute for certain aspects of important interpersonal relationships. A skilled therapist is unlikely to become a mere substitute for a drug, but having formed a good and supportive relationship with a patient is able to use it to identify and alter intrapsychic processes using techniques of insight, restructuring of belief systems, cognitive reframing and challenging of unhelpful beliefs, so that patients learn to see themselves and their problems more clearly and have the desire and the ability to cope with them.

It should also be remembered that many drug-dependent individuals have significant psychiatric problems, especially in the areas of depression and anxiety. Drug use and abuse may result from attempts to medicate these problems and it is therefore not surprising that psychotherapy, which can often help to alleviate depression and anxiety, may indirectly cause a reduction in drug use too.

Supportive, expressive psychotherapy

As the name suggests, this is an analytically orientated psychotherapy, in which special attention is paid to the meanings that patients attach to their drug dependence and in which, using supportive techniques, the patient is helped to identify and work through problematic relationships.

Group psychotherapy

Group psychotherapy is the technique of treating patients in groups rather than individually. The same group of individuals meets regularly, for example weekly or more often, with a trained leader who, depending on the type of group, may actively direct its focus. One of the aims might be to improve the ability of individual members to control their social behaviour – a skill in which some are deficient – and to this end, the behavioural interactions between the members of the group are the subject of examination. Members of the group are confronted with observations about their own behaviour and become aware of their effect on others and of the effect of others on themselves. They learn to listen to interpretations of their behaviour and to deal with the resultant anxiety, which may be difficult and painful at first, so that techniques of circumvention are employed. If group membership remains stable over several months, the group becomes a cohesive structure and its members identify positively with each other and with the group. In this supportive environment, individual growth is possible and the experience gained within the group can be transferred to life outside the group.

Other groups focus on the belief systems held by different members, eliciting errors of thinking (e.g., 'I've made a mess of my life so far, therefore I will always be a worthless person') or unhelpful beliefs ('the only time I can ever enjoy myself is when I'm drunk'). With the help of the therapist, the group is able to challenge beliefs and restructure them, using a number of techniques. Other groups focus on behavioural and cognitive skills for managing emotional states, anger control, and skills for dealing with lapses and for avoiding relapse. These groups are sometimes run along the line of educational courses, with behaviour rehearsal and group role-plays included among the techniques. 'Relapse prevention', on which some groups focus, is based on social-learning theory from psychology, and assumes that the road to relapse or continued abstinence follows a number of choice points; therapy in groups tends to include behavioural and cognitive techniques for dealing with the more common 'choice points', although a skilled therapist will be able to be flexible according to the needs of the group.

Superficially, group therapy is an attractive treatment option because it seems to be a cost-effective method, compared with individual psychotherapy, of offering professional help to drug abusers. However, effective group therapy may require regular attendance by all members and drug abusers may be unreliable and not good at keeping regular appointments, often for legitimate social reasons. Furthermore, effective group therapy requires a high level of disclosure and some drug abusers, who may have been involved in criminal activities, may not be sufficiently reassured about the confidentiality of the proceedings to be frank and honest. Finally, it is easy for group therapy with drug abusers to degenerate into a complaints session about aspects of treatment policy and for the group to exert pressure for change in this policy. These factors, together with poor attendance rates, make it very difficult to direct the group into therapeutic interactions and a very skilful therapist is essential.

Group therapy for drug abuse is not a substitute for individual treatment but is an adjunct to it, aiming to foster individual development and growth. Those most likely to benefit from dynamic group therapy, and most suitable for it, usually have a long history of drug abuse, with only limited success in attaining periods of abstinence. They may also have interpersonal difficulties. In the UK, many of these patients are on long-term (usually for a year) treatment contracts and receive maintenance prescriptions for opiates. However, membership of a group and attendance are voluntary, and should not be made a condition of any treatment contract, and it is customary that the group therapist does not prescribe for the patients. Lack of motivation to achieve abstinence should not be a bar from the group.

Family therapy

The use of family therapy in the treatment of drug abuse is particularly appropriate because, as has long been recognized, the family as a whole may profoundly influence the behaviour of its individual members, including their use, or non-use, of drugs. It is beyond the scope of this chapter to describe and discuss the underlying philosophy and nature of family therapy, but it is important to understand that the family is a relatively stable system that tends to resist change, and that drug abuse may have powerful adaptive consequences that help to maintain that stability. For example, parents on the brink of divorce may remain united to cope with the recurrent crises of a drug-abusing child, and parents who cannot cope with the departure of their adolescent child from the family home may overtly or covertly encourage the drug abuse that keeps the child dependent on them.

Whatever the individual family scenario, the reaction of family members to the drug abuse of one of them often seems to be to maintain the drug-taking behaviour, whether or not they played a predisposing causal role in its initiation. Members of the family, albeit unconsciously, may actually encourage or reinforce drug taking, and may seriously undermine any treatment programme, especially at the stage when the patient is showing progress and drug abuse is declining. Thus, in family therapy terms, the drug abuse of the patient is really that of the family as a whole, and it is logical to include the whole family in the treatment approach. Even when the drug abuser is a young adult who has left home, and even when that adult is married (with or without children), it is often the family of origin that continues to have a powerful influence on drug taking and is the focus for family intervention.

The first problem is to persuade the families of drug abusers to participate in treatment. They may feel, for example, that being invited for family therapy implies that they are in some way to blame for the patient's drug problem. It is therefore essential to stress their potential helpfulness in the treatment process and it may be useful if they know in advance the period of treatment to which they are committing themselves. They may, after all, have had several previous experiences of 'failed' treatments and be unwilling to engage themselves in what seems like another gimmick.

In some types of family therapy the therapist will try to help the family to solve its problems and the individual family members to relate to each other in more positive and constructive ways. To do so, the therapist must 'join' the family group, initially by supporting the family and behaving according to its rules – adopting its style and affect. A new family system is thus formed, consisting of the old family plus the therapist who must establish a positive relationship with each member and establish a leadership within the family group. By joining the group in this way, the therapist can experience at first hand, and participate in, the behavioural interactions that have become the family's response to a particular problem. Often these habitual responses are maladaptive and a series of interventions may then be planned, using the therapist's skills to restructure the family's patterns of interactions, in order to implement change. Tasks may be assigned to individual family members to perform at home before the next session. This provides more 'practice' at better interpersonal relationships and increases the influence of the therapist, whose presence is felt in the family home even during everyday activities.

Of course, a typical and understandable expectation on the part of the family is that it is the identified patient who should change or be changed by treatment. However, the drug-abusing individual does not live and behave in isolation, but interacts with the family group; his/her drug abuse is maintained because the family participates in maladaptive responses and interactions, and treatment is therefore targeted at the whole family. Nevertheless, it should be remembered that the goal of therapy is not the exploration of past events, but the alteration of the present situation. The symptoms of the identified patient should never be lost sight of, and the primary aim of treatment is to influence the rest of the family to help the patient with this problem.

A variation on family therapy is multiple-family therapy in which a number of drug addicts' families are treated conjointly. It is found that the families are able to support each other because of their shared experiences and that they learn to recognize and understand what is happening in their own family by observing similar phenomena in other families. The support offered by the group is particularly helpful at the very difficult time when parents begin to detach themselves from the problems of their drug-abusing child.

Drug counselling

Drug counselling at its simplest level is an advisory service. This deals with the realities of the patient's present situation, but the advice that is given is backed up by the practical help of a professional counsellor. Sessions occur regularly, by appointment, rather than on a casual, drop-in basis, and their frequency varies according to the particular needs of different patients. Counselling entails assessing the specific needs of individual patients and then providing or directing the patient towards the services that meet these needs.

The first step is to 'engage' the patient, and this is often best done using non-directive 'Rogerian' counselling. The key principles of this include taking a non-judgemental approach, with the counsellor having an 'unconditional, positive regard' for the client; the essential skill is 'active listening', which will include summarizing and reflecting back to the client what he/she is saying. Once the counsellor has gained the trust and confidence of the client, and the client has been able to articulate his/her problems and concerns, then the counsellor will help the client to establish realistic goals, which may encompass not just drug taking but also school, work, leisure-time activities, and relationships with family and friends. The available options are presented to the patient, who is helped to decide the best course of action – and then helped to follow the chosen course.

It is important throughout that the patient perceives him/herself as having choices and is in the 'driving seat', accepting that any improvements or slips are due to his/her own efforts. The patient is essentially treating him/herself with the help of a counsellor, rather than being the passive recipient of treatment. Progress in achieving the stated goals is monitored by seeing the patient regularly, and problems can be appropriately dealt with as they arise by a counsellor who becomes well known to the patient and trusted.

Many kinds of problems are dealt with in counselling sessions. When appropriate, specific treatment options can be discussed, such as specific psychological techniques, in-patient, out-patient or community de-toxification, maintenance treatment, drug-free therapeutic communities, etc., and the necessary arrangements for their implementation can be initiated. However, many areas of daily living may also be susceptible to advice and counselling. In particular, ways of avoiding encounters with other drug abusers and drugs should be explored so that essential changes in lifestyle are made. If, for example, drug use always occurs in a particular situation with a particular group of friends, that environment should be avoided at all costs; involvement in a different activity with non-drug users may be a sensible way of avoiding this problematical situation, but simple advice is unlikely to be effective. There must, in addition, be practical help aimed at engaging the drug abuser in new ways of passing leisure time. Similarly, it may be essential for some drug abusers to move house, away from their drug-taking environment, but again they may need positive help before this can be achieved. Thus, drug counsellors often liaise with other agencies on the drug user's behalf and the value of this active, practical support should not be underestimated.

Counselling, insofar as it offers the drug abuser a supportive relationship with a trained counsellor, can of course be considered psychotherapeutic in its own right. Usually, however, no attempt is made to mediate intrapsychic processes or to engage in specific psychotherapeutic techniques.

Motivational interviewing

A variation on counselling using Rogerian reflective listening is 'motivational interviewing', when the therapist does not just reflect back the patient's words, but selects certain comments and feeds them back in a subtly altered form with the purpose of increasing dissonance. The patient is subtly encouraged to persuade the therapist that there is a drug problem and that change is necessary. This permits the introduction of various treatment options for discussion, with the therapist offering various strategies for change and helping the client to identify appropriate goals and ways of achieving them. In other words, the therapist is clandestinely directing the course of treatment, while at the same time letting the client believe that all the decisions have emerged naturally and are his/hers alone.

Behavioural techniques

A completely different approach to the management of drug abuse and dependence is the systematic application of behavioural intervention techniques. This approach focuses on drug abuse as a disorder of behaviour, which it aims to modify. There is no attempt to identify its causes, which might or might not be amenable to treatment, nor to trace the history of the condition. Instead, current behaviour, emotions and beliefs, as they exist when the patient presents, are recognized as the pressing problem to be treated.

Drug abusers, however, often have other problems too, such as poverty, unemployment and homelessness, and it can be argued that it is pointless to try to deal with the drug abuse without first, or simultaneously, dealing with the associated problems – an approach that implies that these problems are the cause of the drug abuse. On the other hand, it can be argued that it is the drug abuse which has led to the other difficulties. If a behavioural approach is adopted there is no reason to be concerned about cause and effect. The principle is to find out which behaviour should and can be changed, to decide what change is wanted and to devise a way of effecting this behavioural change. In more technical terms, before behavioural therapy can be initiated, a behavioural analysis must be carried out so that current behaviours are understood, goals are identified and the ways of achieving these goals are defined. According to the individual behavioural analysis, the resultant programme may be narrow, focussing only on the problem of drug abuse, or broad, encompassing a range of related problems and dealing with various aspects of the individual's behavioural repertoire.

The term 'behavioural intervention' includes many different techniques, some of which are as old as the hills. Rewarding good behaviour, punishing bad and making bitter medicine taste sweeter are all ploys that are used routinely, often automatically, in many therapeutic situations. Their conscious and systematic application to all aspects of treatment, so that every therapeutic situation becomes a positive learning experience, is the basis of behavioural intervention.

Cognitive behavioural psychotherapy

This is an 'active, directive, time-limited treatment' that focuses on identifying a person's thoughts, beliefs, attitudes and assumptions that may be impeding positive behavioural change. Beliefs and assumptions that the person holds may be distorted (during childhood and learning experiences as an adult) and, as a result, the person may have negative interpretations of themself, their future or the world around them which predispose, for example, towards low self-esteem, depression or anxiety, or the continued use of substances. Patients can learn, with the help of a therapist, to correct negatively biased attitudes and beliefs based on faulty assumptions and, as a result, learn to cope without drugs.

Contingency management

This is a procedure based on the principles of behaviour modification, or 'operant conditioning' as it is sometimes called. The starting point is the principle that the consequences of a behaviour will affect the frequency and strength of that behaviour. If the consequence is positive, then the behaviour will increase in frequency and/or strength if the consequence is received, and decrease if it is not (positive and negative reinforcement respectively). If the consequence is negative, then the behaviour will decrease if the consequence is received, and increase if it is not (punishment and negative reinforcement respectively). There are numerous complications to these simple rules, such as the influence of the frequency of the consequence occurring. Thus, positive reinforcement which is received every time leads to rapid conditioning which is then quickly 'unlearned' once the reward stops; paradoxically, positive reinforcement which is received intermittently leads to behaviours which take longer to get rid of. Other complications include the effects of the delay between the behaviour and the consequence, and the association of other stimuli or 'cues' with the behaviour. Complex 'stimulus-response' chains are present in all but the simplest of behaviours, and with the majority of human behaviours any one response is likely to be under the control of many interacting stimuli and reinforcers.

Translated into helping a drug user, it is possible to have specified rewards and privileges which are made contingent upon continuation or initiation of agreed behaviour. This can be thought of as the modern application of the well-known 'carrot and stick' approach, but with several important differences, the main one being that the desired (target) behaviour is defined and explained first, together with the contingent reward, before the procedure is initiated, rather than the individual learning by trial and error what is expected and what the price of failure/success is going to be. Another difference is that the procedures are based on scientific theory which allows for clear predictions to be made, again as opposed to trial and error.

In practice, contingency management utilizes positive reinforcers which are both ethically acceptable and under the control of the therapist. Punishment and negative reinforcement are never used as part of a therapeutic programme, nor is it ethical to use positive reinforcers to which the patient has a right of access. In consequence, the therapist is restricted but, nevertheless, may have a variety of reinforcers that can be utilized for contingency management. For example, with an opiate-dependent individual who is attending a clinic regularly and frequently for a prescription for methadone (or heroin), reinforcers might include methadone take-home privileges (rather than having to take the methadone under supervision at the clinic), frequency of clinic attendance, time of appointment, access to counselling and other 'helping' services, and advantageous holiday arrangements, all of which can be made contingent upon certain behaviours. In practice, similar systems may already exist but in an informal and unrecognized way which makes consistency of approach unlikely. Thus, if patients ask for special arrangements to be made for opiate prescription while they are on holiday, their request is more likely to be granted if they have been 'doing well', i.e., attending regularly with no evidence of illicit drug abuse, etc. Planned contingency management, however, means that drug abusers learn much more directly and therefore more easily and more quickly, exactly what is expected of them.

One way of introducing contingency management into the treatment of drug dependence is to utilize a written contract between the medical staff and the patient. This defines the drugs (if any) to be prescribed, the dose reduction schedule, the duration of prescribing, the frequency of attendance at the clinic, other treatment approaches in which the patient will participate, the consequences of non-attendance and, in particular, the consequences of abusing illicit drugs, etc. Usually, if patients fail to keep their side of the contract and particularly if they continue to abuse illicit drugs, the prescribed dose of drug is quickly reduced.

Although contingency management is theoretically simple, there are certain practical problems peculiar to its application to the treatment of drug abuse. For example, it is often quite difficult to find out quickly whether patients have been abusing illicit drugs, because the results of urine tests may not be available for several days, or even a week or more. The inevitable delay before contingent measures can be implemented unfortunately impairs their efficacy.

However, the use of positive reinforcement, as well as having a therapeutic effect on individual patients, may also have a wider effect on the social and therapeutic atmosphere of the whole clinic by reducing confrontation between staff and patients. Relationships between staff and patients at such clinics are often difficult – patients are often manipulative and threatening in their attempts to obtain their drug of abuse or larger quantities of it, and the staff, frustrated and disheartened by recidivism, develop coercive attitudes towards patients. It is all too easy for the clinic appointment, far from being a therapeutic occasion, to become little more than a time for bargaining about a prescription.

The deliberate adoption of contingency-management procedures helps patients to achieve defined and realistic goals for which they can be rewarded, rather than being punished all the time for failure to make progress towards undefined targets. Equally, positive and non-punitive attitudes on the part of the staff are more likely to attract patients to treatment and to retain them in it. Many clinics already have rules which effectively act as contingencies to control behaviour, although if they are not applied systematically, maximum benefit is not achieved.

It should be apparent that where drug abusers are resident, either in hospital or in a therapeutic community, many potential reinforcers can be controlled and made contingent upon desired behaviour. For example, access to additional recreational facilities, better food, extra visitors, etc. can all be made contingent on a target behaviour identified both by the patient and the therapy staff. A further refinement is to develop this into a points economy system, whereby points are given to patients contingent on desired behaviour, and taken away contingent on maladaptive behaviour. These points can then be exchanged on the ward for a variety of goods and services. All of the transaction 'rates' are clearly defined at the start and are recorded in personal booklets. An advantage of this system is that while some components are applicable to all residents, others can be personalized for the specific treatment needs of individual patients. It is important to understand, however, that among the most potent reinforcers available to staff are staff attention and time, which tend to be contingent on problematic or undesirable behaviour and thus may, unwittingly, increase these behaviours. An awareness of this and their use in a structured behavioural programme has obvious benefits for overcoming these problems.

It has been suggested that contingency-management procedures are little more than 'training' and that their efficacy lapses when contingent rewards and punishments are discontinued. This can be avoided firstly by manipulating the schedule of reinforcement (gradually reducing the frequency of reinforcement), and secondly by replacing the 'artificial' reinforcers of the ward with the 'natural' reinforcers which maintain behaviour in the outside world. However, although it is true that undesirable patterns of behaviour, including drug abuse, may recur when treatment stops, this should be seen as yet another instance of relapse due to the severity of drug dependence and not necessarily as a failure of treatment. Undoubtedly, contingency management, carried out in a structured, systematic and comprehensive way, provides a firm and consistent structure for the drug abuser's life, and it may be the first time, or the first time for a long while, that he or she has experienced this. It provides the patient with an opportunity to learn the boundaries of acceptable behaviour, and even if relapse occurs the learning experience will not have been wasted. One way to improve the long-term efficacy of contingency management is to involve the family, because it may have in its control many social and material reinforcers which can be made contingent on desired behaviour long after the patient has stopped attending hospitals and clinics.

Other behavioural approaches

Contingency management is a very direct approach to the treatment of drug abuse. Other types of behavioural intervention may be appropriate in certain cases. Many individuals resort to self-medication with psychoactive drugs when they feel tense and anxious, and the relief that they experience reinforces this behaviour and may contribute to relapse. Teaching patients to be aware of the situations that induce these feelings and to recognize their own emotional reactions is the first stage of teaching them how to respond in a healthier way. Training in techniques of relaxation may be of long-term value to these patients, reducing nervous tension, providing a natural way of dealing with stress, insomnia and life's challenges and inducing a feeling of general well-being. Some individuals with specific fears or phobias may be helped by desensitization, and others may benefit from training in problem solving, in assertiveness or in social skills. The need for these very specific kinds of behavioural intervention becomes apparent in the course of the assessment procedure, which should establish if there are underlying or associated psychological problems that are amenable to intervention and treatment.

Cue exposure

It has long been recognized that, in addition to the primary reinforcing and dependence-producing properties of many drugs, environmental stimuli associated with drug taking may contribute to the continuation of drug-taking behaviour. Exposure to these stimuli – or cues – which cannot always be avoided in everyday life, may lead to a variety of physiological (increased heart rate, decreased skin temperature, other signs of autonomic activation) and subjective responses long after a drug user has become abstinent and usually cause craving for the drugs. However, carefully planned and executed programmes of exposure to these cues, either in reality or via video- or audiotapes, under conditions of close supervision or in a protected environment with no access to drugs, diminish both the physiological and subjective responses to them (classical or Pavlovian extinction). In theory, therefore, a drug abuser who experiences severe craving at the sight of drug-taking paraphernalia such as syringes and needles can be helped to overcome this by being shown them in situations where he/she cannot then take drugs. Although extinction of conditioned responses has been demonstrated in opiate addicts, it is not yet clear whether this approach has a long-term clinical effect and actually helps to prevent relapse.

Relapse prevention

During the last decade there has been a growing interest in techniques developed specifically to prevent relapse. Typically, these methods involve the identification of high-risk situations, when there is an increased likelihood of drug-taking behaviour. These may be caused by negative emotional states, interpersonal conflicts or direct/indirect social pressures, and the patient is encouraged to record their use of drugs, identifying the factors that may have triggered relapse. With the help of the therapist they can then analyse these situations and develop ways of dealing with them ('coping strategies') in future – perhaps by purposefully avoiding or preventing high-risk situations, or by using structured problem-solving techniques together with role playing. Some approaches advocate graded exposure to environmental cues; others utilize rapid exposure (flooding), with or without the use of beta-blockers to alleviate the inevitable symptoms of anxiety that ensue. On those occasions when craving to take drugs develops, techniques such as 'urge-surfing' are advocated – allowing craving full rein, in the knowledge that it will, eventually, subside – or the

'Samurai' approach – in which the drug taker treats the urge to take drugs as an enemy that can be resisted by being prepared for the attack.

An important element of relapse prevention may be the distinction between lapse and relapse, so that if resolution fails and drugs are taken, the individual does not feel that all is lost, but is able to regain control before relapse into full-blown problem drug taking develops again.

Vocational rehabilitation

Vocational rehabilitation is a treatment modality aimed at helping patients to acquire job-related skills. These may be specific skills, related to specific jobs and/or the interpersonal skills needed to obtain and retain employment. It should be noted in passing that there is actually no firm evidence to relate vocational rehabilitation and its ultimate goal of employment with treatment outcome, although there is a widely and strongly held belief in the therapeutic efficacy of work. This can, of course, become a self-fulfilling argument if being employed becomes a measure of treatment outcome. On behavioural grounds it can be argued that because drug abuse is just one component of an individual's total behavioural repertoire, intervening to encourage and develop desirable behaviour (i.e., obtaining a job), may lead to reduction of the undesirable behaviour (i.e., drug abuse) by direct competition – a sort of 'Satan finds work for idle hands' theory.

Whatever the theory, it is undoubtedly true that unemployment rates may be very high among drug abusers and particularly among young drug abusers, and that they may be very receptive to help in this area of their lives. Delinquent adolescent behaviour and drug taking may have interfered with their basic education. They may have extremely limited vocational skills and may be saddled with poor employment records. At times of high unemployment, particularly, it may be impossible for them to get a job without specific intervention and help.

The first step is an assessment of the patient's motivation, expectations and goals and of his/her existing skills and qualifications. A vocational plan can then be drawn up, with short- and long-term goals including, as appropriate, remedial education and specific academic and vocational skills. Knowing how to complete application forms is also important and, in particular, how to handle sensitive information about drug taking and criminal history and how to emphasize positive aspects of previous employment. In addition, the acquisition of interview skills is vital; this may include learning relaxation techniques to reduce anxiety before the interview, good entrance and exit techniques, general behaviour during the interview with positive presentation of self, and how to cope with hostile interviewers. Role playing and the use of video cameras may be useful preparation for these occasions. In particular, the problem of whether or not to tell the truth about drug taking needs to be discussed. There is considerable prejudice against abusers and some employers may specifically try to find out about drug abuse through questioning and/or urine tests. Big companies with a high turnover of unskilled staff are most likely to be tolerant on this point.

The fear and anxiety of being rejected must also be dealt with, so that self-esteem, which may already be low, is not further impaired if the job application is unsuccessful. If successful however, the ability to retain the job becomes very important and may rest equally on the particular ability to do the job competently and the possession of the interpersonal skills necessary for the workplace.

Vocational rehabilitation therefore encompasses a whole range of skills which contribute to the individual's ability to go out and get a job and keep it. Many of the problems of drug abusers are no different to those of other long-term unemployed, and referral to professional agencies may be valuable. However, schemes for vocational rehabilitation can also be incorporated into residential programmes for drug abusers and can be located in out-patient clinics. Access to vocational counselling, which may be eagerly sought, can be made contingent on desirable behaviour, such as desisting from the abuse of illicit drugs, and vocational goals may be included in the treatment contract between staff and patient.

Therapeutic communities

It has long been recognized that detoxification does not solve drug dependence, that the severity of drug dependence often leads to relapse and that it takes time for drug abusers to learn to live without drugs. For many people, the necessary change in their lifestyle is difficult or impossible if they remain in an environment where drugs are easily available, where they are among old friends who continue to take drugs and where a moment's craving can be translated too easily into drug abuse and relapse.

Therapeutic communities developed as one response to this situation. There are different types of community with different underlying philosophies. All insist on their residents being drug free, although often for only a short period (24 hours), before admission and some provide medical supervision of detoxification. Some have a democratic structure, others are unstructured, offering accommodation and time for those who want to explore the options that are open to them. Programmes last for varying lengths of time (3–15 months); they may offer group or individual psychotherapy which may be compulsory. Some will accept residents who are on bail and conditions of bail; and some offer vocational training.

Christian-based communities emphasize the importance of divine intervention in bringing about change, and Christian worship and Bible study form an important part of their therapeutic programmes.

Community-based hostels integrate their residents into the local community from the start, teaching them to live in the 'outside' world without resorting to drugs.

Concept houses

Perhaps the best-known type of therapeutic community is the concept house. The first of these was Synanon which was established in California in 1959. Others followed (Phoenix House, Daytop Village, Odyssey House), differing in the details of their organization, the degree of professional involvement and the therapeutic techniques used, but with obvious similarities to each other.

All are drug-free communities and are residential, so that their inmates are within the therapeutic environment for 24 hours a every day. At first, residents are completely isolated from their former life and are not permitted to have visitors, letters or telephone calls. Daily life within the community is very structured, with residents spending most of their time in organized group activities and with little opportunity for doing anything alone. This forces interaction with other residents and permits constant scrutiny of their behaviour by their peers, and appropriate outspoken criticism.

Concept houses have a rigid social hierarchy with an autocratic leadership. Newcomers have very low status – they have few privileges and may be assigned menial household tasks. Those who remain abstinent, participate fully in community life and show personal growth in terms of honesty and self-awareness, move up the hierarchy, assuming greater responsibilities and enjoying increased privileges, so that senior residents become models for new residents. There is also a defined system of rewards and punishments, 'good' behaviour being rewarded with greater privileges, while breaking any of the community's rules is followed by punishments such as severe verbal reprimands, job demotion and loss of privileges.

A variety of group therapies may be employed, but the most important is encounter-group therapy. This involves a small group of community members meeting three times a week or more. The composition of the group changes from session to session so that there is no opportunity for tacit or deliberate collusion between any members, and to emphasize the need for all residents to communicate with all other members of the community and not just with the few in a static group. The group leader may be formally appointed, may emerge from the group or may be the most senior resident there. At an encounter group there are aggressive verbal attacks upon individuals to confront them with their observed behaviour and attitudes within the community, and sometimes complaints about an individual are submitted before the group meets. Total honesty is expected, both in the verbal attacks and the responses, and shouting and swearing, far from being discouraged, are seen as manifestations of basic and honest 'gut reactions' that cut through the usual more intellectual defences. Uninhibited responses such as these are only permitted within the encounter group meeting: at other times or places in the community such uncontrolled behaviour would be punished. An encounter-group meeting may last for several hours: its violent, emotional assault can be very exhausting and supportive measures are often necessary afterwards for those who have been the focus of confrontation.

Selection of patients suitable for a therapeutic community

Residence in a therapeutic community may be a useful option for chronic drug abusers whose previous attempts at abstinence have failed. It is suitable for young people in whom there is room and time for personality growth and development, and many therapeutic communities have an upper age limit of 35 years. Those who lack social skills, including those who have problems of socialization and problems of assertiveness, are particularly likely to benefit from community life. The rigid, structured system of the concept houses is often helpful for the development of impulse control in young, risk-taking addicts, but it is unwise to expose anyone with a history of psychosis to the intense emotional experience of the encounter group.

Evaluation of the effectiveness of therapeutic communities is notoriously difficult, but generally, those drug abusers who 'stay the course' and complete the programme subsequently do well. It is not surprising, however, that many who enter concept houses cannot endure the lifestyle and leave early: for this reason, some houses now have a more flexible induction programme to encourage more residents to stay longer. Some of those who 'graduate' successfully from therapeutic communities and remain drug abstinent subsequently find work in services for drug abusers if they still find it difficult to separate completely from the world of drugs and drug dependence. However, it should be remembered that residents of therapeutic communities usually have a long history of drug abuse and dependence and a correspondingly poor prognosis. The success rate of the therapeutic communities, however small, is therefore especially creditable and valuable.

Hostels

The risk of relapse is high if newly abstinent drug-dependent individuals return to their old haunts and lifestyles, and hostel accommodation provides the opportunity for them to consolidate the success of withdrawal. Many of the pressures of daily life are reduced by staying in a hostel, and help and counselling is readily available if problems arise. However, there is little direct supervision, so that the residents regain responsibility for conducting their own lives in preparation for living independently. Thus, hostels often act as a halfway house or stepping stone between more supportive, residential treatment and ordinary life in the outside world. It is essential that rules about not bringing drugs or alcohol into the hostel are strictly enforced, so that those who are still vulnerable to relapse into drug abuse and dependence are not exposed to increased risk prematurely.

A very different approach is adopted by the Roma Drug Project (Rehabilitation of Metropolitan Addicts) which caters specifically for drug users notified to the Home Office and receiving a regular prescription for opiates from a drug-treatment clinic or GP. It provides counselling, group therapy and outside activities, and a secure environment for those taking opiates on a long-term, maintenance basis, helping them to establish a settled lifestyle while still taking drugs.

Self-help groups

The concept of self help, in the sense of mutual help within a community, is a traditional and valued approach to many problems. With the changing structure of society, due to increased mobility and the loosening of family ties, this type of community support seems to occur less easily and more rarely, and more formal self-help groups (SHG) have emerged to fill the void.

Nowadays, an SHG is a group of individuals with similar problems who meet together voluntarily to help each other to help themselves. In the field of substance dependence, the best known SHG is Alcoholics Anonymous (AA), followed by Narcotics Anonymous (NA) (founded in 1953) (see p. 190). Since then, a host of other groups have been formed in response to a variety of drug problems, such as tranquillizer dependence, opiate dependence, solvent abuse and cigarette smoking. They aim to help the drug-dependent or drug-abusing individual become abstinent.

These groups often begin due to the energy and enthusiasm of one or two individuals in a particular locality, and sometimes because of the absence (whether real or perceived), inadequacy or irrelevance of professional services for the particular problem. There is often an underlying philosophy that it is impossible for the individual to overcome the drug problem alone, but that this can be achieved with the help of the group. The common theme of all SHGs is of mutual aid – of individuals helping each other by offering friendship and sharing common experiences. They provide group support, social acceptance and social identity for individuals who may have become very isolated because of their drug problem. Furthermore, an established group possesses a wealth of experience and develops skills and expertise that may be of genuine practical help to those trying to cope with a drug problem. Because those who have come off drugs usually continue to attend the group for a while, new members are able to meet and identify with abstinent individuals. This, in itself, may be a novel and very valuable experience for those who have been involved in a drug subculture for a long time and they may, for the first time, become aware that recovery is an attainable goal.

Because SHGs often develop where and because professional services fail to meet the needs of drug abusers, it is easy to understand why some have 'anti'-professional attitudes. Equally, some professional health-care workers feel very threatened by these groups, which sometimes attract a lot of attention from the media. However, there need not be and should not be any conflict between the two 'systems'. Professional health-care and SHGs should not compete but should complement each other, and professionals should recognize the value of SHGs in their area and reinforce their activities. They should encourage patients with drug-abuse problems to attend them and should not hesitate to refer patients to them. However, it is essential that professionals should not become directly involved in SHGs; if they do, the groups are no longer 'self help', but just another professionally organized service, with a consequent loss of their unique kind of support and help.

In addition to SHGs for drug abusers, there is a complementary range of SHGs for their parents and families. These meet a need which is largely ignored elsewhere, and help families to cope with the strains of living with a drug abuser. Particularly in the early stages of a drug-taking career, parents may want to keep the knowledge of the drug problem within the family, and therefore find it difficult to seek help. They may be frightened by unpredictable mental states and unpredictable, sometimes aggressive, behaviour. They may be anxious about their own legal status if drugs are being taken in their home. Living with a drug abuser can thus be a very stressful experience and the support of others in the same predicament is usually a great relief. As the strength of the family unit as a whole is a very positive asset for the drug-abusing individual, any support given to the family may beneficially affect the outcome of the underlying drug-abuse problem.

Narcotics Anonymous

Narcotics Anonymous (NA) is an international fellowship or society for recovering addicts who meet regularly to help each other to stay off drugs. It is open to anyone with any type of drug problem, and the only require-ment for membership is the desire to stop using drugs.

NA has a 'Twelve Step' programme for achieving abstinence. The 12 steps taken by every NA member include:

1   admitting that one is an addict and powerless over one's drug-taking;

2   acknowledging that only a power greater than oneself (God) can help, and turning one's life over to Him;

3   making a fearless moral inventory, recognizing defects of character and asking God to remove them;

4   admitting previously committed wrongs and trying to make amends for them;

5   carrying the spiritual message of NA to addicts and practising its princi-ples in all aspects of daily life.

In addition, the 'Twelve Traditions' of NA safeguard the freedom of the group by outlining the principles that guide its organization and adminis-tration: NA groups are autonomous and self-supporting and decline outside contributions; they are non-professional and do not become involved in any issue or enterprise that may divert them from their primary purpose. Above all, the rule of anonymity is considered para-mount because it ensures that principles remain more important than individual personalities.

Members of NA attend meetings regularly. There is often a discussion based on the Twelve Steps and great stress is placed on complete openness and honesty with other members of the group, the single, shared common problem creating strong bonds between individuals. The composition of the group changes, often from meeting to meeting, and the constant flow of new members is valuable because the necessary reiteration of the basic tenets of NA is reinforced for more long-standing members. New members are encouraged to look for a sponsor within the group, a particular person to turn to at times of great need, and the responsibility of being a sponsor can be rewarding and helpful for the person concerned.

An important component of the NA programme for staying off drugs is the adoption of limited objectives. It recognizes that it is difficult (and sometimes impossible) for a drug-dependent person to envisage the rest of life without drugs, and so the addict is advised to promise him/herself not to use drugs just for 1 day – something that many have done willingly or unwillingly in the past and is therefore known to be possible. Having abstained for 1 day, the addict renews this short achievable contract on a daily basis. If a day is too long, the promise of an even shorter time span without drugs (say 5–10 minutes at a time) can prevent the first resumption of drug use that signals relapse. This strategy focuses the addict's attention on the immediate problem of not taking drugs and undermines the practised excuses and rationalization for drug taking offered by experienced addicts. In addition, attainable and attained objectives are immediately rewarding and therefore reinforce the desired behaviour.

The strong spiritual component of NA may be off-putting to some potential members, but the assertion that divine help is always available is necessary to counterbalance the admission, in the first of the Twelve Steps, that one is powerless over one's addiction. Those who are willing to 'try' NA should be advised and encouraged to go to as many meetings as possible and even to attend the meetings of more than one group. Time spent at NA is time spent in a drug-free environment, away from all the secondary reinforcers of a drug-taking lifestyle, and is positively therapeutic in its own right.

Families Anonymous

Families Anonymous (FA) is an organization allied to NA and aims to help the relatives of drug-dependent individuals. FA meetings, like NA meetings, are based on openness and honesty and provide an opportunity for the families of drug abusers to meet others in the same situation as themselves and to share experiences which may never previously have been divulged. These meetings offer social acceptance and, for many families, a relief from social isolation, and the accumulated experience of the members means that they are able to offer constructive advice and help in dealing with particular situations and problems.

Attending FA meetings can help to heal the emotional damage inflicted on the families of drug-abusing individuals and in some relationships this may be crucial to the success of attempts at drug abstinence. For example, some family members may become accustomed to a particular role which they may be reluctant to relinquish when the drug taker becomes abstinent, and they may unconsciously sabotage any hope of recovery. FA helps its members to be aware of the changes that occur within the family and to understand their own responses and, in this way, may make a very positive contribution, albeit indirectly, to the recovery of the drug-dependent individual. Members of the family of drug addicts may attend FA meetings even if the drug abuser is not attending NA.

Supportive groups

In addition to SHGs and groups that are conducted according to group analytical principles, there are a number of other groups, primarily supportive in nature, for drug abusers with particular needs. They differ from SHGs in being organized and run by a 'professional', but otherwise offer a similar caring and non-critical environment. For example, there is an increasing number of drug-dependent individuals who are parents, and they and their children have special needs which can be catered for – to a certain extent – in an informal group setting. This facilitates mutual support between the members by providing them with a time and a place to meet. They can chat about general child-care matters and other topics, exchange and share baby clothes and equipment, and the children can play with toys provided for the occasion. Clearly this resembles the ordinary 'Parent and Toddler' playgroup meetings which are attended by many new parents and which provide them with much needed support. Drug-abusing parents need this support too and perhaps more than those who do not abuse drugs – but may be reluctant to attend an 'ordinary' playgroup because of anxiety about their drug problem. Thus a family group may fill a void in their lives and relieve their very serious problem of social isolation. This in turn may have a beneficial effect on other areas of their lives, including their drug taking.

A supportive group may also be helpful to those who have just come off drugs and who are still at risk of resuming drug use. Those who are near the end of a detoxification programme (e.g., taking less than 10–15 mg methadone daily) may also attend this group, and the example of those who have successfully become abstinent acts as an example and encouragement for members of the group.

Groups such as these are frequently organized as part of the total programme of services of a drug-dependence treatment clinic. In addition, they are often organized by voluntary agencies as one component of a community, 'street-level' response to a local drug-abuse problem.

Minnesota method

The term 'Minnesota method' is very misleading, implying as it does a distinct method or way of treating substance dependence that is different to other methods. In practice, the Minnesota method integrates many of the treatment approaches described in this chapter into a programme that is tailored according to individual needs. It involves a multidisciplinary team that includes doctors, nurses, social workers, counsellors, psychologists, etc. who can provide a wide range of professional services.

Treatment may be as an out-patient or as an in-patient and begins with a thorough assessment, and detoxification if necessary. An individual treatment plan is then developed. In-patient treatment, when deemed appropriate, lasts for 4–6 weeks. There are regular individual counselling sessions and group therapy twice daily. There is an education programme for patients, with lectures, giving advice about ways of achieving recovery, and organized exercise and relaxation sessions which improve general mental and physical health, as well as providing opportunities for social interaction. Families are also involved in the treatment process by family therapy or family counselling.

Perhaps the unique feature of the Minnesota method, if there is one, is the integration into the individual treatment programme of the NA philosophy. Patients participate in NA self-help groups while in the primary stage of treatment, and continue to do so when discharged to after-care. Because many patients find the idea of God and divine intervention in their recovery off-putting, the spiritual component of the philosophy is stressed rather than the religious component. The 'higher power' can be interpreted as the collective power of the whole group, so that it is to the care of the group, rather than to God, that the patient surrenders his/her will and life.

After a period of in-patient treatment, some patients may be discharged home, but continue to attend NA meetings. Others may require several months in a more structured environment, such as a hostel, where counselling and group therapy can continue, and where integration into the wider community can be achieved gradually, while involvement with the local NA group is developing.

Making attendance at NA a regular component of the treatment programme right from the beginning perhaps increases the likelihood of long-term involvement, which in turn may be a significant factor in the reported success of the Minnesota method.

Crisis intervention

Crisis-intervention centres are usually staffed by nurses and social workers with a doctor on call for medical emergencies. They offer temporary shelter and social support to drug abusers at times of crisis, when they may be more receptive to help and more motivated to tackle their drug problem.

A crisis-intervention centre is a particularly useful facility for those who abuse barbiturates and other sedative hypnotics and who arrive at hospital accident & emergency departments (A & E) in a state of chronic intoxication. They cannot be discharged in this condition, but they are unwelcome patients on any conventional medical ward because their behaviour is often very disruptive. If they are referred and taken to a crisis-intervention centre, their detoxification can be supervised by trained personnel, and when they are sufficiently recovered, the process of counselling can begin. Primary health-care can also be offered to drug abusers who are unable to obtain it (or unwilling to seek it) elsewhere.

Crisis intervention provides a humane response at a time of great need. It is unlikely to have much rehabilitative value unless the staff succeed in referring the drug abuser onwards to a longer-term programme. In so doing, crisis intervention proves its value as an acceptable entry point into treatment for many people who would otherwise not be helped.

In-patient care

A patient may be admitted for in-patient care for a variety of reasons:
1   for assessment of the state of dependence;
2   for stabilization on opiates;
3   for stabilization and subsequent detoxification of opiates, barbiturates, benzodiazepines or other sedative hypnotics;
4   for detoxification of alcohol-complicating drug dependency;
5   for treatment of the secondary complications of drug abuse, for example, abscesses, hepatitis, septicaemia, HIV infection, AIDS, etc.;
6   for the general sorting out of the chaos that severe dependence on drugs can cause;
7   assessment of mental state.

A multipurpose drug-dependence in-patient unit is therefore likely to have, at any one time, patients with a wide range of problems and who present a number of different and often difficult problems of management. It is fair to say that this is not an 'easy' group of patients. Although they come into hospital voluntarily (drug abuse and drug dependence do not constitute grounds for compulsory admission), they do not always comply with the prescribed treatment regime and may often go to extraordinary lengths to obtain extra drugs. This apparently wilful behaviour should be recognized as a manifestation of the severity of their dependence and, indeed, as a group they are usually the most severely dependent, many with a past history of failed attempts at detoxification. Some patients have another condition that makes their drug dependence more difficult to manage (e.g., pregnancy, psychosis, brain damage), and many have severe disorders of personality. However, the difficulties should not be exaggerated. Many patients are well-motivated, comply with the treatment regime and successfully complete the detoxification schedule for which they were admitted.

Ideally, the in-patient unit provides a structured and therapeutic environment in which specific and general treatment interventions can be implemented. A variety of activities should be organized on a regular basis to form a well balanced timetable of events in which the patients are expected to participate. These include various group sessions, some of which may be conducted on group analytical lines, or use motivational interviewing techniques or focus on relapse prevention, while others deal with the practical problems and difficulties associated with drug dependency. The latter are primarily supportive, rather like self-help groups, and may tackle issues such as the problems people have in relating to others, their attitudes, behaviour and responsibilities. Specialist speakers may be invited to talk about topics of special concern such as AIDS, rehabilitation units, etc. There may also be a range of activities aimed at improving the patient's general health with sessions or classes in physiotherapy, relaxation, yoga, keep fit, etc. Recreational activities may be organized including different sports, games and arts and crafts.

It is hoped that patients in hospital, in this therapeutic environment, will start to develop a way of life and a daily routine that is not centred on drugs and drug taking, and which they find more fulfilling. It would be naive, however, to pretend that it is easy to bring about these changes in lifestyle and underlying attitudes.

The first essential is, obviously, that the ward should be drug free – except for medically prescribed drugs. Although patients are admitted voluntarily, their motivation may fluctuate or they may be on the unit for reasons other than receiving treatment for their drug dependency. To ensure a drug-free environment, an in-patient unit for drug abusers is necessarily often a locked ward; patients are only allowed to leave if escorted, and visitors are restricted to a few named and trustworthy individuals for each patient. If drugs are still smuggled in, it may be necessary for all gifts to patients to be inspected by the nursing staff, and for gifts of food to be restricted to unopened cans and packets. These measures seem, and indeed are, draconian. They have to be enforced because if just one person succeeds in introducing illicit drugs to the unit, the temptation to share them may prove too great for other patients whose treatment regime is therefore sabotaged. Before admission, patients may be asked to sign a contract indicating that they understand the rules of the ward and agree to comply with them.

Failure to keep to the rules usually means that the patient will be discharged, but this apparently straightforward consequence may be difficult to implement in every case. Sometimes there is no definite evidence that illicit drugs have been consumed – merely a strong suspicion on the part of the nursing staff. Confirmation of drug taking by a positive urine test may take so long that the result is irrelevant and discharge merely punitive, if in the interim period the patient has not taken illicit drugs and has participated fully in the treatment programme. In addition, there may be overriding medical reasons for not immediately discharging an in-patient who has been abusing illicit drugs – if, for example, the patient is pregnant, or severely ill, or in the middle of a sedative detoxification regime.

Aggressive behaviour is another problem that requires careful and sensitive management. It is not, of course, confined to drug-dependence treatment units, but is perhaps more likely to occur there than on some other wards because of the high incidence of 'personality disorder' among drug-dependent in-patients, and sometimes because of intoxication with drugs. Undoubtedly, many patients find it difficult to tolerate the environment of a closed ward, particularly if they cannot resort to drug taking, as they would undoubtedly like to. They may express their frustration by verbal and/or physical aggression. It is to be hoped that the professional skills and expertise of the staff minimize the risk of this, but patients should understand, before they are admitted, that violent or aggressive behaviour will not be tolerated. If it arises, the patients concerned may incur loss of privileges and visiting rights, or may be discharged immediately. On some occasions, however, even if there are good reasons to discharge a violent patient, there may be overwhelming medical reasons for not doing so.

The difficulties faced in the management of illicit drug taking and of violent behaviour highlight the problems of caring for drug-dependent patients. They undoubtedly require firm and consistent handling, and this is essential if they are to learn that manipulative behaviour is not useful. At the same time, the desire on the part of professionals to be firm and consistent should not lead to a stereotyped response for every deviation, or a punitive attitude towards the very behaviour for which the patient is seeking help.

References and further reading

Advisory Council on the Misuse of Drugs (1988). *AIDS and drug misuse: Part 1*. HMSO, London.
Advisory Council on the Misuse of Drugs (1989). *AIDS and drug misuse: Part 2*. HMSO, London.
Beck AT (1976). *Cognitive Therapy and the Emotional Disorders*. International Universities Press, New York.

Boudin HM, Valentine VE, Ruiz MR & Regan EJ (1980). *Contingency contracting for drug addiction: an outcome evaluation.* In: Sobell L, Sobell MC & Ward E (eds). *Evaluating Alcohol and Drug Abuse Treatment Effectiveness.* Pergamon Press, New York.

Callahan EJ, Price KA & Dahlkoetter J (1980). Behavioural treatment of drug abuse. In: Daitzman R (ed.) *Clinical Behaviour Therapy and Behaviour Modification.* Garland Press, New York.

Cook CH (1988). The Minnesota model in the management of drug and alcohol dependency: miracle, method or myth? *British Journal of Addiction,* **83**, 625–634.

Department of Health, Welsh Office & Scottish Home and Health Department (1991). *Drug Misuse and Dependence: Guidelines on Clinical Management.* HMSO, London.

De Leon G & Rosenthal MS (1979). Therapeutic communities. In: Dupont RL, Goldstein A & O'Donnell J (eds). *Handbook on Drug Abuse.* National Institute of Drug Abuse, Washington DC.

Emrick CD, Lassen CL & Edwards MT (1977). Non-professional peers as therapeutic agents. In: Gurman AS & Razin AM (eds). *Effective Psychotherapy: A Handbook of Research.* Pergamon Press, Oxford.

Farmer R & Ghodse AH (1993). Therapies for substance misuse. In: Granvill-Grossman K (ed.) *Recent advances in clinical psychiatry.* Churchill Livingstone, Edinburgh.

Gossop M, Johns A & Green L (1986). Opiate withdrawal: inpatient versus outpatient programmes and preferred versus random assignment to treatment. *British Medical Journal,* **293**, 103–104.

Gossop M & Strang J (1990). Treatment and Management. In: Ghodse AH & Maxwell D (eds). *Substance Abuse and Dependence,* 131–148. Macmillan Press, London.

Hirsch R & Imhoff J (1975). A family therapy approach to the treatment of drug abuse and addiction. *Journal of Psychedelic Drugs,* **7**, 181.

Jameson A, Glanz A & Macgregor S (1984). *Dealing with Drug Misuse. Crisis Intervention in the City.* Tavistock, London.

Kaplan SR & Razin AM (1978). The psychological substrate of self-help groups. *Journal of Operational Psychiatry,* **9**, 57.

Kaufman E & Kaufman P (eds) (1979). *Family Therapy of Drug and Alcohol Abuse.* Gardner Press, New York.

Melamed BG & Siegell J (eds) (1980). *Behavioural Medicine: Practical Applications in Health Care.* Springer, New York.

Pinkerton SS, Hughes H & Wenrich WW (eds) (1982). *Behavioural Medicine: Clinical Applications.* Wiley, London.

Platt JJ & Metzer D (1985). The role of employment in the rehabilitation of heroin addicts. In: Ashery RS (ed.) *Progress in the Development of Cost-Effective Treatment of Drug Abusers,* 111–121. NIDA Research Monograph 58. Department of Health & Human Services, Rockville.

Stitzer ML, Bigelow GE & McCaul ME (1985). Behaviour therapy in drug abuse treatment: review and evaluation. In: Ashery RS (ed.) *Progress in the Development of Cost-Effective Treatment for Drug Abusers.* NIDA Research Monograph 58. Department of Health & Human Services, Rockville.

Wells B (1990). Treatment and management. In: Ghodse AH & Maxwell D (eds). *Substance Abuse and Dependence,* 149–175. Macmillan Press, London.

Woody GE, Luborsky L, McLellan AT *et al.* (1983). Psychotherapy for opiate addicts: does it help? *Archives of General Psychiatry,* **40**, 639–645.

6

Specific methods of treatment

Opiates

By the time that they seek help for their drug problem, most of those who abuse opiates have an established dependency and are seeking some sort of pharmacotherapy. They may want to come off drugs but fear the abstinence syndrome too much to attempt it alone, or they may be hoping for a long-term prescription for opiates because they are finding it increasingly difficult to maintain their drug habit from illicit sources.

Before any decision is made about detoxification using opiates or long-term maintenance treatment, it is essential to be sure that the patient is indeed genuinely physically dependent on opiates. This diagnosis is based on information acquired during the assessment period (Chapter 4); it relies on the history of drug taking, with attention being given to whether the financial means of the patient adequately account for the drug use claimed, and the patient's familiarity with the drug scene. A careful physical examination, looking particularly for signs of opiate withdrawal (Chapter 3) and of self-injection, and the results of several urine tests are also very important. If the out-patient assessment of physical dependence is equivocal, the patient should be admitted to hospital for more careful observation.

Detoxification – opiate withdrawal

Detoxification is the process of coming off drugs, of ridding the body of the drugs by withdrawing them, usually by giving gradually decreasing doses. The final goal is drug abstinence and there are many ways of achieving it. Detoxification can be carried out as an in-patient or as an out-patient; it can take days, weeks or months; it usually involves the prescription of opiate drugs – but this is not essential, and other drugs and other treatment modalities may be helpful too.

The choice of detoxification programme depends on what has been found during the assessment period: the severity of physical dependence, the nature of drug-related problems, and previous experience of detoxification are some of the factors to be taken into account. The aim is to match the patient to the most appropriate course of detoxification. For example, a long-standing addict may need a few months on a stable dose of methadone to permit a general sorting out of all drug-related problems before a very gradual reduction of dosage is made. At the opposite end of the spectrum, those with only minimal physical dependence may be able to tolerate detoxification without opiates, but using other drugs to alleviate the symptoms of withdrawal.

If a patient has been referred to a specialist treatment unit, the course of detoxification is decided after discussion by the multidisciplinary team. Whenever possible, they take into account and incorporate the patient's wishes and preferences for a particular way of coming off drugs, but because of the very nature of drug dependence, this is not always possible. It is because they are so severely dependent that for some patients the time may never be quite right to attempt detoxification; there seems always to be a reason (an excuse) for delay in starting to come off. In essence, they become trapped by denial and rationalization and, left to themselves, would continue to take opiates probably indefinitely, with a promise to initiate withdrawal always a few weeks away.

It requires patience and skill to cut through these defences, to bring the patient to an acceptance of the realities of the situation and to initiate detoxification. Anyone involved in the treatment of drug-dependent patients needs to be aware of these difficulties and must guard against being manipulated into providing indefinite opiate maintenance by default. Opiate maintenance may, on occasion, be necessary (p. 215), but it should result from a positive decision that is right for a particular patient; it should not be allowed to develop from a situation of ever-postponed detoxification.

This situation illustrates the difficulty of treating drug-dependent patients. Their stated reason for seeking help, that they want to come off drugs, may be at variance with their behaviour, which is drug seeking; they seek help voluntarily but then reject the advice they are given, so that arguing and bargaining about treatment, almost unheard of in other branches of medicine, occur frequently in the DDTUs (drug-dependence treatment units). Such behaviour should be interpreted as a manifestation of the severity of dependence and should be responded to appropriately.

Of course, the patient's treatment aims are not always at variance with those of professional advisers. Some are highly motivated to come off drugs, indeed some (although in practice a minority) may wish to do so far more rapidly than is considered wise or likely to be successful by the professionals. In this situation, where the patient actually wants less opiate than might be prescribed, the choice of detoxification can safely be left to the patient. Any attempt to come off drugs should be welcomed and encouraged, and the belief on the part of the patient that a particular treatment is right, may be crucial to motivation to succeed – if only to prove the professionals wrong. Even if the attempt fails, the patient can always try again and may then be more receptive to advice and counselling.

The opiate abstinence syndrome which develops if opiates are not prescribed during detoxification varies in severity according to which opiate has been taken, for how long and in what dose. It may vary from a mild, 'flu-like illness to a condition in which the patient is very distressed and feels truly wretched (p. 74). Undoubtedly, fear of the abstinence syndrome and consequent anxiety about it can make all the symptoms far worse. In addition, just as different people have different pain thresholds and experience pain differently, so opiate-dependent individuals vary in the way that they experience the abstinence syndrome, even with similar levels of physical dependence. Whatever the differences, fear of abstinence syndrome may be worse than the condition itself and may be a barrier preventing patients from attempting detoxification. All patients should be reassured that their drug withdrawal will be correctly managed to prevent or minimize the symptoms and discomfort of the abstinence syndrome. A confident approach on the part of all involved professionals is essential to allay anxiety and to reassure those who may have heard lurid tales of 'cold turkey'.

Because the symptoms of opiate withdrawal can be (and usually are) prevented by a schedule of gradual dose reduction, there is a tendency for health-care professionals to be dismissive about detoxification: 'Coming off is easy; staying off is the problem' is bandied about. It is true that opiate withdrawal is a straightforward medical procedure and causes no life-threatening medical emergency, but for the person involved it is a difficult step to take and one which requires courage. This should be recognized and respected.

It should also be appreciated that detoxification may need to be repeated: some patients resume illicit opiate abuse while undergoing detoxification and others do so later. Such relapses are not inevitable, and should not be anticipated by a negative approach; nevertheless they do occur and repeated attempts at detoxification are often necessary. Rather than treating relapse as a failure, any worthwhile period of abstinence should be welcomed as a success and the patient's achievement recognized. A positive approach encourages cooperative rather than confrontational attitudes between patients and staff, and in this atmosphere more patients will be prepared to try again.

Finally, it is worth emphasizing that opiate detoxification does not necessarily require referral to a specialist unit and indeed may be managed with no medical supervision at all. The opiate-dependent individual may choose to reduce his/her daily dose gradually, on his/her own. The patient may even choose to stop taking opiates abruptly, thereby causing the dreaded 'cold turkey'. There is no doubt that many addicts do come off drugs on their own and that many may do so repeatedly, sometimes when forcibly detained by concerned parents. On humane grounds, no one would recommend this course of action, but there is no medical contraindication if the individual concerned is otherwise well. Certainly, this approach is reasonable for young users with a fairly short (6 months to 1 year) history of daily use, who take only small amounts of heroin (25 mg per day). They can be cared for at home during the withdrawal period, as if they are suffering from 'flu', with simple analgesics such as paracetamol being given to relieve muscular aches and pains. The major drawback of 'going it alone' is the consequent lack of professional help, guidance and counselling and of the specialized treatments than can help to reduce the risk of relapse.

If general practitioners are asked to help in such cases, they may prescribe antispasmodics (dicyclomine hydrochloride, hyoscine) to relieve colicky abdominal pains, diphenoxylate or loperamide for diarrhoea, or neuroleptic drugs such as phenothiazines. If they find that they have insufficient time available to offer an appropriate level of counselling, a collaborative approach with a local drug advisory service or community drugs team may prove helpful. The type of case that may be managed in a primary care setting, without referral to a specialist agency, includes young drug-dependent individuals, particularly those with only a short history of dependence, and who will have good support from non-using family and friends during the difficult early days of withdrawal. For these patients there are substantial advantages to being managed in the community, with fewer opportunities for becoming enmeshed in the sub-culture of established users who attend the specialist agencies. (Conversely, some patients are not suitable for detoxification in a primary care/ community care setting. These include older users with a long history of substance misuse, who often obtain their drugs from multiple illicit sources and who have unsettled or even chaotic lifestyles.)

Detoxification using non-opiate drugs

Detoxification using non-opiate drugs can be started before full assessment of all the patient's problems has been completed and without the need to establish a firm diagnosis of physical dependence. Assessment of related problems can then continue during the detoxification procedure. Being able to start treatment quickly may be very helpful in engaging the patient in

treatment because many lose interest and motivation during a long period
of assessment.

Indications

1   Some patients may request assistance with opiate detoxification but do
not want to take opiate drugs any more.
2   These regimes may be useful if there is any lingering doubt about
whether the patient is really physically dependent on opiates or not. It must
be remembered that taking opiates regularly during stabilization and in
detoxification may be sufficient to cause dependence in a casual, previously
non-dependent opiate abuser, and that non-opiate 'detoxification' is a safer
alternative for these patients.
3   In many countries, doctors are not permitted to prescribe opiates in the
treatment of drug dependence, not even temporarily for the purpose of
detoxification. In this situation, non-opiate drugs are the only way to provide
some symptomatic relief during opiate abstinence, although they rarely, if
ever, successfully relieve the subjective distress of withdrawal or craving.

Choice of non-opiate treatment programme – general principles of management

There are a variety of treatment approaches, none of which is noticeably
better than any other. Opiate abstinence is not a life-threatening condition
and the choice of treatment can be made according to what 'suits' individual patients, their particular circumstances and symptomatology. As
detoxification often has to be repeated, some patients find that certain
symptoms are very distressing and that a particular treatment regime may
be helpful.

Whenever possible, the drugs chosen to alleviate the symptoms of opiate
withdrawal should have little or no dependence liability of their own. There
is no point in treating one kind of dependence by creating another and the
individuals concerned have a proven vulnerability to the dependence-
producing properties of psychoactive drugs.

Patients should be warned not to abuse any other drugs while undergoing detoxification because of the risk of drug interaction. They should be
told specifically not to increase the dose of the prescribed drug on their own
initiative. As a group who are very used to increasing the dose of drugs to
gain increased effect, they are likely to do so with the drugs prescribed for
detoxification if they seem to be controlling the symptoms of opiate withdrawal inadequately. Patients should be told that in this situation they
should return for further assessment and help.

Despite these warnings, patients may present in an intoxicated state during their detoxification programme. The response to this situation depends on the circumstances and, in particular, on why the patient resumed drug abuse. If drugs were taken because the symptoms of opiate withdrawal were intolerable, it may be appropriate to increase the dose of prescribed drugs, to prescribe an additional drug, or to introduce a different type of treatment. If this does not prevent further episodes of intoxication, or if drug abuse is occurring for other reasons, such as an inability to stay away from the black market, it may be wiser to taper off the dose of prescribed drugs more quickly than planned. This will reduce the risk of drug interaction and of further episodes of intoxication and may discourage the patient from abusing illicit drugs in future.

Non-opiate treatment regimes

Neuroleptic drugs

Neuroleptic drugs such as the phenothiazines are particularly suitable for the management of the opiate abstinence syndrome because they have anti-emetic, sedative and anticholinergic effects; the latter help to reduce abdominal cramps which may be a very distressing symptom of opiate withdrawal. Phenothiazines should be avoided if the patient has hepatitis and used cautiously if liver function tests are abnormal in any way.

Thioridazine (Melleril) is often chosen because it has a low incidence of extrapyramidal side-effects. A suitable dose regime would be thioridazine 25 mg twice daily, with 50–70 mg at night, for a period of 1–2 weeks; the dose should be tapered at the end of this time.

Diphenoxylate, loperamide

Diphenoxylate and loperamide are very mild opioid drugs with low dependence liability used for symptomatic relief during the opiate abstinence syndrome, and particularly if severe diarrhoea is a prominent symptom. Diphenoxylate is available in combination with atropine as co-phenotrope (diphenoxylate hydrochloride 2.5 mg; atropine sulphate 25 μg). Two tablets should be taken four times daily for 3–4 days, and then the dose should be gradually reduced. The dose of loperamide is 2 mg four times daily. Both of these drugs can be used if necessary as an adjunct to other non-opiate treatment regimes, such as thioridazine or clonidine.

Beta-adrenoreceptor blocking drugs

The use of beta-adrenoreceptor blocking drugs in the treatment of opiate withdrawal was originally based on an observation that propranolol abolished the euphoric effect of heroin in dependent individuals and that it reduced craving after heroin withdrawal. Propranolol may be helpful for patients with a high level of somatic anxiety, manifested by raised pulse rate, high blood pressure, etc. The effect of propranolol should be monitored and the dose adjusted according to the patient's response. A daily dose in the range of 80–160 mg, in divided doses, is usually effective and may be prescribed for a 2–3-week period. Oxprenolol may also be used. Beta-blockers should be avoided if the patient suffers from asthma.

Clonidine

Clonidine is an alpha-adrenergic agonist drug that acts on the locus coeruleus, suppressing the withdrawal overactivity of noradrenergic neurones and therefore reducing the release of noradrenaline. Thus it effectively suppresses some of the autonomic signs of opiate withdrawal, but is less effective at suppressing the subjective discomfort of withdrawal. Unfortunately, the partial symptomatic relief provided by clonidine carries undesirable side effects – sedation and hypotension, and detoxification using clonidine is best carried out in hospital where blood pressure (standing and lying) can be monitored regularly. Because of these side-effects, clonidine treatment is unsuitable for patients with cardiac or renal problems, who should not be exposed to the risk of hypotension; it should also not be used for pregnant women (see Chapter 8).

In hospital, treatment with clonidine should start with 200–400 μg daily, in divided doses, increasing gradually to a maximum of 1.2 mg daily, in divided doses (three times per day). Many patients cannot tolerate such a high dose because of postural hypotension, and if the blood pressure is less than 90/60, administration of clonidine should be postponed until the blood pressure has risen to this level. Treatment should continue for 5–6 days for heroin users and for 7–10 days for methadone users. Because of the theoretical risk of hypertension on sudden cessation of clonidine treatment, it should be withdrawn gradually.

Clonidine may be used on an out-patient basis, if arrangements are made to monitor blood pressure every day, for carefully selected patients who can be relied on to take the drug strictly in accordance with medical directions. In such cases, the maximum dose should not exceed 400 μg taken in divided doses (100 μg taken four times daily).

A new innovation is the introduction in the USA of clonidine patches, applied on a weekly basis and which permit transdermal absorption of the drug.

Lofexidine

A structural analogue of clonidine, lofexidine, can also be used for the alleviation of symptoms in patients undergoing opiate withdrawal. It appears to act centrally in the same way as clonidine, reducing sympathetic tone. Although it may be less sedating and less hypotensive than clonidine, it may also be less effective at suppressing the signs of withdrawal.

Treatment should be initiated with doses of $200\,\mu g$ twice daily, increasing as necessary (for symptom control) in steps of $200-400\,\mu g$ daily to a maximum of 2.4 mg daily. Treatment should continue for 7–10 days and then the dose should be gradually reduced over a period of 2–4 days.

Clonidine in conjunction with opiate antagonist drugs

Traditionally, the severity of the opiate abstinence syndrome has been minimized by withdrawing opiates gradually. A different approach is to attempt to compress the abstinence syndrome into as short a time as possible on the principle that a short period of very severe symptoms may be less distressing or easier to cope with than a more prolonged period of milder symptoms. One way of obtaining sudden intense withdrawal is to give an opiate antagonist drug, such as naloxone, which displaces opiates from the receptors by competitive antagonism. Intramuscular or intravenous naloxone is given repeatedly, at frequent intervals, for a few days, until further injections have no effect and the patient is then considered detoxified. The abstinence syndrome induced in this way can be treated with a variety of drugs including neuroleptics, propranolol and atropine.

More recently, treatment regimes have been developed using opiate antagonists and clonidine. An example of such a regime is:

day 1: clonidine $100\,\mu g$ three times a day;

day 2: clonidine $200-300\,\mu g$ three times a day (according to effect and blood pressure); naloxone 0.2 mg intramuscular, then 0.4 mg intramuscular 2 hourly for four doses;

day 3: clonidine – same dose as day 2; naloxone 0.8 mg intramuscular; five doses at 2 hourly intervals;

day 4: if necessary, the completeness of detoxification can be demonstrated by a naloxone challenge: naloxone 0.4 mg intramuscular should

produce no effect; naloxone 0.8 mg intramuscular 1 hour later should
not cause any withdrawal response either.

Alternatively, naltrexone, an opiate antagonist with a longer duration
of action than naloxone, can be used in conjunction with clonidine.
Following a naloxone challenge test (0.8 mg naloxone intramuscular),
clonidine 100–300 μg is administered orally to relieve withdrawal symptoms. Naltrexone 12.5 mg is given later on the first day, followed by 25 mg
on the second day, 50 mg on the third day and 100 mg on the fourth day.
Clonidine 100–300 μg is given three times a day for the first 2 days, with a
total dose of 300–900 μg per day which is reduced to 300–600 μg on day
3 and to 300 μg or less on day 4, all in divided doses. The dose of clonidine
should be adjusted according to the intensity of withdrawal symptoms and
any evidence of hypotension.

An advantage of this treatment regime is that because of the long duration of action of naltrexone, once-daily administration is sufficient, so that
out-patient treatment is facilitated. However, all patients should be carefully
monitored, especially at first, in case they develop hypotension.

Sedative drugs

If opiates cannot be prescribed for the purpose of detoxification, severe symptoms due to the opiate abstinence syndrome can be treated by the administration of a sedative drug (e.g., diazepam, chlormethiazole). It should be
appreciated that this course of action is not the treatment of choice: sedative
drugs do not relieve the distress of opiate withdrawal nor the craving for
opiates, although they do reduce associated anxiety. A further drawback to
their use is that they have a dependence-producing liability of their own
which makes them unsuitable for administration to individuals who are vulnerable to drug dependence. However, in some countries, doctors are not
permitted to prescribe opiates to dependent individuals, and in this situation
sedatives may be helpful for those with a moderate or severe degree of physical dependence on opiates. A short course is all that is required and suitable
dose schedules are shown in Tables 6.1 and 6.2.

Acupuncture

The use of acupuncture in the treatment of drug dependence is a comparatively recent innovation. It followed the incidental observation in 1973 by
doctors in Hong Kong (Wen and Cheung) that electro-acupuncture being
employed for analgesia satisfactorily relieved the symptoms of heroin withdrawal. At first the acupuncture needles were inserted in the ear, in two

Table 6.1 Use of diazepam in opiate detoxification

Day	Dose (mg) administered orally	Total
1–3	10, four times daily	40
4	10, three times daily	30
5	10, twice daily	20
6	5, twice daily	10
7	5, once daily	5
8	–	–

Table 6.2 Use of chlormethiazole in opiate detoxification

Day	Dose (capsules) administered orally	Total
1–3	2, four times daily	8
4	2, three times daily	6
5	2, twice daily	4
6	1, twice daily	2
7	1, daily	1
8	–	–

Note each capsule (192 mg chlormethiazole base) = 5 ml elixir (250 mg/5 ml chlormethiazole edisylate).

points near the wrist and in the hand, but the technique was modified, with no reduction in effectiveness, so that now only the 'lung' points of the ear are used. The needles are electrically stimulated for 40 minutes with a gradually increasing current (bipolar spike wave form; AC current; pulse width 0.6 ms; frequency up to 111 Hz or cycles per second). Comfortable detoxification can be achieved with acupuncture alone if treatment can be given more or less continuously for the first 3–4 days after drug withdrawal.

According to traditional theories, acupuncture helps the process of detoxification by releasing blockages of energy flow (chi) induced by the suppressive actions of opiates. The discovery of the endogenous opiate-transmitter system gave acupuncture some scientific respectability. For example, the reversal of acupuncture-induced analgesia by naloxone implies that endogenous opiates and opiate receptors are involved in acupuncture-induced analgesia. It was also found that a strain of mice, deficient in opiate receptors, had a poor analgesic response to acupuncture. In addition, heroin-dependent individuals treated with acupuncture were found to have raised concentrations of an endogenous opiate met-enkephalin in the cerebrospinal fluid.

Acupuncture appears to have no harmful effects and thus there is no reason to deny it to those patients who believe that it is the key to their successful detoxification. However, in the absence of carefully designed and controlled trials, the usefulness of acupuncture remains unproven, so that it is a treatment only for those who specifically request it and who have great faith in it.

Neuro-electric treatment (NET)

Experimentation with different methods of electroacupuncture revealed that the acupuncture needles were unnecessary and that electrical stimulation could be transmitted adequately transcutaneously using blunt electrodes. This eliminates any pain associated with skin puncture and the risk of infection by contaminated needles. In addition, because the treatment can be self-administered by the patient, it can be used much more frequently and even while the patient is asleep, so that withdrawal symptoms can be effectively prevented.

The electrodes are hoop-shaped and have a conducting area of diameter 2.5 mm. They are attached to a headset, worn either on top of the head or round the neck, and are held on to the concha of the ear by tension. Electrode jelly improves the skin contact. A neurostimulator has been developed which can deliver a variety of wave forms and parameters of current. Opiate-dependent individuals are said to respond best to square wave electrical stimulation with pulse width 0.25 ms and within the frequency range 75–300 Hz, but the choice of frequency depends on the drug of abuse: 2000 Hz is used for those dependent on cocaine and amphetamine, and 30–49 Hz for those dependent on sedative hypnotics. The current is gradually increased, usually by the patient, until it can be felt in the ears (approximately 1–2 mA). Side-effects (nausea, headache) are reported only rarely and can be reversed by reducing the current or by having more frequent short periods of treatment; polarity may also be important and the negative electrode should be attached to the left ear. The patient may be treated continuously for the first 3–5 days after drug withdrawal and then receives 2–5 hours treatment per day for the next 10–21 days.

Like acupuncture, the effectiveness of NET is unproven scientifically; nevertheless, it seems to help some patients when used in conjunction with other treatment methods, and it may obviate the need for additional psychoactive drugs.

Alternative medicine

In common with other chronic conditions for which there is no obvious and universally accepted 'cure', drug dependence has been (and still is) treated by a wide variety of methods, some of which seem bizarre to those trained in scientific medicine. These unconventional approaches, including herbalism, vitamin and mineral supplements, bathing, breathing and exercise, are usually harmless, although megadoses of vitamins are not. They often have a holistic emphasis on good health and a healthy lifestyle, both mental and physical, which can be very therapeutic. As these treatment methods are unproven, doctors can hardly recommend them to patients but, in the absence of a conventional 'cure' for drug dependence, the doctor need not attempt to dissuade a patient from pursuing an alternative approach. If a particular patient really wants to do this, the doctor should admit his/her own ignorance and advise the patient to consult a recognized practitioner in the chosen field. The patient's faith or belief in a particular approach may be just sufficient to spark and maintain the elusive quality of motivation, and achieving detoxification is more important than the route by which it is attained. Therefore, there should be no conflict or antagonism about the patient's choice of treatment, so that there is no barrier to the patient's returning to more conventional treatment if and when he/she wants and needs to.

Detoxification using opiates

If a diagnosis is made of physical dependence on opiates, and if the decision is taken to prescribe opiates, at least in the short term, in reducing dosage for detoxification, the first step is to stabilize the patient on a pharmaceutical preparation of an opiate.

Choice of opiate for stabilization and detoxification

On pharmacological grounds, the choice of opiate for stabilization and detoxification is theoretically unimportant. Because of cross-tolerance, any opiate will prevent or relieve the abstinence syndrome caused by the withdrawal of any other opiate. Whichever drug is chosen, the aim is to maintain the blood opiate level between the dependence level and the tolerance level (see Fig. 6.1). If the blood opiate level falls below the dependence level, the symptoms of the opiate abstinence syndrome develop. If the tolerance level is exceeded, the patient will experience euphoria. Between these two levels is a 'therapeutic' range for blood opiate level, in which the dependent individual feels well, appears normal and is generally considered 'straight'. The therapeutic range is not fixed, but varies according to the individual severity of dependence. It is different in different people and at different times in a drug-taking career, and this explains why the stabilization dose varies from patient to patient and must be assessed on an individual basis.

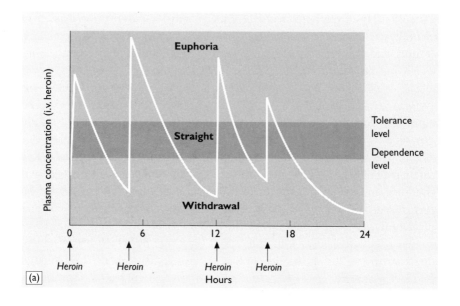

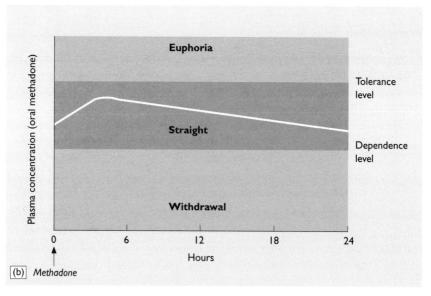

Fig. 6.1 Schematic diagram of (a) heroin and (b) methadone use.

Methadone is an ideal drug for opiate stabilization. It has a long duration of action (24–36 hours) so that a single daily dose maintains blood opiate levels within the desired range. The patient experiences neither euphoria nor the abstinence syndrome, but is maintained in a 'normal' physiological state.

It can be taken orally so that the complications of injection are avoided, and when dispensed for oral consumption it is in the form of a syrupy liquid which, even if diverted to the black market, is not suitable for injection.

These factors have led to its widespread acceptance as the drug of choice when opiates are to be prescribed to opiate-dependent individuals. Interestingly, when heroin syrup was compared with methadone syrup for stabilizing in-patient opiate addicts, the drugs were found to be equally effective on subjective and objective scores of withdrawal. Moreover, the addicts had no better than random chance of identifying which opiate they had been given. In the UK, methadone is prescribed as methadone mixture BNF (1 mg/ml).

Although much of the ensuing discussion focuses on the use of methadone for opiate detoxification and maintenance treatment, some doctors are unwilling to use it, often because of the strict legal requirements associated with its prescription (see p. 341). *Codeine* and *dihydrocodeine*, which are also opiates, offer an alternative that may be particularly suitable for the less severely dependent, with a fairly short history (less than 2 years) of daily use, but whose withdrawal symptoms are not adequately treated with non-opiates. It should be emphasized, however, that both of these drugs are widely abused and treatment regimens utilizing them should be managed just as carefully as those using methadone or heroin.

A total daily dose of 240–360 mg dihydrocodeine is adequate for most opiate-dependent individuals for whom this approach is suitable. This is eqiuvalent to 8–12 tablets (30 mg) of dihydrocodeine which should be taken in divided doses. Withdrawal is achieved by reducing the total dose by one tablet at agreed time intervals. Because codeine is available without prescription, some non-medical agencies have advised clients who do not wish to consult a doctor to achieve withdrawal using 'over the counter' codeine, and have helped them to draw up their own detoxification schedule. In such cases it is essential to ensure that these drugs do not become just another source of supply for a drug-dependent individual.

Dose of opiate for stabilization

The dose to be prescribed is that which will adequately suppress the manifestations (signs and symptoms) of opiate withdrawal over a 24-hour period, but which does not produce intoxication. As most patients abuse illicit heroin of uncertain purity it is not possible to establish the appropriate dose from the history alone. Even for patients who abuse pharmaceutical opiates, it is unwise to prescribe the equivalent dose of methadone suggested

by the history alone because of the uncertain reliability of this information. Thus, although 'conversion' tables exist, which give the methadone
'equivalent' of other opiates, it is much safer to establish the necessary
daily dose of methadone on an individual basis by a formal stabilization
procedure. Although the underlying principle is the same, the practical
details of stabilization vary according to whether it is carried out on an
out-patient, in-patient or day-patient basis.

Out-patient stabilization

Out-patient stabilization is effected by daily appointments, with an incre-
mentally increasing dose of opiate given under supervision and followed by
a period of observation to ensure that intoxication does not occur.

On the first day the patient is given 10–20 mg methadone, according to
clinical judgement of the severity of physical dependence. This dose must be
drunk in front of the doctor or nurse. It is very unwise to give more than
20 mg methadone as an initial dose, in case the patient has exaggerated the
severity of his/her dependence and cannot really tolerate a high dose. The
patient is then observed for 1 hour for any evidence of intoxication (especially drowsiness or pin-point pupils) but, if well, is permitted to leave.

When the patient returns, 24 hours later, he/she is assessed for any
evidence of physical withdrawal such as feeling unwell, insomnia or muscle
cramps, and objective signs such as pupil dilatation, yawning, sniffing, restlessness, gooseflesh, etc. If any of these symptoms or signs are present, even
if only mildly, the daily dose of methadone should be increased by 10 mg,
which is again consumed under supervision and the patient is observed for
the necessary 1 hour. This procedure is repeated daily until the patient no
longer exhibits any evidence of the opiate abstinence syndrome. The dose
prescribed on the previous day is then the baseline dosage which should be
repeated daily thereafter.

The prescribing doctor should appreciate that there is no need to be
excessively 'frugal' (or mean) about the dose of methadone. If the procedure described above is carried out, there is no risk that the patient will
become intoxicated and the precise dose on which the patient is finally
stabilized is unimportant as far as future management is concerned.
Indeed, if the dose of methadone is not increased, because symptoms are
felt to be 'too mild', it increases the likelihood of the patient seeking illicit
opiates, thereby sabotaging the stabilization process and increasing the
risk of intoxication.

The patient should be warned that the stabilization process will be
adversely affected if he/she abuses illicit opiates during this period and that

this leads to difficulty in assessing the correct dose. If opiates are taken illic-itly, the following procedure should be adopted.

1   If there is evidence of the opiate abstinence syndrome at the time of attendance, the usual increment of 10 mg methadone can be made.

2   If there is no evidence of the opiate abstinence syndrome, the previous day's dose should be repeated. The patient can be told that if this is insufficient, leading to the emergence of withdrawal symptoms, he/she should attend again (on the same day) to receive a 10 mg dose of methadone, rather than seeking relief from an illicit source.

Patients will therefore learn that the dose to be prescribed cannot be manipulated merely by their claiming that they had been forced to resort to illicit drugs. The daily dose of methadone will be increased only if there is clinical evidence at the time of attendance of the opiate abstinence syndrome.

In-patient stabilization

In-patient stabilization can be achieved more rapidly because the patient is under constant observation and supervision. After admission to hospital the patient is given no opiate until clinical observation reveals the symptoms and signs of the withdrawal syndrome. Methadone 10–20 mg is then administered and the patient is observed for evidence of intoxication. Methadone 10 mg is given as necessary through the day whenever evidence of the opiate absti-nence syndrome recurs. The total dose of methadone required in the 24 hours from the onset of signs is thus calculated, and is the baseline dose which can be continued on a daily basis, usually divided between two doses per day.

One advantage of in-patient stabilization is its rapidity: patients quickly reach the baseline daily dose which ensures physical comfort. They are spared the early days of out-patient stabilization when the prescribed dose is small and when they may find it hard not to resort to illicit drugs. The indications for in-patient stabilization are:

1   if patients request it – usually because they feel that they would be unable to comply with the out-patient procedure;

2   if previous attempts at out-patient stabilization have been unsatisfac-tory due to non-compliance;

3   if out-patient assessment has been equivocal and the diagnosis of dependence is still uncertain.

Day-patient stabilization

Out-patient stabilization can be achieved more rapidly if it is possible for the patient to attend a day-care facility, hospital, clinic or doctor's surgery on a day-patient basis. In this situation, methadone can be administered as-necessary, throughout the day, as long as the final dose is given no later than 1–2 hours before the patient leaves for home.

Alteration of stabilized dose

Once the baseline daily dose has been reached, either as an out-patient, or as an in-patient, it cannot be increased merely at the patient's request. Occasionally, however, within a short period of stabilization, it may be necessary for an adjustment to be made, either increasing the dose if the patient is seen to be manifesting continuing signs of opiate withdrawal, or decreasing the dose if there is evidence of intoxication after the accumulation of several doses of methadone.

Dose reduction regimes

Detoxification using decreasing doses of opiates can be carried out as slowly or as quickly as desired. A general principle is that at higher dose levels, the daily dose reduction can be greater, because it represents a smaller percentage of the total, and that as the daily dose falls, reduction should be more gradual. For example, if the stabilization dose is more than 40 mg daily, the dose can be reduced by 5 mg daily until 40 mg/day has been reached; thereafter the dose should be reduced by 5 mg every other day. Alternatively, a patient who has been stabilized on methadone 60 mg daily could be detoxified in 30 days by reducing the dose by 2 mg each day. Detoxification in hospital can proceed more rapidly than on an out-patient basis.

Drug withdrawal can be carried out on a blind or open basis. With the latter, the patient is aware of the dosage reduction schedule, but if withdrawal is 'blind', the reductions are made without the patient's knowledge; this may help patients whose anxiety about drug withdrawal makes the procedure more difficult than it need be. Sometimes patients prefer to prepare their own detoxification schedule, which should be discussed with staff and, if necessary, amended before the start.

Fixed-term opiate-treatment contract

A much slower and therefore more prolonged reduction of opiates may be appropriate for some patients. In this situation, opiates are prescribed for a predetermined period, usually of 6 months, but sometimes for 1 year. At the same time, the patient and the staff work towards attaining and maintaining a constructive and healthy lifestyle. A complete treatment plan is worked out describing the opiate dose regime, the treatment aims and the activities and treatment approaches in which the patient is expected to participate. This is formally presented to the patient as a contract, which is signed by the patient and the key health-care professional, and which is filed in the case notes where it can be referred to if necessary. The contract is conceptually a 'contingency-management' contract and includes rewards for progress and sanctions for relapse and other undesirable behaviour. It provides a framework for the individual patient to take an active part in treatment, reduces dissent between patient and staff and ensures continuity of treatment even if staff change.

Because the expressed goal is to work towards abstention within a definite if prolonged time period, it is against the philosophy and purpose of the contract for it to be used as a form of indefinite opiate maintenance. The contract should not be renewed immediately or continuously if the patient relapses, although he/she may still be offered treatment. Similarly, extension of the contract should be occasional rather than customary, and should only occur after full review of the situation by the whole multidisciplinary team (if the patient is attending a specialist treatment clinic).

It should be apparent that a contract such as this, in which opiates are prescribed for several months, is unsuitable for those whose dependence status is doubtful or who have only a mild degree of physical dependence. It should be reserved for those patients who have not been able to achieve long-term abstinence after several attempts at detoxification, both as an in-patient and as an out-patient. For many of these individuals, whatever the original cause(s) of their drug dependence, it seems to have become the core of their other problems, and they have a better chance of breaking into this cycle if they have a guaranteed supply of their drug. Freed from the need to seek and buy opiates illicitly, they can attempt to resolve coexistent problems, and the consequent reduction of stress may make it easier for them to give up taking opiates.

Opiate maintenance

An alternative to detoxification is maintenance treatment, which means the legal supply to the dependent individual of a daily dose of opiate sufficient to prevent the onset of the abstinence syndrome. Having achieved stabilization (p. 209), the patient is subsequently maintained on the baseline daily dose of opiate for a prolonged period, and perhaps indefinitely. This should never be offered as a first line of treatment, except perhaps for an elderly patient or for an individual with AIDS, but it could be considered for patients who have relapsed several times during or after detoxification.

Thus it is suitable for those who can lead a more or less normal life when they take opiates in a stable and non-escalating dose, but who cannot do so if opiates are withdrawn.

To spare the patient the temptation of having large quantities of drug available for personal consumption or to sell, methadone should be made available in quantities sufficient only for 1 day at a time. If the patient cannot attend the clinic every day to receive and consume the drug under supervision, arrangements can be made with a local pharmacist for the prescription to be dispensed on a daily basis, with a double ration on weekends. The special arrangements and requirements associated with prescribing controlled drugs to addicts are described in Chapter 11.

Maintenance or withdrawal?

Undoubtedly, if the treatment regime is observed, methadone maintenance will keep the patient in a physiologically normal condition, able to work and earn a living. It removes the need to obtain drugs illicitly, it 'saves' the patient from the black market, it eliminates the need for injection, with all its potentially hazardous consequences.

However, a serious cause for concern is that long-term opiate maintenance is not really treatment in any meaningful sense of the word. It offers no chance or hope of cure, but is only a way of maintaining the dependent state. It encourages drug-dependent individuals towards a passive acceptance of their condition, and for the thousands of young drug abusers of today it is a severe penalty for youthful errors.

A subtle implication of such a policy, if it becomes routine, is that it is so clearly the 'end of the road' that some opiate-dependent individuals may be unwilling to present for a treatment which is the final confirmation of the hopelessness of their condition and of the impossibility of change. Instead of coming foward for help at an early stage of their drug-taking career, they continue with illicit drug abuse and the advantages of early intervention are lost.

It is often suggested that drug withdrawal will only be successful if the patient 'wants' to come off drugs, and until that time arises, he/she should be provided with a maintenance prescription. Undoubtedly, motivation for abstinence is very important and may be crucial to the long-term success of detoxification. For some patients, motivation is triggered by the legal, social or medical consequences of their drug abuse and dependence; many patients, for example, have given up drug taking because of fear of AIDS. For others, any latent motivation that they may have to become abstinent is counteracted by the profound psychological dependence induced by opiates, by their intense craving and need for drugs, which becomes more severe the longer they take opiates (illicit or prescribed). Thus, lack of motivation can be seen as a symptom and as an indication of the severity of dependence, and waiting for motivation to 'happen' may be a comfortable collusion with the patient that nothing can or should be done to interrupt their drug-dependent condition.

Of course, patients cannot be forced to accept detoxification, but if when they seek help, this does not include the option of maintenance for which perhaps they had hoped, they may be persuaded by the positive attitudes of health-care professionals towards attempting detoxification. If opiate main-tenance is routinely available as a treatment option, it is understandable and to be expected that many will opt for it rather than face the anxieties of being without their drug, and the chance of achieving abstinence is lost – at least for a while.

In summary, therefore, long-term methadone maintenance should be regarded very much as the last resort in the management of opiate depend-ence, particularly for the young addicts of today. Withdrawal should be attempted and repeated, if only to establish that it cannot be tolerated or that the addict's life without drugs becomes increasingly chaotic. There are a few patients – and it is only a small proportion – who will do better if they receive a regular prescription for opiates; they will have a more stable lifestyle and will cease the use of illicit drugs.

Oral or intravenous? Heroin or methadone?

The theoretical basis of opiate maintenance is simple – so simple that the prac-tical problems of implementing it as a treatment modality may be overlooked by those who are unfamiliar with drug-dependent individuals and their lifestyle. Problems arise because a patient on maintenance treatment cannot be isolated from a world with a drugs black market, where opiates and injectable drugs command a high premium. This situation means that when opiates are prescribed to a patient either for stabilization or maintenance, every effort must be made to ensure that the legally prescribed, pharmaceuti-cally pure drugs do not become diverted to the black market. The aim, there-fore, is to prescribe the opiate with the least black market value and potential, and to prescribe the 'right' (minimum) dose, so that the patient has to take it all, personally, to prevent the onset of withdrawal symptoms and has no surplus to produce euphoria or to sell. Methadone mixture which has ideal pharmacokinetic properties for opiate maintenance fulfils these criteria too.

However, many patients want more than to be kept in a state of physio-logical normality by oral methadone. They crave the 'rush' or 'high' that follows injection and, rejecting methadone maintenance, turn to the black market for the heroin they prefer. Others accept the methadone and obtain illicit heroin as well. Many abuse a variety of other psychoactive drugs, according to availability and personal whim.

Self-injection may be an important component of this drug-taking behaviour. It may have started because the effect of injected drugs was preferred, but there are often sound economic reasons too: the cost of a drug habit increases in step with the increase in tolerance, and administration by injection delivers the whole dose directly into the bloodstream, for maximum effect without any waste. By association with the rewarding properties of the drug, injection acquires secondary reinforcing properties of its own and many addicts are reluctant to relinquish it. For some individuals (the true 'needle-freaks'), the act of injection is as important as any drug that they inject.

Of course, every effort should be made to persuade and encourage these patients to accept maintenance opiates in oral form. Some do settle down with an oral drug, provided a regular supply is guaranteed, but others remain unwilling to give up injection, often suspicious about the effectiveness of oral drugs.

Such behaviour can be interpreted as a manifestation of the severity of their dependence, and in this situation, rigid adherence to a policy of only prescribing oral methadone effectively excludes the most severely dependent patients from treatment. It may therefore prove necessary to prescribe injectable drugs, trying after a few weeks or months to gradually change over to an oral substitute. For the transition period, patients may receive part of their opiate in injectable form and part in oral form.

The justification for prescribing injectable opiates is that for a certain group of patients it may be the only way to engage them in treatment at all, and that without this 'lure' they will remain out of reach of all the interventions (counselling, psychotherapy, behaviour therapy, social work intervention, etc.) that make up the totality of treatment for drug dependence.

If injectable opiates are prescribed, methadone is still the drug of choice because one daily administration maintains the patient free from withdrawal symptoms, whereas heroin requires more frequent administration. In practice, the advantage of methadone over heroin is less clear-cut, because many who receive the former prefer to divide the dose and have several smaller injections so that they can experience the 'high' after injection more often. Injectable heroin is prescribed to some patients if it is felt that this is the only way that they can be engaged in treatment.

The prescription of injectable drugs to severely dependent individuals may also be a way of reducing the harm that these patients do to themselves. The black market heroin that they otherwise use is of variable and unknown purity, and the syringes and needles used to inject it are often scarce and are frequently shared. The user is at risk from infection, from overdose and from the effect of injected adulterants. In contrast, pharmaceutically pure opiates, injected in a known and appropriate dose using a sterile syringe, are much safer. Those receiving injectable drugs should be educated in the correct procedure for sterile injection and advised about the least harmful route for injection (subcutaneous or intramuscular in preference to intravenous), and the safest sites (arm, rather than jugular vein). Once again, however, the advantage of prescribed over illicit drugs is often more theoretical than real. For severely dependent patients, involvement in the black market becomes an integral part of their drug-taking life and lifestyle. It is not surprising, therefore, that buying and selling of illicit drugs does not always cease when, or because, the individual concerned is given a maintenance prescription for opiates; the clinic is just one source among several for obtaining drugs. In some cases therefore, opiate maintenance, even if injectable drugs are prescribed, fails to bring the promised order and stability to the lifestyle of the opiate-dependent individual. In this situation, it may be felt that prescribing injectable opiates is serving no useful purpose at all and a change is made to oral opiates; the knowledge that they may lose their guaranteed supply of pure opiate may encourage some patients to desist from black market activity and to participate fully in the treatment process.

High dose methadone maintenance

A very different approach to opiate maintenance has been adopted at some centres in the US, where the policy is not to give the minimum dose of methadone, but a high dose achieved by stepwise increments.

The rationale is that at low doses of prescribed methadone the patient requires only a small quantity of 'extra', usually illicit, opiate to reach and exceed the blood opiate level at which euphoria is experienced (tolerance level, see p. 209). As the maintenance dose of methadone increases, the proportionate increase in the tolerance level is much greater and it takes proportionately more supplemental opiate to exceed it. With a maintenance dose of 80–90 mg it becomes pharmacologically impossible (it is said) for the patient to experience euphoria. However much illicit opiate is consumed, the patient does not get a 'high'. When taking these large doses the patient should not experience any craving for opiates, and even if illicit opiates are tried, their euphoric effects are blocked. Because they are no longer rewarding, opiate-seeking behaviour should cease because of extinction of a previously conditioned response.

A disadvantage of high dose methadone maintenance is that unless methadone consumption is supervised every day at the clinic, there is a risk that part of the large doses prescribed may be sold to the black market and other drugs bought instead. In common with all maintenance programmes, it prolongs the state of dependence in individuals who might otherwise become abstinent. Finally, increasing the daily dose of methadone to this level worsens the severity of physical dependence on opiates, even if certain aspects of daily life, such as attending school, getting a job, desisting from crime, improve.

Laevo-alpha-acetylmethadol

A major concern about opiate maintenance treatment is that prescribed drugs may be diverted to the black market. One approach to this problem, adopted in the US, is that the patient attends the clinic daily and consumes methadone under supervision. This is inconvenient for the patient and time consuming for clinic staff, who have less time for counselling, etc. The use of laevo-alpha-acetylmethadol (LAAM; methadyl acetate) is a way of reducing these problems because the patient only needs to attend the clinic three times a week.

LAAM is a synthetic opiate which suppresses the opiate abstinence syndrome for 48–72 hours, this extended pharmacological action is due to its biotransformation to an active metabolite, noracetylmethadol. When administered orally three times weekly, LAAM provides safe and effective maintenance, with no evidence of the opiate abstinence syndrome despite the long gaps between treatment.

Because patients attend for treatment less frequently, their lives can become less medication and clinic-orientated. It is felt that they thus become less psychologically dependent on medication and identify more easily with a drug-free lifestyle.

Because of its long duration of action, induction of treatment with LAAM and dose stabilization should be carried out slowly, starting with a dose of 20 mg, three times weekly and increasing by 10 mg every other dose, until the maintenance dose is achieved. Although the slower pace of stabilization may be difficult for a few patients, once it is achieved the smooth therapeutic action of LAAM eliminates the daily 'highs' and 'lows' that occasionally occur with methadone, so that patients feel healthier, more alert and 'normal' on LAAM. Some patients may require a slightly higher dose than usual at the weekend, so that they have no withdrawal symptoms during the 72 hours before the next clinic attendance.

Patients should be warned of the delayed onset of action of LAAM so that they do not take additional opiates (or other central nervous system sedatives) and precipitate a serious overdose. If this occurs, high doses of naloxone are required and may need to be repeated for up to 72 hours.

Opiate antagonists

Once opiate detoxification has been achieved, the individual remains at risk of relapse for some time and may, if exposed to a situation previously associated with drug taking, experience severe craving and even the symptoms of opiate withdrawal. He/she may then succumb to this need and take opiates, and in a similar situation is even more likely to take them again; he/she is then well on the way to relapse.

It has been argued that if opiates had no effect and specifically did not relieve the symptoms of abstinence, their use would not then be repeated; the individual would 'learn' that opiates were not useful. In more technical terms, opiates would have been robbed of their reinforcing effect and eventually, opiate-seeking behaviour should cease as a result of extinction of a previously conditioned response.

The clinical use of opiate antagonists rests on these suppositions. They are drugs that block or counteract the effects of opiates so that if an 'ex-addict' – an opiate-dependent individual who has become abstinent – is maintained on an antagonist and then takes an opiate drug, he or she experiences none of its effects.

Naloxone is a pure opiate antagonist, but is unsuitable for relapse prevention because it has low oral efficacy and its short duration of action necessitates frequent administration. Naltrexone is more suitable; it can be taken orally and because it blocks the effects of opiates for up to 72 hours, it requires administration only three times a week. If naltrexone is given to an individual who is still physically dependent on opiates, it precipitates withdrawal symptoms which are protracted because of the long duration of action of naltrexone. It should not therefore be administered until 7 days after the last dose of heroin or 10 days after the last dose of methadone. It should be preceded by a naloxone challenge test: naloxone 0.4 mg is injected intramuscularly and the patient is observed for 1 hour for evidence of the opiate abstinence syndrome; if there are no symptoms, the injection is repeated once and observation continues. If withdrawal symptoms appear, they will be short-lived (2 hours) because of the short duration of action of naloxone, and can be relieved, if necessary, by opiate administration. If there is no evidence of the opiate abstinence syndrome after naloxone, it is safe to initiate treatment with naltrexone. The initial dose is 25 mg, and if there are no symptoms of withdrawal, a regime of 50 mg per day can be initiated the following day. However, because of the drug's long duration of action, administration three times a week is common, with 100 mg on Monday and Wednesday and 150 mg on Friday.

Although the use of opiate antagonists is theoretically simple, it requires a high degree of motivation on the part of the patient to take naltrexone regularly, because it has no reinforcing effect of its own and because it robs opiates of their pleasurable effects. It should be administered under supervision either by a close family member or at the clinic to ensure that it is taken. Those who do best on naltrexone form a fairly small group, usually with a history of stable relationships and employment. It may, for example, be particularly suitable for 'professional' (e.g., doctor) addicts. It is also useful in the management of female patients who have just given birth to a child whom they fear may be taken from them if they resume drug abuse and who are therefore highly motivated to remain abstinent.

To improve patient cooperation, external reinforcers such as payments have been tried and longer-acting antagonists, such as depot preparations of naloxone which extend opiate blocking for up to 60 days, are also being tested. These would have the practical advantage that once the injection had been given, patient non-compliance could not occur.

For individuals such as these, naltrexone provides not a cure but some protection against becoming dependent again, and this protective effect can be enhanced by concurrent psychotherapy, family therapy, behaviour therapy, etc. Indeed, naltrexone should only be considered an adjunct to other forms of support and treatment for patients who have recently come off opiates, rather than a treatment in its own right. There is a clear relationship between time spent on naltrexone and opiate-free status but, of course, naltrexone cannot provide permanent protection. Nevertheless, after cessation of treatment, it can be resumed if the patient relapses (but before dependence develops), or feels vulnerable to relapse, and may prevent occasional illicit use progressing quickly into regular and compulsive use.

Because there is concern that naltrexone, even in therapeutic dosage, may be hepatotoxic in some patients, it is only given to patients with normal liver function, and this should be monitored regularly throughout treatment.

Patients should be warned that the blockade effect of naltrexone is competitive, and that although it is possible to overcome the block with very large doses of opiates, it is extremely dangerous to attempt to do so because of the risk of overdose. Patients on naltrexone should be given a 'caution card' issued by the drug manufacturers; this states the nature of their medication and explains that if they have an accident, for example, and require opiate analgesia, they will need much larger doses than usual. It should be made clear to the patient that naltrexone has no effect in preventing abuse of other classes of drugs.

Sedative hypnotic drugs

Sedative hypnotic drugs cause physical dependence and an abstinence syndrome which may be of life-threatening severity. Maintenance treatment – i.e., the legal prescription of the drug in sufficient dosage to prevent the onset of the abstinence syndrome – might therefore seem a reasonable treatment option. However, because tolerance to the effects of sedative hypnotics is limited, their continued consumption in high dosage keeps the patient in an unacceptable state of intoxication, often incapable of leading a useful life. It is for this reason that maintenance on sedative hypnotic drugs is not a helpful or practical response and should not be adopted.

Drug withdrawal

Patients who are dependent on sedative hypnotic drugs can generally be regarded as falling into one of two groups – those who are dependent on prescribed drugs, and those who obtain their drugs illicitly and who often abuse other drugs and alcohol too. The management of these two groups is different.

'Therapeutic' sedative dependence

Those who are dependent on prescribed sedatives (frequently benzodiazepines) have often been receiving long-term prescriptions from a single prescriber. The dose may be within or above the normal therapeutic range and may be a stable dose or one that has been increasing at a fairly gradual rate. These patients are not usually part of a drug sub-culture, they are not involved in other forms of drug abuse, nor are they dependent on drugs of other classes.

Many of these patients can be treated on an out-patient basis with a very gradual reduction of dosage over several weeks or perhaps even months – usually from the same, single prescriber. As a rule of thumb, benzodiazepines can be withdrawn in steps of about 1/8 (range 1/10–1/4) of their daily dose every fortnight. Patients who are taking short- or medium-acting benzodiazepines may find withdrawal particularly difficult because of the rapid alterations in blood concentrations that occur and the consequent variations in symptomatology. In such cases they should be transferred to an equivalent dose of diazepam, which should preferably be taken in a single dose at night (see Table 6.3). The dose of diazepam can then be reduced in fortnightly steps of 2–2.5 mg. If withdrawal symptoms occur, the dose should be maintained until they improve, when reduction can be resumed, if necessary in

Table 6.3 Approximate doses of benzodiazepines equivalent to diazepam 5mg

Drug	Dose
Diazepam	5 mg
Chlordiazepoxide	15 mg
Loprazolam	0.5–1.0 mg
Lorazepam	500 μg
Lorametazepam	0.5–1.0 mg
Nitrazepam	5 mg
Oxazepam	15 mg
Temazepam	10 mg
Triazolam	125–250 μg

smaller fortnightly steps. In general, prescriptions should only be for 1 week at a time because larger quantities, to last for a longer period, may prove too great a temptation for someone who is finding withdrawal very difficult.

Adjunctive treatment such as group or individual anxiety-management programmes can also be offered, but continuing psychological support is the most important element and the patient should be seen at least weekly. During withdrawal, and afterwards, the patient may attribute all untoward symptoms – both physical and psychological – to drug withdrawal, and may have unrealistic expectations about the outcome of treatment. Advice about non-pharmacological approaches to symptom management is therefore important and this can be helped by the patient keeping a diary of severe symptoms. Beta-blockers may lessen some symptoms but should only be tried if other measures fail, and never as the first response. Antidepressants should only be used if clinical depression is present.

Some patients may need or request in-patient withdrawal treatment, either because the prescribed dose is very high or because the patient prefers a more rapid detoxification which would be too risky on an out-patient basis.

Non-therapeutic sedative dependence

Sedative hypnotic drug abusers who are abusing drugs of other classes (polydrug users) and those who take sedatives obtained illicitly (sometimes obtained from several medical practitioners), are usually taking very high doses and are part of the addiction sub-culture.

Previously, this group mainly abused barbiturates, often intravenously. Nowadays, barbiturate abuse has lessened and has largely been replaced by abuse of benzodiazepines and chlormethiazole (with or without alcohol). These drugs are less toxic than barbiturates and there is a reduced risk of serious overdose necessitating intensive medical intervention. However, heavy sedative drug abusers continue to have serious legal, social and medical difficulties.

Out-patient detoxification is seldom appropriate for these patients, who are unlikely to comply with the planned programme and who are at risk of suffering serious withdrawal phenomena such as convulsions or toxic confusional states. Very occasionally, an opiate-dependent individual who also takes a stable dose of benzodiazepine (within or near the therapeutic dose) may be suitable for out-patient withdrawal of sedatives with a fixed-term reduction schedule over 2–4 weeks.

In-patient detoxification is the treatment of choice and is strongly advised for patients who are dependent on sedatives. It can be divided into four phases:
1 observation;
2 stabilization on sedatives;
3 detoxification; and
4 post-withdrawal observation.

Observation

The patient is observed from the time of admission for signs of sedative withdrawal (such as tremor, agitation, tachycardia, postural hypotension). Sedatives are not given unless there is evidence of physical dependence. However, as the later signs of sedative withdrawal are dangerous, it is important that the earlier signs are not missed.

In the case of patients who are abusing long-acting benzodiazepines, signs of withdrawal may not appear for several days and it is necessary to be alert to the possibility that a patient may need to start a sedative schedule as long as 5–7 days after admission. Usually, however, evidence of withdrawal is obvious much earlier than this.

Stabilization on sedatives

If the patient shows signs of sedative abstinence, a suitable sedative drug should be administered. Theoretically, because of cross-tolerance, any sedative drug can be used, but it is customary to choose a drug from the same group as the patient's drug of abuse. Furthermore, long-acting drugs are preferable because the more stable blood levels prevent rapid swings in symptomatology. Thus, diazepam is prescribed for those whose principal drug of abuse is a benzodiazepine and phenobarbitone for those who abuse barbiturates; chlormethiazole is prescribed to alcohol abusers.

The stabilization dose should be adjusted according to individual need. The history of drug consumption (which drug, what dosage) may be helpful but is not always reliable, so that safe stabilization relies heavily on careful observation of symptoms. The aim is to maintain the patient, temporarily, in a condition of very, very mild intoxication, manifest by slight sedation, so that the patient feels comfortable and there is no risk of serious withdrawal events. Stabilization regimes are described below for diazepam, phenobarbitone and chlormethiazole; that for diazepam is described in most detail, but exactly the same principles apply whichever drug is selected. It must be emphasized that these regimes are intended only as guidelines. Decisions about the frequency of administration of drugs and the necessary dose depend on clinical judgement of observed symptoms and signs. It should be remembered that lower dosages of drugs may be required in patients with severe liver disease.

Diazepam. If diazepam is chosen as the drug for stabilization, 20 mg is given orally and the patient is observed. If after 1 hour the symptoms of withdrawal persist, this dose may be repeated. Usually, however, and certainly after a total dose of 40 mg, symptomatic relief is obvious. Thereafter, observations continue and diazepam 20 mg is given if and when symptoms re-emerge. In any case, diazepam 20 mg should be given after 6 hours and repeated at 6-hourly intervals. However, care must be taken not to over-sedate the patient; excessive drowsiness, confusion, ataxia, slurred speech and nystagmus are warning signs that the patient is becoming intoxicated, with a serious risk of respiratory depression. If three or more of these symptoms are present, the next dose of diazepam should be omitted. Mild symptoms of intoxication can be managed by dose reduction rather than omission. In practice, most patients will be satisfactorily stabilized on diazepam 80–100 mg daily, in divided doses.

Rarely, the patient may be suffering nausea and vomiting as a result of drug withdrawal, or be so agitated that oral administration is initially impractical. In this situation 10–20 mg diazepam can be given intravenously, at a rate of 5 mg/min, until the patient is calm. This can be repeated if necessary after 30–60 minutes. Subsequent doses can then be given orally according to the clinical situation.

For patients with severe liver disease it may be more appropriate to select a different benzodiazepine, with a shorter half-life. Oxazepam (15–30 mg four times daily) or lorazepam (1–2 mg four times daily) are possible alternatives.

Phenobarbitone. The initial dose is 120 mg orally which can be repeated after 1 hour if necessary. This dose, equivalent to 1.8 mg/kg, is satisfactory for a patient of 'normal' weight (70 kg), but may require adjustment in obese or underweight patients. Phenobarbitone 120 mg should be administered 6 hourly unless clinical observation of intoxication suggests that a dose should be reduced or omitted (see above); if signs of withdrawal emerge, the dose may need to be increased. Phenobarbitone too, if necessary, can be given by intramuscular or intravenous injection (1.75 mg/kg).

Chlormethiazole. Two or three capsules of chlormethiazole should be given in the first instance, and may be repeated after 1 hour if necessary. The usual dose for stabilization is two or three capsules, 6 hourly, unless observation of symptoms of withdrawal or intoxication (see above) suggest otherwise. Chlormethiazole can also be used for acute withdrawal stages; 30–50 ml (240–400 mg) of a 0.8% solution should be given at a rate of about 4 ml (60 drops)/min until the patient is mildly drowsy. The rate of administration should then be reduced to 10–15 drops/min and adjusted according to the patient's response.

Once the patient has been satisfactorily stabilized, this dose is maintained for 3–7 days. Three days is sufficient for those dependent on barbiturates, but those who have been abusing predominantly long-acting sedatives, such as diazepam, should receive the full stabilization dose for 7 days before any dose reduction is initiated. Observation continues throughout this period of stabilization and appropriate adjustment of the dose may be necessary. If withdrawal signs re-emerge the dose should be increased, and if intoxication develops the dose should be reduced.

Some patients abuse a mixture of benzodiazepines, alcohol and barbiturates. The choice of detoxification agent is not critical in these cases, although it is probably better to use one with a greater anticonvulsant action. In all cases, only a single drug is prescribed.

Detoxification schedule

Daily incremental reductions of the dose are made over a period of 14–21 days. Larger incremental reductions can be made at the beginning of the detoxification schedule, when they represent a small percentage of the total daily dose, and smaller reductions at the end. Examples of typical withdrawal schedules are shown in Tables 6.4–6.6.

Adjustment of the stabilization dose or of the rate of reduction is made only on the basis of clinical indications to do so and not merely at the patient's request. The purpose of treatment is to withdraw the patient safely from a toxic agent rather than to perpetuate the use of drugs. Increasing the dose or slowing the rate of dose reduction according to the patient's whim undermines this philosophy, while accelerating the process increases the risk of withdrawal convulsions.

Chapter 6

Table 6.4 Benzodiazepine withdrawal schedule, showing dose of diazepam (mg) administered orally

Day	Time of dose administration				Total
	08.00	12.00	17.00	22.00	
1–7	20	20	20	20	80
8	20	10	20	20	70
9	20	10	10	20	60
10	10	10	10	20	50
11	10	10	10	10	40
12	10	5	10	10	35
13	10	5	5	10	30
14	5	5	5	10	25
15	5	5	5	5	20
16	5	–	5	5	15
17	5	–	–	5	10
18	5	–	–	5	10
19	–	–	–	5	5
20	–	–	–	5	5
21	–	–	–	–	0

The starting dose must be determined individually and the detoxification schedule should be modified accordingly.

Post-withdrawal observation

After completion of sedative withdrawal, a minimum period of observation in hospital is recommended before the patient is discharged in case there are delayed manifestations of the abstinence syndrome, such as convulsions. Barbiturate-dependent individuals should stay in hospital for at least 2–3 days after completing drug withdrawal, but those dependent on benzodiazepines should stay for 7–10 days.

Patients should be strongly discouraged from discharging themselves during any phase of sedative withdrawal. If there is evidence of mental disorder at the time of threatened self-discharge, then consideration can be given to compulsorily detaining the patient for his or her own safety under Section 5(2) of the Mental Health Act 1959. Patients who refuse to continue with the detoxification schedule should be advised to remain in hospital for a minimum period of 2 days after the last dose, to minimize (though not eliminate) the risk of convulsions after leaving hospital.

Table 6.5 Barbiturate withdrawal schedule, showing dose of phenobarbitone (mg) administered orally

Day	Time of dose administration				Total
	08.00	12.00	17.00	22.00	
1–3	150	150	150	150	600
4	150	120	120	150	540
5	120	120	120	120	480
6	120	90	90	120	420
7	90	90	90	90	360
8	90	60	60	90	300
9	60	60	60	60	240
10	60	45	45	60	210
11	45	45	45	45	180
12	45	30	30	45	150
13	30	30	30	30	120
14	30	15	15	30	90
15	15	15	15	30	75
16	15	15	15	15	60
17	15	–	15	15	45
18	15	–	–	15	30
19	–	–	–	15	15
20	–	–	–	–	0

The starting dose must be determined individually and the detoxification schedule should be modified accordingly.

Convulsions (during/after sedative detoxification)

If a sedative detoxification procedure such as that outlined above is adhered to, it is unlikely that convulsions will occur. However, although infrequent, they may arise even in the course of the best managed schedules, and sometimes even when the patient is being prescribed sedatives. The emergency treatment is sodium amylobarbitone 250 mg intramuscular. If convulsions occur during the periods of stabilization or detoxification, this suggests that the stabilized dose is too small or that the rate of withdrawal is too rapid, and an appropriate adjustment of the daily dose of sedative should be made. If they occur when withdrawal has been completed, sedatives should be reintroduced and withdrawn again at a slower rate.

It should be noted that phenytoin and other anticonvulsants are ineffective in preventing withdrawal fits and are not effective substitutes for gradual sedative detoxification. Phenothiazines and other drugs with epileptogenic properties should be avoided during sedative withdrawal.

Table 6.6 Chlormethiazole withdrawal schedule, showing dose of chlormethiazole (capsules) administered orally

	Time of dose administration				
Day	08.00	12.00	17.00	22.00	Total
1–3	3	3	3	3	12
4	3	2	2	3	10
5	2	2	2	2	8
6	2	1	1	2	6
7	1	1	1	2	5
8	1	1	1	1	4
9	1	–	1	1	3
10	1	–	1	1	3
11	1	–	–	1	2
12	1	–	–	1	2
13	–	–	–	1	1
14	–	–	–	–	0

Each capsule (192 mg chlormethiazole base) = 5 ml elixir (250 mg/5 ml chlormethiazole edisylate).
The starting dose must be determined individually and the detoxification schedule should be modified accordingly.

Intoxication

If sedative intoxication develops while the patient is taking the standard stabilization dose, this may indicate that the initial diagnosis of sedative dependence was incorrect and that the patient has not developed tolerance to these drugs. Alternatively, it may suggest that the patient is simultaneously abusing illicit drugs. Whatever the cause, reduction of dose is necessary but careful observation should continue.

If intoxication develops during the period of drug withdrawal, this is probably due to illicit sedative abuse. Doses should be omitted while the patient is intoxicated, but otherwise the detoxification schedule should be adhered to.

LSD and cannabis

There is no specific treatment for those who abuse or are dependent on LSD or cannabis. Physical dependence, if it occurs, is only slight and the abstinence syndrome, if it develops, is correspondingly mild and does not cause significant distress. There is therefore no need to prescribe alternative psychoactive medication, and this should be avoided so that the patient learns how to cope without resorting to pharmacological solutions.

Cocaine and amphetamine

Until recently, no specific treatment was recommended for stimulant abuse on the grounds that the abstinence syndrome, if it developed, was self-limiting and not dangerous. Now, however, due to the easy availability of very pure cocaine in the form of 'crack', there are many more cases of very severe dependence with a correspondingly very distressing abstinence syndrome. It has thus become apparent that a more active approach to treatment may be necessary to help severely dependent individuals through their detoxification, otherwise the severity of their symptoms may prevent their ever becoming abstinent.

However, unlike the treatment of dependence on opiates or sedative hypnotics, gradual detoxification by means of step-wise reduction of dosage is not recommended, because it is not successful. Drugs should therefore be stopped abruptly. The consequent psychiatric symptoms which may require pharmacological treatment are as follows.

1   Dysphoria with agitation. This can be treated with diazepam, either orally or intravenously. Propranolol may also be helpful (40–160 mg/day).

2   Severe depression. This is usually transient, but while it lasts it may be of suicidal intensity. A number of drugs have been used including tryptophan, pyridoxine, l-tyrosine, phenothiazines and tricyclic antidepressants (TCAs). Unfortunately, there are no controlled studies to prove the efficacy of any particular treatment regime.

3   Psychotic symptoms. These usually resolve within a few days; a phenothiazine drug or haloperidol may sometimes be necessary.

It is worth noting that some patients show considerable resistance to phenothiazines and benzodiazepines so that larger doses than usual may be necessary. Clonidine is said to be effective for the treatment of associated anxiety and tachycardia but hypotension may occur.

Those who are consuming large quantities of stimulants and who are severely dependent may require in-patient detoxification. This is indicated if there have been repeated attempts at out-patient detoxification, or if drug withdrawal leads to severe depression or prolonged psychotic symptoms. Admission enables complete dissociation from sources of drugs and from drug-using situations and also permits more attention to be paid to the patient's general health and nutritional status which may have suffered severe neglect. However, this can only provide a temporary respite and the high relapse rate after discharge from hospital emphasizes the extreme importance of all the general measures of intervention outlined in Chapter 5.

The particularly severe problems associated with dependence on cocaine have prompted research into new approaches to treatment to facilitate abstinence. These have tended to focus on two areas: firstly, the treatment of underlying disorders for which the cocaine abuser may have been attempting self-medication; and secondly, identifying drugs that will block the effects of cocaine that may reinforce its use. At this stage, however, such treatments can only be considered experimental, and scientific, double-blind trials are needed urgently. The following drugs are being studied.

1   TCAs, desimipramine. Animal research has demonstrated long-term effects on neurotransmitters and receptors following chronic cocaine use, that may be reversible by TCAs. In a double-blind, placebo-controlled clinical trial, desimipramine was found significantly to reduce craving for cocaine and significantly to increase abstinence rates.

2   Bromocriptine. It has been suggested that chronic cocaine abusers suffer from dopamine depletion and that it is this neurochemical abnormality that accounts for their craving for cocaine. In theory, therefore, dopamine agonists such as bromocriptine and amantadine should be helpful and experimental studies with bromocriptine suggest that it does reduce post-cocaine symptomatology and craving. Once again, double-blind controlled studies are necessary.

4   Methylphenidate (Ritalin). Because methylphenidate produces euphoria that is indistinguishable from that caused by amphetamine and cocaine, it has been suggested that it could be used to 'maintain' cocaine-dependent individuals on a controlled dose of a legally prescribed drug so that they do not need to resort to cocaine. This (like maintaining heroin-dependent patients on methadone) would have all the supposed advantages of reducing black market associations, providing economic stability and so on. Reduced abuse of cocaine and an attenuation of its effects was reported in one small-scale study of methylphenidate, although abstinence from cocaine was not sustained. Experience in the UK suggests that problems caused by methylphenidate are no less severe than those caused by other stimulants, including cocaine. In particular, the consequences of self-injection with methylphenidate are very serious.

References and further reading

Arif A & Westermeyer J (eds) (1990). *Methadone maintenance in the management of opioid dependence: an international review.* Praeger Publishers, New York.

Department of Health, Welsh Office & Scottish Home & Health Department (1991). *Drug Misuse and Dependence: Guidelines on Clinical Management.* HMSO, London.

Devenyi P & Saunders SJ (1987). *Physicians' Handbook for Medical Management of Alcohol and Drug-Related Problems.* Addiction Research Foundation, Toronto.

Dole VP & Nyswander MA (1965). Medical treatment for diacetylmorphine (heroin) addiction. *Journal of the American Medical Association*, **193**, 645–656.

Gossop M, Bradley B, Strang J & Connell PH (1984). The clinical effectiveness of electro-stimulation vs oral methadone in managing opiate withdrawal. *British Journal of Psychiatry*, **1144**, 203–208.

Kleber HD & Gawin FH (1984). Cocaine abuse: a review of current and experimental treatments. In: Grabowski J (ed.) *Cocaine: Pharmacology, Effects and Treatment of Abuse*, 111–129. NIDA Research Monograph 50. Department of Health & Human Services, Rockville.

Kleber HD, Riordan CE, Rounsaville BJ *et al.* (1985). Clonidine in outpatient detoxification from methadone maintenance. *Archives of General Psychiatry*, **42**, 391–394.

Morgan JR (1990). Treatment and management. In: Ghodse AH & Maxwell D (eds). *Substance Abuse and Dependence*, 98–130. Macmillan Press, London.

Newman RG (1979). Double blind comparison of methadone and placebo maintenance treatments of narcotic addicts in Hong Kong. *Lancet*, **ii**, 485–488.

Patterson MA (1975). *Addictions Can be Cured. The Treatment of Drug Addiction by Neuro-electric Stimulation*. Lion Publishing, Berkhamsted.

Riordan CE & Kleber HD (1980). Rapid opiate detoxification with clonidine and nalox-one. *Lancet*, **i**, 1079–1080.

Sellers EM (1984). Diazepam tapering in detoxification for high dose benzodiazepine abuse. *Clinical Pharmacology and Therapeutics*, **36**, 410–416.

Smith MO (1979). Acupuncture and natural healing in drug detoxification. *American Journal of Acupuncture*, **7**, 97–106.

Spitz HI & Rosecan JS (1987). *Cocaine Abuse: New Directions in Treatment and Research*. Brunner/Mazel, New York.

Wen HI & Cheung SY (1973). Treatment of drug addiction by acupuncture and electrical stimulation. *Asian Journal of Medicine*, **9**, 138–141.

7

Complications of drug abuse and their treatment

Those who abuse drugs may suffer many physical and psychological problems as a consequence of their behaviour. Some problems can be directly related to the pharmacological effects of the drugs, but many are associated with the methods of drug administration and more specifically with self-injection. Some drug abusers inject subcutaneously ('skin-popping') and some do so intramuscularly, but the most favoured route is intravenous – because this delivers the whole dose, with no wastage, directly into the bloodstream, producing the maximum effect with minimum delay, although increasing the likelihood of a toxic overdose. Whatever complications ensue, their management and the ultimate prognosis is adversely affected by the poor general state of health of many of those who are severely dependent on drugs, resulting from poor social conditions, malnutrition and self-neglect.

No attempt has been made in this chapter to cover all the possible complications of drug abuse, but to address instead those situations that are most frequent and cause particular problems. The emphasis throughout is on the practical aspects of diagnosis and patient-management.

Infective complications of injection

Whatever route is chosen, injection carries a high risk of infection. Needles and syringes are often used several times and may be shared with others. Sterilization of injection equipment, if it is attempted at all, is usually inadequate and therefore ineffective, and the skin is rarely cleaned before injection takes place. Dirty injection habits cause local infection at the site where the needle penetrates the skin and the underlying vein and more generalized illnesses which may be of life-threatening severity. Some infections, notably hepatitis and HIV/AIDS, are transmitted directly from one drug abuser to another as infected blood contaminates shared syringes and needles.

Cellulitis and abscesses

These are local infections occurring at the site(s) of injection. Cellulitis is a spreading infection of the subcutaneous tissues. The affected area is red, swollen, painful and warm, with ill-defined borders, whereas an abscess is a localized collection of pus in a cavity. They may be caused by skin-popping or main-lining, and may be complicated by local thrombophlebitis (inflammation and clotting of a vein) and by the irritant effects of injected drugs (e.g., barbiturates). The local lymph nodes, in the axilla or groin, become enlarged and the patient usually has a fever.

Cellulitis and abscesses are very common complications of self-injection, and drug abusers often seek treatment for them in accident and emergency departments. The affected part – usually the arm or leg – should be rested and elevated whenever possible. It should be cleaned and dressed and abscesses drained, if necessary. Swabs should be taken for bacteriological culture (aerobic and anaerobic), and sensitivity and antibiotic treatment should be initiated. The majority of infections are caused by a penicillinase-resistant *Staphylococcus*, so flucloxacillin is an appropriate choice of antibiotic (or erythromycin if the patient is allergic to penicillin) while awaiting the results of bacteriological examination. The first dose should be given by intramuscular injection.

Chronic skin infection, associated with skin-popping, may be complicated by amyloidosis, that is a major cause of renal damage (nephropathy). Deep abscesses may extend to underlying joints causing a septic arthritis. Bone infection (osteomyelitis) may also occur, most often in the vertebrae, and is usually due to septic emboli from a distant abscess.

Admission to hospital is indicated if the infection is severe or if the patient has toxic symptoms. The decision to admit the patient is often influenced by the knowledge that some drug abusers may not return regularly for further dressings and may be unreliable about taking a full course of antibiotics. It is often safer to admit the patient to hospital (if he/she consents to this), so that treatment can be properly supervised and further complications prevented.

Endocarditis

Endocarditis is one of the most severe forms of infection in humans, in which the smooth lining of the heart valves – the endocardium – is infected and destroyed by bacteria. In those who do not inject drugs this process only occurs if the endocardium has been previously damaged, but in injecting drug abusers it can develop in a previously normal heart.

Infection causes the heart valves to become distorted by crumbling masses of blood clots and bacteria ('vegetations'), bits of which (emboli) break off and are borne away by the bloodstream to other organs, where they act as septic foci. At the same time the vegetations prevent normal closure of the valves of the heart which then cannot function properly. This process is accentuated by the gradual destruction of the valve. In the majority of drug abusers with endocarditis, the infection is localized to the tricuspid valve, which is unusual in non-drug users.The organism (*Streptococcus viridans*) that usually causes endocarditis is comparatively rare in drug abusers, in whom 'unusual' organisms are more likely to be responsible for the illness. For example, the majority of cases are caused by *Staphylococcus aureus*, perhaps because those who regularly inject themselves appear to have a high carriage rate of *Staphylococcus aureus* in the nose, throat and the skin of the antecubital fossa. Sometimes the source of infection may be a cutaneous abscess or septic thrombophlebitis. Other organisms that are occasionally responsible include Gram-negative bacteria such as *Pseudomonas* and *Klebsiella*. The yeast fungus, *Candida*, can also cause endocarditis in drug abusers, although for this and other organisms of low virulence it may be necessary for there to have been prior valve damage before infection could occur. Such damage may develop as a result of bombardment of the endothelial surface with particulate matter present in the injected material.

Endocarditis should be suspected in any patient with a fever and a changing heart murmur, and the characteristic cutaneous manifestations (petechiae, subungual-splinter haemorrhages and Osler's nodes) are present in up to 50% of patients. Staphylococcal endocarditis in particular is characterized by an acute onset and fulminant course, with many septic and embolic complications. Heart failure develops in severe, untreated cases. Diagnosis depends on positive blood cultures that should be carried out as soon as there is any suspicion of endocarditis, as a favourable outcome depends on the early initiation of appropriate antibiotic therapy. Two-dimensional echocardiography can be very useful in identifying and documenting the valve lesion and may sometimes demonstrate vegetations.

Treatment follows the same lines as for the general population and a combination of antibiotics is chosen according to the sensitivities of the bacteria identified on blood culture. Treatment should continue for a minimum of 4 weeks and, certainly at first, should be by continuous intravenous infusion, so that adequate blood levels of antibiotic are maintained.

'Blind' prescribing, before the results of blood culture and sensitivity tests are available, is very difficult because of the wide range of possible organisms. If it is absolutely essential because of the patient's clinical condition, an aminoglycoside (e.g., gentamicin) in combination with a penicillin, or a cephalosporin alone should be used, but specialist (bacteriological) advice should be sought. Surgical intervention (valve excision and replacement) may sometimes be necessary for patients with progressive cardiac failure that is unresponsive to medical management and when it proves impossible to eradicate the infection from the valves with antimicrobial agents.

Septicaemia

Almost any organ can become infected during drug abuse by injection so that arthritis, osteomyelitis, nephritis and bacterial pneumonia may all occur in those who use contaminated syringes and needles. Any of these localized bacterial infections may, in turn, give rise to septicaemia, in which actively multiplying bacteria are no longer confined to the affected organ, but are present in the bloodstream too.

The most common cause of septicaemia in drug abusers is *Staphylococcus aureus*, but *Streptococcus, Pneumococcus, Salmonella* or *Candida* – or indeed almost any microorganism – may, on occasion, be responsible for this very serious, life-threatening infection.

Septicaemia should be suspected if the patient is suffering from fever with hypotension or unexplained confusion, impairment of consciousness, renal failure or liver failure. Once suspected, the condition must be investigated by sending specimens of blood for culture (aerobic and anaerobic) to see if bacteria are present and, if they are, to establish their sensitivity to antibiotics. A successful outcome depends on the early initiation of appropriate antibiotic treatment, and while waiting for the results of sensitivity tests, it is usually necessary to start treatment 'blind' – a cephalosporin, or an aminoglycoside together with a penicillin, would be a suitable choice in this situation. Antibiotics should be given by intravenous infusion. Intensive supportive therapy is also required.

Acquired immune deficiency syndrome

Acquired immune deficiency syndrome (AIDS) is caused by infection with a retrovirus, human immunodeficiency virus (HIV) Once inside the body, HIV is attracted to T-helper (T4) lymphocytes that play a crucial role in mobilizing the body's immune system. HIV invades these cells and replicates within them, thereby preventing them from carrying out their normal functions. Thus, the infected individual's ability to fight infection is impaired and he/she becomes vulnerable to a wide range of opportunistic infection.

Infection with HIV stimulates the body to produce antibodies that, unusually and unfortunately, appear to have little or no ability to neutralize HIV. The detection of this antibody forms the basis of the HIV-antibody test. If positive, it denotes prior infection with HIV, but does not necessarily mean that the patient has AIDS or will contract it. It does imply, however, that the patient is carrying the virus and can transmit it to others. A negative HIV-antibody test probably means that the patient has not been infected with HIV, but the latent period between infection and the development of a positive antibody test can be as long as 3 months, so a single, negative test may lead to a false sense of security. So far, two strains of HIV have been identified. The second form of the virus, HIV-2, appears to be similar in effect and action to HIV-1, and most laboratories test simultaneously for both viruses.

In an infected individual with AIDS, HIV antibody can be detected in high concentration in the blood and, in males, in semen. It has also been detected in low concentration in other body fluids, such as saliva, tears, urine, spinal fluid, cervical secretions and breast milk. However, unlike many other viruses, HIV is fragile and survives poorly outside the body, so that transmission is only by three routes and requires close contact:

Transfusion or inoculation of infected blood

The risk of infection from the transfusion of blood and blood products is now small in countries with high standards of screening donor blood. Drug abusers who share injection equipment are, however, a very high risk group, and rates of HIV infection among injecting drug users have been reported at 30% in Amsterdam, between 30% and 40% in Rome, and between 40% and 60% in some Spanish cities. In the UK, the known level of HIV infection in injecting drug abusers remains low, at less than 2% in most areas, with the exception of Edinburgh (25%), Dundee (25–30%) and London (8%). Because of the high risk of infection with HIV, injecting drug users are at high risk of contracting AIDS, accounting for 25% of all AIDS patients in the USA. In Europe the picture is, at present, rather brighter, with only 8% of all AIDS patients being drug injectors, although again there are wide regional differences.

Sexual contact

Transmission of HIV can occur through both hetero- and homosexual genital contact. This is an important route of transmission from drug abusers to the general population, since some drug abusers may turn to prostitution to finance their habit.

Materno–fetal spread

HIV may be transmitted across the placenta from an infected, pregnant addict to the unborn child. Infection may also occur at the time of birth, either during vaginal delivery or by Caesarean section. Currently, it appears that there is a 13% risk of transmission from mother to baby.

Clinical features of HIV and AIDS

Infection with HIV does not mean that the individual inevitably contracts AIDS. However, it has become apparent that the most important factor in developing AIDS is the length of time since infection, and cohort studies now suggest that 50–75% of infected individuals may progress to symptomatic disease within 10 years. Patients present with a variety of constitutional and non-diagnostic symptoms as well as rashes and swollen lymph nodes. Later, there may be specific findings in the lungs, gastrointestinal tract or the central nervous system. Because of the impaired immune response, opportunistic infections are common. There is a tendency for these to recur and when there is deep organ involvement with fungi or parasites, this is difficult to eradicate.

Examples of common infections in those with HIV include infection with a yeast-like organism, *Candida albicans*, that may cause persistent thrush in the mouth and throat; a serious pneumonia caused by *Pneumocystis carinii*; and an otherwise rare skin tumour, Kaposi's sarcoma, that develops in 25% of people with AIDS.

The following clinical classification system used by the US Centers for Disease Control (CDC) has gained general acceptance for describing HIV infection, allowing identification of different subgroups for scientific study.

1 Group I: acute infection. An acute illness may occur at the time of seroconversion to the HIV-positive state, although this may be asymptomatic. There may be fever, malaise, enlarged lymph nodes, headache and rash, lasting for several weeks before resolving spontaneously.

2 Group II: asymptomatic seropositive. This phase may last for months or years. The individual, although HIV-positive, is well with no signs or symptoms of HIV or AIDS.

3 Group III: persistent generalized lymphadenopathy (PGL). Although otherwise well, the patient has enlarged lymph nodes for more than 3 months, in the neck, armpit or groin, for which there is no explanation other than HIV.

4 Group IV: HIV with disease. This group has been further subdivided into the following categories.

(a) Constitutional disease. Chronic active viral infection with constitutional symptoms such as weight loss, diarrhoea etc., lasting for more than 1 month.

(b) Neurological disease. This is due to the direct effect of HIV on the brain and spinal cord, e.g., dementia.

(c) Secondary infectious disease. (i) Specified secondary infectious diseases, specified in the CDC surveillance definition of AIDS e.g., *Pneumocystis carinii* pneumonia, extrapulmonary cryptococcosis, Kaposi's sarcoma. (ii) Other specified secondary infectious diseases.

(d) Secondary cancers including those in the CDC AIDS definition.

(e) Other conditions. These are other conditions that are indicative of a defect in cell-mediated immunity.

It should be appreciated that while many people are infected with HIV and develop a range of conditions as a consequence (from which, indeed, they may die), they do not all contract AIDS. In order to achieve worldwide consistency of surveillance and reporting of AIDS, there are now clearly defined criteria that must be fulfilled before this diagnosis can be made. These criteria can be summarized as follows:

1   without laboratory evidence of HIV infection, the presence of any of 12 specific conditions (e.g., *Pneumocystis carinii* pneumonia, Kaposi's sarcoma) is diagnostic of AIDS, provided that there is no other reason for immunodeficiency;

2   if the HIV test is positive, any of these 12 diseases or any of a further list of 12 other indicator diseases may be defined as AIDS;

3   if the HIV test is negative, AIDS can still be diagnosed as long as all other causes of immunodeficiency have been ruled out, if the patient is suffering from *Pneumocystis carinii* pneumonia or if one of the other 12 indicator diseases is present, together with a low T-helper lymphocyte count (less than 400 mm^3).

HIV testing of drug abusers

HIV testing is available at most drug-dependence treatment units. Although testing is not a compulsory condition of treatment, patients at high risk (e.g., those who inject their drugs and those at risk because of their sexual behaviour) should be encouraged to have the test.

The aim of pre-test counselling is to ensure that the individual is fully informed and prepared for the implications of either a positive or negative result; and to provide the individual with the necessary harm reduction advice, regardless of the result of the test. It therefore includes the following.

1   Education on viral transmission, the manifestations of HIV infection and the nature of the test. If the patient decides to be tested, it should be emphasized beforehand that two blood samples may be required.

2   Education on ways of reducing the risk of infection, such as 'safer sex' and of giving up injecting or, failing that, of never sharing injection equipment.

3   Education on the implications of positive and negative results.

(a) Positive result. This means that the patient has been infected with HIV and could transmit it to others. No further test is available to predict the future course of events, so the patient found to be HIV-positive has to live with that knowledge, but in ignorance and in fear of the eventual outcome. The ability of the patient to cope with this degree of uncertainty and with the knowledge that they have been in contact with a life-threatening virus should be explored before the test is done. If the patient is pregnant, the risks to her and to the fetus should be explained.

(b) Negative result. This does not exclude the possibility of prior infection because seroconversion (presence of detectable antibodies) may take 3–6 months. Therefore, to be absolutely sure of freedom from HIV, a second test has to be carried out a few months later. A negative result is in itself no safeguard against infection in the future; just because a drug abuser has been 'lucky' up until the time of the test and has not been infected with HIV, it does not mean that the same risky practices can be continued.

4   Discussion of confidentiality. Drug-dependence treatment units need to have established policies regarding the disclosure of HIV test results, e.g., within the multidisciplinary team and to the general practitioner, and the patient should be fully informed of this before testing.

5   The possible social and financial implications of the test – whatever its result – should be fully explained to the patient, who should understand that in some situations (life insurance, mortgage applications, employment) merely having had the test (even if the result is negative) may be disadvantageous, because of the implication of an 'at-risk' lifestyle. There should also be some discussion about the implications a test result may have for their relationship with their partner(s), and the patient should be encouraged to talk to their partner(s) about this in advance. At the same time patients should be warned to be cautious about telling friends and acquaintances the result of the test because they may later regret the lack of confidentiality.

After discussion of all these points, patients should be allowed and encouraged to take enough time to think about testing and to come to a final decision. Some may feel that, whatever the result, their future behaviour will be the same: if HIV-negative, certain measures will have to be adopted to prevent their becoming infected; if HIV-positive, the same measures will have to be adopted to prevent them transmitting infection. They may conclude, therefore, that there is no point in having the test, given that this in itself may jeopardize their future in an unpredictable way. Others, however, cannot tolerate such uncertainty and would prefer to know, one way or the other, regardless of any potential disadvantages. HIV testing may be very important for drug abusers who are unwell, to enable a diagnosis to be made, and is vital for women who are thinking of becoming pregnant or who are pregnant (see Chapter 8).

The fact that HIV counselling has been given and the patient's decision about testing should be clearly recorded in the case notes.

Post-test counselling

The result of HIV testing should be given to the patient face to face, preferably by the pre-test counsellor. Informing the patient by telephone or in writing is not appropriate.

1   Negative HIV-test result. The pre-test education and counselling about risk reduction should be emphasized again and a further test should be offered for about 6 months later.

2   Positive HIV test result. The psychological impact of a positive result should not be underestimated and the patient must be allowed time to express their initial reactions. They should be reminded that a positive result does not mean that they have AIDS or will necessarily get it. However, education on reducing the risk of transmission of HIV should be repeated. Patients may welcome an offer of assistance in informing their partner(s) of the test result and they should be informed of support groups such as the Terrence Higgins Trust and Body Positive. A referral should be made to the appropriate local clinic dealing with HIV-positive patients.

Much of the information covered during post-test counselling will be forgotten in the shock of discovering that the test was positive. The patient should be offered another appointment within a week or so, to provide an opportunity to repeat the information and to talk more calmly about the implications of the test result. The patient should have ready access to a keyworker or doctor for support.

Preventive measures – advice to patients

The risk of sharing injection equipment should be explained to all drug abusers. Those who are HIV-positive should understand their responsibility not to infect others, and should also be aware that their own risk of developing AIDS will be reduced if they stop exposing themselves to the infections carried by contaminated equipment and illicit drugs. Those currently HIV-negative put themselves at the risk of AIDS every time they share injection equipment. Indeed, it should be pointed out to all drug abusers that stopping injecting completely is the only safe behaviour, because drug abusers who inject are always at the risk of wanting a fix on impulse and of deciding to share someone else's equipment.

It should not be forgotten that drug abusers, although a high-risk group for AIDS because of their injection practices, can transmit HIV and be infected by it by other routes too. They should be advised about how to change their sexual behaviour to minimize the risk of transmission of the infection into the non-drug-abusing population. They should also be warned of the risk of sharing razors and toothbrushes which often come into contact with blood. Drug abusers who are HIV-positive should be taught how to clean up spillages of blood or urine.

Treatment of HIV and AIDS

A large number of antiviral drugs have been tried in the treatment of AIDS and there has been some relaxation of the otherwise extremely lengthy testing process for new drugs so that AIDS sufferers can have the benefit of new developments as soon as possible. The antiviral drug, zidovudine (formerly AZT), a reverse-transcriptase inhibitor (an enzyme that enables the RNA of HIV to be transformed into the DNA of the host cell) has received most attention and has demonstrated immunological, virological and clinical benefits in patients with fulminant HIV infections. However, it has serious side-effects, most notably bone-marrow suppression, and it is very expensive. It is important to appreciate that zidovudine only delays progression of the disease; it does not cure it by eradicating the infection and 20–30% of those who take it for over 2 years develop resistance to its effects. Hopes that its use in the early stages of HIV infection, in asymptomatic individuals, would delay or prevent the development of AIDS, appear to have been unfounded.

In the absence of an effective specific treatment for HIV and AIDS, efforts to improve the general health of the individual by a holistic approach to lifestyle assume greater importance. In addition, opportunistic infections should be diagnosed and treated promptly. It is also essential that the need for psychosocial counselling for patients, families and friends is recognized.

Hepatitis

Hepatitis is also very common among drug abusers who inject themselves, again because they may often share injection equipment and thus transmit infection from one to another. It does not matter whether injection is intravenous, intramuscular or subcutaneous; once the skin has been breached by a contaminated needle, the infection can be introduced.

Hepatitis B

The variety of hepatitis most likely to be associated with drug abuse is caused by the hepatitis B virus (HBV) that can be detected in the body by various markers or antigens to which the body responds by producing specific antibodies. After infection there is a long incubation period of 2–6 months, and during this time the patient is asymptomatic, although capable of infecting others. The virus replicates itself inside the cells of the liver and this may or may not result in acute hepatitis. The illness begins insidiously, usually with loss of appetite, nausea, tiredness and general malaise. There may be vomiting and abdominal distension and discomfort; a loss of desire for cigarettes by smokers is said to be a classic symptom; and skin rashes, joint pain and severe headaches may also occur. There may or may not be a fever which subsides when jaundice becomes apparent. The liver enlarges and becomes tender and there are abnormalities of liver function: serum glutamic oxalo-acetic transaminase (SGOT) and serum glutamic pyruvic transaminase (SGPT) are raised and the SGOT : SGPT ratio is usually less than 1 (less than 1 or 2 in alcoholic liver disease).

In the UK, acute clinical hepatitis B is a notifiable disease and between 1975 and 1980, about 18% of reported cases each year occurred in drug abusers (about 200 cases per year). After a slight increase in 1981–83 in the total number of cases, there was a sharp rise in 1984 in both the total number of cases and in the number of drug-abuse-associated cases, followed by an equally sharp decline to much lower levels than previously. Various explanations have been offered for this reversal in the trend, but it is hoped that it is due, at least in part, to reduced sharing of injection equipment. Other factors, such as increased immunization rates and a reduced number of users who inject may also be significant.

Chronic hepatitis

Usually, viral replication ceases as antibodies develop to the viral surface antigen (HBsAg) and these antibodies confer lasting immunity, so that reinfection with HBV cannot occur. In about 10% of cases, however, viral replication does not stop and the virus remains in the liver, usually for the rest of the patient's life. Persistent, chronic infection may not be associated with liver injury and the patient may be asymptomatic, but still capable of transmitting infection to others This situation is recognized by the persistence of HBsAg in the blood. Persistent HBV infection may result in chronic hepatitis which is defined as liver inflammation (recognized by elevation of transaminases) persisting for longer than 6 months. Two types of chronic hepatitis have been described: chronic persistent hepatitis, which is relatively benign, and chronic active hepatitis, which is progressive. This in turn may lead to cirrhosis, in which the liver becomes irreversibly damaged. Many drug abusers, already vulnerable to liver damage from viral hepatitis, also damage their livers by excessive consumption of alcohol. It has recently been shown that chronic, asymptomatic carriers of HBV are at greater risk of developing liver injury from alcohol than non-carriers, and consequently, they should be strongly advised not to drink alcohol. It should be noted that chronic hepatitis B infection is now the most common cause of primary hepatocellular carcinoma – cancer of the liver. The risk of developing this cancer is estimated to be 250 times greater for chronic carriers of HBV than for those who are uninfected.

Hepatitis C

The occurrence of multiple episodes of hepatitis in drug abusers used to be attributed to infection with hepatitis A virus (HAV) or to exacerbations in a chronic carrier. However, specific antigens and antibodies have now been identified, indicating that other viruses are involved. These were previously known as non-A, non-B hepatitis agents (NANB), but hepatitis C virus (HCV) has now been separately identified as being responsible for many episodes, not only in drug abusers, but also in haemophiliacs and other recipients of blood transfusions and blood products. Antibody testing indicates a very high level of exposure to HCV in drug users, but because the initial illness is commonly mild, many patients deny any knowledge of having had hepatitis, despite the presence of antibodies. The implications and long-term prognosis of HCV infection, in terms of the frequency of occurrence of chronic active hepatitis, cirrhosis and hepatocellular carcinoma is still uncertain. However, given that in some areas, 60–80% of injecting drug abusers have HCV antibodies, the concerns regarding long-term morbidity are high. It is known, for example, that a persistent carrier state may develop, although the test to establish this is not yet readily available.

Delta virus

During the last decade another hepatitis virus, the delta virus, has been the subject of considerable investigation and research. It is now known that it is a unique but defective transmissible virus and that infection with it can only occur if the individual is simultaneously infected with HBV, or is a chronic carrier. Two basic categories of delta infection have therefore been identified. 'Co-infection' occurs when there is simultaneous infection with both HBV and delta virus. Most of such cases run a fairly benign course, similar to that caused by HBV alone, with progression to chronic B+D hepatitis occurring in only 2% of cases. 'Superinfection' with delta virus occurs when the patient first became infected with HBV some months earlier, or if he/she is already a chronic carrier. In these situations, HBV is already replicating vigorously and the delta virus can begin to replicate immediately, resulting in a very severe infection. Delta superinfection is therefore associated with fulminant hepatitis and a high rate of progression to chronic active hepatitis. It is not associated with a greater risk of liver cancer, perhaps because of the high early-mortality rate.

Treatment

There is no specific treatment for acute hepatitis. Bedrest, according to how the patient feels, a well-balanced, normal diet with an adequate intake of calories and abstinence from alcohol are probably the most important points. Admission to hospital for a few days may be necessary if the patient is ill and/or domestic circumstances do not permit adequate care at home. Fulminant hepatitis and death occur in less than 1% of cases. In severe cases, opiate withdrawal itself may be hazardous and can precipitate hepatic failure. Detoxification must therefore be very gradual and must be closely supervised. Prothrombin time should be measured three times a week, any prolongation suggesting that hepatic failure may be imminent.

Special antiviral drugs such as interferon and vidarabine have been tried in some cases with persistent hepatitis-B viraemia with delta infection. The decision to use interferon is based on evidence of HBV replication in the serum and in the liver detected by the presence of specific antigens. Interferon is administered subcutaneously for a 16-week course and the success of treatment depends on the duration of infection and on the integrity of the immune response. Non-compliance with the arduous treatment regime may preclude some patients being offered treatment with interferon, which is unlikely to be effective if the patient continues to take opiate drugs by injection.

As indicated above, asymptomatic chronic carriers of HBV should be advised to stop drinking alcohol.

Prevention of transmission

HBsAg has been detected in all body fluids, so there is a theoretical risk that hepatitis can be transmitted other than by parenteral infection. It can undoubtedly be spread by sexual intercourse. Perinatal transmission can also occur (see p. 271). The measures for preventing the transmission of hepatitis B and C are identical to those recommended for HIV: there should be no sharing of injection equipment and 'safer' sexual practices should be adopted. Clinical and laboratory staff are at risk of contracting hepatitis from drug abusers in the same ways that they are at risk from HIV infection. Indeed, at present there is a greater risk of hepatitis, both because more drug abusers are infected with HBV and HCV than with HIV, and because the hepatitis viruses are more resilient to destruction outside the body. The stringent procedures which have been adopted since the threat of AIDS was identified will also prevent the transmission of hepatitis. They should be routine when handling any specimen from any drug abuser who injects drugs.

Screening

In the UK and other countries where the prevalence of HBV is low, screening for hepatitis is not cost-effective. However, high-risk populations, such as drug abusers who self-inject, should be screened, and, if negative, be offered immunization. Antibody to hepatitis B core antigen (anti-HBc) is the best prevaccination screening test.

Active immunization against hepatitis B

The development of a vaccine for hepatitis B has proved difficult because of repeated failure to grow the virus in tissue culture. A vaccine of alum-absorbed, inactivated HBsAG was eventually prepared from the serum of chronic, symptomless carriers. The vaccine is safe and effective, although expensive, but is unacceptable to many people because of a perceived (but unproven) risk of transmission of HIV and/or other infections. A more recent development has been to apply genetic engineering techniques. Genetic material (DNA) from HBV is introduced into yeast cells so that they possess some of the antigenicity of HBV and can stimulate antibody production. Any possibility of disease transmission is ruled out because only part of the genetic material from HBV is used.

The availability of an absolutely safe vaccine means that a policy of active immunization for those at risk from infection with HBV can be implemented. Immunization should be offered to drug abusers who inject, to the staff at drug-dependence treatment units and to others who are in regular contact with, and give treatment to, drug abusers who self-inject. Sexual contacts and family members in close contact with patients infected with HBV should also be immunized.

For both types of vaccine, a course of three doses is required, with the second dose being given 1 month after the first and the third 5 months later. Booster doses are recommended every 5 years, but should be repeated earlier if antibody levels are low following immunization, because this indicates continued susceptibility to hepatitis B.

Passive immunization against hepatitis B

A single, acute exposure to HBV may occur if someone is accidentally pricked with a needle used by or for a patient with hepatitis B, and this is an indication for passive immunization. Hepatitis B immunoglobulin should be given as quickly as possible, and preferably within the first 48 hours after exposure. A dose of 3 ml (200 iu of anti-HB/ml) is usually administered and repeated 30 days later. Alternatively, active immunization with vaccine can be combined with simultaneous administration of hepatitis B immunoglobulin, given at a different site.

Immunization against hepatitis C and delta virus

As yet there is no vaccine for hepatitis C or delta virus. However, as the clinical course of HBV infection is much more severe if the patient also has HCV, vaccination against HBV is especially recommended for those with HCV antibodies but no evidence of immunity to HBV. Immunization against hepatitis B also protects against delta virus because this virus only replicates in the presence of hepatitis B infection.

Pulmonary complications

Pulmonary complications are common among drug abusers who inject their drugs because of the introduction into the venous system of particulate matter – either from crushed tablets or the insoluble adulterants of illicit drugs. These particles (microemboli) become trapped in the tiny arteries of the lungs, which they obstruct, causing those areas of the lung that are deprived of their blood supply to die (pulmonary infarction). Areas of inflammation – granulomas – may surround these microemboli, and the occlusion of the pulmonary arterioles may sometimes be so severe and widespread that there is an increase in pulmonary artery pressure (pulmonary hypertension). This should be suspected in a patient who complains of fatigue, breathlessness or angina. Later, there may be oedema and the patient may cough up blood. Little can be done to improve the situation and the prognosis is poor.

Psychiatric complications

The abuse of potent psychoactive drugs does not always produce the desired and sought-after psychic effect but may, on occasion, lead to an abnormal and unwanted mental state. Sometimes the drug-abusing individual becomes unconscious (or drowsy), and sometimes he/she becomes very disturbed and may suffer from hallucinations or delusions. These conditions may arise because a single, very large dose of the drug was taken (overdose), or because of excessive consumption over a long period (chronic intoxication), or because the drug-abusing individual is unusually sensitive to the effect of a particular drug and develops an idiosyncratic response. Sometimes the abnormal mental state may be due to a 'flashback' – a recurrence of a hallucinogenic drug experience after the effect of the drug has worn off – and sometimes it may be due to drug withdrawal.

The patient's mental state depends on which drug has been taken and its dose, and on the individual's previous experience with drugs and dependence status. Often, none of these variables is known, so that the doctor or other health-care worker is confronted with a patient in an abnormal mental state, suspected of being due to drug abuse, and has to proceed in ignorance of the underlying cause. Patient care and management is therefore based on sound general principles and there is little treatment that is drug-specific. Certain symptoms and signs are suggestive of particular drugs and sometimes there is a clear history of what has been taken. However, even apparently sound information may be misleading or may only tell part of the story: illicitly obtained drugs are often contaminated with unknown adulterants, some of which are pharmacologically active. Street heroin, for example, is often adulterated with a barbiturate and/or other sedative hypnotics, so that measures to treat a heroin overdose may be only partially effective and recovery may be complicated by an unanticipated withdrawal syndrome. In addition, deliberate polydrug abuse, overdose and dependence is common and may present difficult problems of management.

The acutely disturbed patient

Several drugs of abuse can cause disturbances of behaviour, depending on the dose that is consumed and the sensitivity and dependence status of the individual concerned. Unfortunately, there are no clear-cut psychiatric 'syndromes' to provide an instant diagnosis of the drug of abuse, and the clinical picture may be complicated by polydrug abuse. Some information may be available from the patient, or others, and this may be helpful in diagnostic and treatment decisions.

A rapid assessment of the patient's mental state should be made in all cases, to provide a record of baseline observations, before medication (if any) is started, and to describe precisely the nature of the behavioural disturbance so that emergency treatment is appropriate to the condition. A systematic approach to the description and assessment of the acutely disturbed patient is essential and a suggested format for these assessments is provided below.

1   General behaviour. What is the patient doing? How is the patient behaving? Restless, agitated, tense? Gestures, grimaces? Any repetitive behaviour? Hostile, aggressive?

2   Talk. Talking much or little? Spontaneously or only in answer to questions? Coherent or incoherent? Strange words? Flight of ideas?

3   Mood. Constant or labile mood? Cheerful? Depressed? Frightened, suspicious, anxious, perplexed?

4   Abnormal belief. Ideas of reference? Paranoid delusions? Delusions of bodily change? Delusions of passivity? Thought reading or intrusion?

5   Abnormal experiences. Hallucinations or illusions – auditory, visual, tactile? Depersonalization, derealization?

6   Cognitive state. Attitude to present condition? Aware of possible cause?

On the basis of these observations it should be possible to decide whether the patient is suffering from:

1   a psychotic illness, characterized by hallucinations and delusions in a setting of clear consciousness – often manifesting thought disorder and lacking insight into the nature of the condition;

2   a panic reaction, with fear as the overwhelming symptom;

3   an organic mental state: characterized by confusion (disorientation in time and space, impaired mental functioning), and often accompanied by disorders of perception (hallucinations, illusions). The patient is often perplexed and frightened by these experiences.

Any of these three types of reaction can occur with any drug and it may not be possible to decide on clinical grounds which drug(s) caused the abnormal mental state. A physical examination should be carried out whenever possible, but this may be difficult or impossible if the patient is very disturbed and/or hostile. Pulse rate, blood pressure and body temperature should be recorded and a sample of urine sent for toxicological analysis. The vital signs should be monitored regularly until the patient's mental state is normal. Any evidence of self-injection should be noted and the size of the liver recorded.

Management

The patient should be cared for in a quiet environment with no unnecessary stimulation. Lighting should be moderate and there should be no shadowy areas that might be worrying for a delirious or paranoid patient. Above all, the room should be as safe as possible for the patient and the staff, especially if the patient becomes violent.

The staff should be adequately trained so that they can cope confidently with disturbed patients and remain calm. They should avoid moving too close to the patient, and they should not walk behind the patient, because this may seem very threatening to a paranoid individual. Talking should be quiet, but not whispered so that paranoid and delirious patients do not misinterpret what is being said.

Patients should be reassured about the nature of their experiences. It should be explained that their distressing symptoms are drug-induced and will wear off gradually, as the drug is eliminated from the body. Re-orientation – telling the patient where he/she is and what time it is – and offering positive explanations may all help to calm an acutely disturbed patient. In particular, all procedures such as examining the patient and obtaining blood samples, etc. must be explained before they are undertaken.

Acutely disturbed patients are in a state of high sympathetic arousal. They may have a raised body temperature and may sweat profusely. It is easy for them to become exhausted and dehydrated which in turn may exacerbate the underlying condition. It is important therefore that they are cared for in a quiet room where it is easier for them to rest, and that they are given plenty of fluids and actively encouraged to drink enough.

Gastric lavage and forced diuresis to increase drug excretion are rarely appropriate or possible in acutely disturbed patients. Their use in specific clinical situations is described below. It may be difficult to achieve satisfactory environmental conditions for a disturbed patient in, for example, a busy accident and emergency department. Nevertheless, attention to the measures outlined above is positively therapeutic, reduces the risk of outbursts of violent behaviour and may obviate the need for sedative medication. In general, the best approach is to wait for the effect of the drug(s) that have caused the disturbed behaviour to wear off, rather than to intervene with more and different psychoactive drugs to counteract their effects. The latter approach often complicates the clinical picture, making diagnosis more difficult, and carries a risk of harmful drug interactions.

Drug treatment

Some patients may be so disturbed, however, that general supportive measures are inadequate and treatment with drugs is then necessary. If it has not been possible to make a definite diagnosis about the cause of the patient's mental state, an empirical approach to treatment must be adopted.

In general, chlorpromazine is used when psychotic symptoms are the most prominent feature of the patient's condition. It may be administered orally (100 mg) or intramuscularly (50–100 mg). Chlorpromazine should not be given if intoxication with phencyclidine is suspected (see p. 262).

Diazepam is used for panic states and severe agitation. The dose is 10 mg orally or by slow intravenous injection. The intramuscular route should be used only if oral or intravenous administration is not possible.

If an organic mental state is diagnosed, it is best, if possible, to avoid all psychoactive medication.

Differential diagnosis and specific treatments

Cannabis

When taken in sufficient dosage, cannabis typically causes a toxic psychosis with confusion, disorientation, paranoid symptoms (suspicion, delusions) and hallucinations. The combination of organic features (confusion, impaired concentration and memory) with psychotic symptoms is very suggestive of cannabis abuse. In some individuals this develops when only a small quantity of cannabis has been used, but usually it is a dose-related effect. The patient's eyes are often red, due to injected conjunctivae, and although there may be tachycardia, blood pressure is usually normal.

Sometimes these symptoms are nothing more than a 'bad trip' and subside spontaneously. 'Talking down' by peers who are familiar with such adverse responses may be all that is required while the effects of the drug wear off.

Those suffering from prolonged (more than 5–8 hours) and more severe symptoms are more likely to seek professional help. If their behaviour is very disturbed and they do not respond to simple reassurance, chlorpromazine 25–50 mg im acts as a sedative and as an antipsychotic drug.

Flashbacks may occur after cannabis use and should be treated if necessary, according to the patient's mental state, with chlorpromazine.

LSD and other hallucinogens

Although hallucinations and other abnormal perceptual experiences are the sought-after effects of hallucinogens, they are not always pleasurable, and according to the user's mental state and the setting in which drug use occurred, they may sometimes be so terrifying that they overwhelm the drug taker. Thus the typical adverse reaction to hallucinogen abuse is a state of severe panic caused by uncontrolled hallucinations.

At times the patient may be mute and withdrawn, apparently preoccupied by inner experiences, but mood is characteristically very labile and may swing suddenly to severe anxiety. Depersonalization, confusion and suspicion may also occur.

LSD has sympathomimetic effects and somatic signs of its use include pupillary dilation, tachycardia, raised blood pressure and increased body temperature.

The adverse reaction to LSD usually lasts for 8–24 hours and during this time, trained and experienced staff may be able to 'talk down' a panic-struck patient. This is achieved by helping the patient to regain contact with reality and to relax and to understand the nature of his/her experiences without being overwhelmed by them. However, if the patient is excessively agitated, medication will be necessary. Diazepam 10–30 mg orally is usually effective and can be repeated every few hours, if necessary. Chlorpromazine (50–100 mg) is sometimes used, but only if it can be established with reasonable certainty that anticholinergic drugs have not been taken (chlorpromazine potentiates the effects of anticholinergic drugs and may precipitate hypotension).

Flashbacks, if they occur, are usually self-limiting and short-lived and rarely require treatment. Occasionally they occur frequently and become distressing, in which case treatment is the same as for an acute panic attack. Patients should be warned not to take hallucinogens or cannabis again because this may precipitate further flashbacks. If flashbacks persist and become increasingly troublesome, the patient should be assessed more thoroughly for underlying psychiatric illness.

Stimulants (amphetamine and cocaine)

Chronic abuse of central nervous system stimulants causes a psychotic illness characterized by delusions of persecution, ideas of reference and hallucinations (auditory and visual). The patient is likely to be restless, talkative and irritable and may exhibit a repetitive, stereotyped behaviour.

The highly characteristic, almost diagnostic feature, is the absence of any confusion or disorientation so that the psychotic symptoms all occur in a setting of clear consciousness and it may be difficult to distinguish this drug-induced illness from schizophrenia.

The sympathomimetic effects of stimulant drugs may produce characteristic physical signs – tachycardia, hypertension, sweating, raised body temperature and dilated pupils – but these are very variable because of the development of tolerance in the chronic abuser. There may, however, be evidence of weight loss or of self-injection.

Stimulant psychosis usually arises in the course of chronic abuse, but sometimes occurs after a single (usually large) dose. Cases that present for treatment are more likely to be due to amphetamine use than cocaine because the effects of the latter wear off quickly, before they cause excessive concern. After amphetamine, hallucinations disappear over 24–48 hours, but delusions may persist with reducing intensity for a week to 10 days or longer.

An acutely agitated and psychotic patient should be given chlor-promazine 25–50 mg i.m. or 50–100 mg orally and this is repeated as necessary. Haloperidol is also effective. Antipsychotic medication may only be necessary for the first 24 hours, occasionally for a few days. If agitation and anxiety are the most prominent symptoms, diazepam may be used instead.

The excretion of amphetamine can be increased and the duration of the adverse reaction reduced by keeping the patient well hydrated and by acidification of the urine by intravenous administration of ammonium chloride. Urinary catheterization is then essential and serum electrolytes must be measured frequently.

Hyperthermia (raised body temperature) is a potentially serious side-effect of amphetamine overdose. It is more likely to occur in an inex-perienced user after a large dose of amphetamine than in a chronic user who has become tolerant to the effects of the drug, but body temperature should be monitored in all cases. If it rises rapidly or if it rises above 102°F (39°C), it should be treated promptly by sponging with cold water, ice-packs and fanning. Chlorpromazine (25–50 mg i.m.) can be given, but blood pressure should then be monitored closely in case hypotension occurs. It is important to recognize and to treat hyperthermia vigor-ously because it may be the forerunner of convulsions (see p. 263). Severe hypertension is another serious complication of amphet-amine toxicity, because of the risk of cerebral haemorrhage and of cardiovascular collapse. It should be treated with phentolamine 5 mg i.v., repeated if necessary, or with diazoxide 100–150 mg i.v. repeated after 10–15 minutes if necessary.

It is important that patients recovering from stimulant intoxication should be kept in a peaceful environment, away from unnecessary stimulation. They may sleep for many hours as the effects of the drugs wear off and may later become apathetic and depressed, sometimes suicidally. Antidepressant medication may then be necessary.

Phencyclidine

Phencyclidine consumption leads to bizarre clinical states that pose particular problems of management. In doses such as those that are often obtained at street level (5–10 mg) it produces an acute confusional state with disorientation in time and place. Characteristically, the patient is very agitated and often in a state of severe panic. There may be sudden outbursts of very violent behaviour, when the drug abuser seems to have superhuman strength, alternating with periods of mutism when the individual may respond only by nodding or eye movements. The eyes are often held wide open, giving a staring appearance and nystagmus may be present. There may be severe muscle rigidity and a grossly ataxic gait. Episodes of nausea and vomiting may occur. Pulse, blood pressure, temperature and respiration rate are usually increased.

It is generally agreed that patients intoxicated with phencyclidine should be subjected to as little verbal and physical stimulation as possible, to minimize the risk of provoking violent outbursts. Ideally, they should be cared for in isolation on a cushioned floor in a quiet room. The patient should be constantly observed in case convulsions or unconsciousness occur and pulse, blood pressure and respiration should be monitored. It is best not to give any psychoactive drugs at all, but to wait for the effect of phencyclidine to wear off. Most patients can communicate normally within 2 hours and are apparently fully recovered within 4 hours Monitoring should, however, continue for a further 2 hours. If necessary, diazepam 10–20 mg can be given orally to control violent behaviour that threatens the safety of the staff and/or patient. Haloperidol may also be used, but phenothiazines are contraindicated because they are believed to potentiate the anticholinergic actions of phencyclidine and may produce severe and prolonged hypotension. It may be necessary to restrain the patient physically to protect both patient and staff and this is achieved more safely by using people rather than mechanical restraints.

Sedatives

The chronic abuse of sedative drugs may cause acute behavioural disturbances in two quite distinct ways.

1   Chronic intoxication. Patients who take sedatives regularly become tolerant to their effects and tend to increase the dose. When the limit of tolerance is reached, further increases lead to a state of chronic intoxication in which the patient has slurred speech, staggering gait and nystagmus and is mentally confused. Such patients (particularly those taking barbiturates) are characteristically hostile, aggressive and uncooperative, and are often brought to medical attention because of dangerous, socially unacceptable behaviour. Physical examination often reveals characteristic signs of barbiturate self-injection – thrombophlebitis, ulcers, brawny oedema, etc.

Unfortunately, little can be done except to wait for the effect of the drug to wear off, and although during this time the patient may be extremely disruptive and difficult to manage, he/she cannot be discharged because he/she is in a state of intoxication. Pulse, blood pressure, respiration and temperature should be monitored regularly and the patient's level of consciousness recorded. If the patient falls asleep, he/she should be placed in a semiprone position and observations should continue without fail; an intoxicated, conscious patient may lapse into unconsciousness as more of the drug is absorbed into the bloodstream.

After recovery, patients should be admitted to hospital for supervised sedative withdrawal (see p. 223). Many refuse this option and discharge themselves, against medical advice, to resume their drug abuse. They present to accident and emergency departments with monotonous regularity in an intoxicated condition, and it requires a high degree of professionalism to maintain impeccable medical care in the face of such recidivism. Occasionally patients are receptive to crisis intervention and agree to referral to a specialist unit.

2   Withdrawal. Acutely disturbed behaviour may also arise in the course of the sedative abstinence syndrome. Some patients develop a psychotic illness, similar to the delirium tremens caused by alcohol withdrawal, and characterized by disorientation, hallucinations and delusions. The timing of these symptoms depends on the duration of action of the particular sedative, so that they may arise on the 2nd or 3rd day after the last dose was taken, or at any time in the following 2–3 weeks. The physical signs of sedative abstinence include tachycardia, with an increase in heart rate of more than 15/minute, and orthostatic hypotension (fall in blood pressure) on standing. Patients are usually tremulous and severely agitated and may

make determined efforts to obtain their drug. There may be evidence of barbiturate injection.

Once the diagnosis has been made, treatment must be prompt to prevent the onset of withdrawal convulsions. Pentobarbitone 120 mg or diazepam 20 mg should be given and the patient admitted to hospital for stabilization on sedatives and supervised detoxification.

Solvents

The clinical picture varies according to the severity of intoxication and the drug of abuse. At first, the patient appears as if drunk and may be exhilarated in mood and impulsive in activity. More severe intoxication results in an organic mental state with confusion, slurred speech and staggering gait. Hallucinations and delusions may also occur and the diagnosis is confirmed by the smell of volatile inhalants on the breath and clothes.

Patients with acute disturbance of behaviour due to solvent abuse present for treatment only rarely because the reactions are short-lived and resolve spontaneously, as the effect of the drug wears off. There is no specific treatment, but the patient should be carefully observed during the recovery period.

Compulsory treatment

Although drug abuse and drug dependence *per se* do not constitute grounds for compulsory admission to hospital, a patient may sometimes become so severely disturbed as a result of taking drugs that treatment is essential either to protect the patient, or to protect others from the patient's actions. For example, a patient may be so violent and aggressive that he or she has to be physically restrained from attacking anyone nearby. Under the influence of LSD, patients have been convinced of their ability to fly and have attempted to prove it by leaping from a window. These patients lack insight into their condition and are unlikely to consent to treatment. In such situations compulsory treatment is justified for any patient who is a danger to him/herself and/or anyone else, and is permitted under the 1983 Mental Health Act according to the following sections.

Section 2 is relevant if the patient is seen at home or in the accident and emergency department of the hospital. An application for admission is made, based on the written recommendations of two registered medical practitioners who have examined the patient and have then completed the prescribed form. If possible, one doctor should have previous acquaintance with the patient (usually the patient's general practitioner), while the other should be a doctor approved by the Secretary of State as having special experience in the diagnosis and treatment of mental disorder.

A patient who is admitted to hospital under Section 2 may be detained in hospital for up to 28 days, but no longer. Usually, however, the acute effects of the drug abuse have worn off long before the 28 days have elapsed, so that if a longer period of treatment is considered necessary the patient will probably by then be able to decide whether to agree to the treatment.

Section 4. If the patient is acutely and severely disturbed and in need of urgent treatment, it may not be possible to get hold of two doctors quickly enough. In this case an emergency application may be made under Section 4 of the Mental Health Act, either by a close relative of the patient or by an approved social worker. The emergency application must also be signed by one of the doctors described above (either the general practitioner or the specialist). It lasts, as an interim measure, for only 72 hours, and during this time the second medical recommendation for hospital treatment is sought. If it is obtained, the patient can be detained in hospital for 28 days, if necessary.

Section 5. If a patient who is already in hospital becomes acutely disturbed and refuses treatment and/or tries to leave hospital when it is clear that he/she is a danger to him/herself and/or others, the patient may be detained and treated under Section 5 of the Mental Health Act. The registered medical practitioner in charge of the patient makes the formal application which can be enforced for only 72 hours. If it is not possible for a doctor to come immediately to sign the requisite form, a nurse may detain the patient until the doctor arrives, for up to 6 hours.

The drowsy or unconscious patient

Unconsciousness in the course of drug abuse and dependence is usually due to an overdose of an opiate drug or of a sedative hypnotic drug such as a barbiturate, benzodiazepine or methaqualone. Sometimes drugs of both types are taken together causing a potentiation of their effects; alcohol consumption may also contribute to the clinical picture. Prolonged solvent sniffing can also cause unconsciousness. Indeed, coma may be the consequence of an overdose of almost any drug; if it occurs after drugs such as amphetamine, LSD, cannabis, phencyclidine, etc. it is evidence of a very severe degree of poisoning.

Whatever the cause, the priorities of treatment are the same as for any unconscious patient – to establish an adequate airway and to support the circulation, if necessary. The first step, therefore, is to assess the vital signs.

If there is no pulse, cardiopulmonary resuscitation should be started immediately. If the heart is beating, the patient's breathing should be assessed. Central nervous system depressants cause respiratory depression so that slow, shallow breathing is common and there may even be apnoea (breathing stops). If respiration is absent or inadequate, assisted ventilation by mouth-to-mouth resuscitation or Ambu-bag inflation should be started. In hospital, endotracheal intubation can be performed and the patient established on a ventilator. If intubation and ventilation are not needed, an oropharyngeal airway will prevent the tongue from falling back and obstructing the airway. Oxygen may be administered because these patients are usually hypoxic, but this should be done carefully in case the relief of hypoxia precipitates apnoea. The patient should be nursed semiprone to keep the airway clear and to prevent the aspiration of vomit.

Once urgent first-aid measures have been carried out, a rapid physical examination should be made. The following points should be noted to aid diagnosis and so that appropriate action can be initiated.

1   Blood pressure. Low blood pressure (hypotension) is common after barbiturate overdose. Because a systolic blood pressure of less than 80 mmHg may cause brain and kidney damage, it should be treated promptly: intravenous fluids should be administered, preferably with central venous pressure monitoring to prevent fluid overload. High blood pressure may occur in amphetamine intoxication and can be treated with a beta-adrenoreceptor-blocking drug (e.g., propranolol).

2   Pulse. If arrhythmias occur, ECG (electrocardiograph) monitoring should be initiated so that appropriate treatment can be started.

3   Chest sounds. Severe pulmonary oedema is a life-threatening complication of opiate overdose. It should be treated with positive pressure ventilation. Aspiration pneumonia is common after opiate overdose because of depressed reflexes and opiate-induced vomiting.

4   Pupil-size. Pin-point pupils are (almost) diagnostic of opiate use, but pilocarpine, used in the treatment of glaucoma, also causes miosis. Pupillary constriction may be absent after opiate use if large amounts of amphetamine or cocaine were taken at the same time. Prolonged hypoxia, caused by respiratory depression and leading to cerebral (brain stem) anoxia, produces fixed, dilated pupils. In other words, the absence of pin-point pupils does not rule out the possibility of opiate overdose.

5   Breath odour. This may indicate consumption of alcohol or solvent sniffing.

6   Evidence of trauma. Note especially any head injury that may be contributing to unconscious state.

7   Evidence of injection. Needlemarks, abscesses, fibrosed veins etc.

suggest long-term drug abuse and probable dependence. The possibility of the emergence of an abstinence syndrome should be borne in mind.

8   Liver size. Enlarged liver and/or presence of jaundice suggests impaired liver function. All resuscitative measures should be planned to minimize the risk of precipitating hepatic failure.

9   Body temperature. Hypothermia is common in patients who have been unconscious for a long time, and particularly after barbiturate (or phenothiazine) overdose. It is easily missed unless the temperature is taken (rectally) using a low-reading thermometer. The patient should be wrapped in blankets to conserve heat and not exposed unnecessarily for examination and investigation. Hyperthermia (after stimulant overdose) should be treated promptly with sponging, ice-packs and fanning.

10   Investigations. Blood should be taken for toxicological analysis, for blood sugar, urea and electrolyte estimation, and for a blood count. Emergency management cannot wait for the results of these tests, but they establish a baseline which may be helpful for future decisions about treatment.

11   Additional measures. If hypoglycaemia is suspected, administer 50 ml of 50% glucose solution. According to the general condition of the patient (level of consciousness, pulse, blood pressure, respiration) the following measures may be necessary.

(a) An intravenous line can be established to provide rapid access to the circulation, if this proves necessary.

(b) An indwelling urinary catheter may be inserted to monitor urinary output and 50 ml of urine sent for toxicological analysis as soon as possible. Because drugs are concentrated in the urine, they are more likely to be detected there than in the blood sample.

(c) Cardiac monitoring can be initiated.

(d) Gastric lavage may be appropriate if the drug is known to have been taken orally within the previous 4 hours. It should only be done if the heart rate and circulation are stable and should only be attempted in an unconscious patient if there is a cuffed endotracheal tube in place to prevent the aspiration of stomach contents.

Specific measures

Opiate overdose

If unconsciousness is thought to be due to an overdose of an opiate drug, the opiate antagonist, naloxone, can be given. It should be administered intravenously in a dose of 0.4 mg (1 ml), and this can be repeated at intervals of 2–3 minutes until sufficient naloxone has been given to reverse the effect of the opiate overdose Respiration (rate and volume) increases, systolic blood pressure increases, the pupils dilate and the level of consciousness improves. The total dose of naloxone that is required to achieve this improvement varies, according to the dose of opiate that was taken and on pre-existing physical dependence on opiates. There is usually some response after two or three doses, but more may be needed for the full effect.

The duration of action of naloxone is shorter than that of many opiates, so that there is a risk that the patient may slip back into unconsciousness as the effect of naloxone wears off. It is essential, therefore, that the patient should remain under observation after he/she regains consciousness, so that repeated doses of naloxone can be given if necessary. This is especially important if the overdose is of methadone or of the even longer-acting l-alpha-acetylmethadol (LAAM), when monitoring should continue for at least 72 hours. In such cases, continuous intravenous infusion (2 mg naloxone diluted in 500 ml saline) obviates the need for repeated injections and the rate of infusion can be adjusted to maintain level of consciousness, respiration and blood pressure at satisfactory levels.

The response to naloxone in cases of opiate overdose is so reliable that a lack of response implies that opiates have not been taken, or are not the cause of the patient's present state. Up to 10 mg naloxone (in divided doses) can be given to establish this point, and as naloxone has virtually no effect when administered alone, this therapeutic trial has no adverse effect if the patient's condition is not due to opiate overdose (but see below).

Naloxone should be administered cautiously to those who are (or are suspected of being) physically dependent on opiates. Once the respiratory depression has been counteracted, 'surplus' naloxone precipitates the opiate abstinence syndrome. This is short-lived (because of the short duration of action of naloxone) and although not hazardous for the patient, is uncomfortable and distressing. If it occurs, the patient should be reassured that it will not last long, but no attempt should be made to overcome it by giving opiates.

Later, when the effects of the overdose have completely worn off, an opiate-dependent individual will manifest signs of opiate withdrawal. This should be managed by re-stabilizing the patient on methadone, using the procedure described on p. 213.

Naloxone is generally considered to be a pure opiate antagonist, devoid of pharmacological activity except for its reversal of opiate effects. It may, very rarely, cause hypertension, pulmonary oedema and cardiac arrhythmias (usually only in those with an underlying cardiac abnormality). The risk of these serious adverse effects is so small that naloxone continues to be recommended for the treatment of opiate overdose.

Sedative hypnotic overdose

There is no antagonist for the treatment of sedative overdose so that the keynote of treatment is good supportive care. Forced alkaline diuresis used to be advocated for patients in deep coma, but this procedure is not without risk and it is now recognized that it is useful only for severe phenobarbitone poisoning. Charcoal haemoperfusion is used for patients with severe barbiturate poisoning whose condition fails to improve or who deteriorate despite good care.

Particular problems may occur when those who are dependent on sedative hypnotic drugs take a larger than usual dose and become unconscious. Their initial management is the same as for any patient with a sedative overdose, but when the effect of the drug wears off, the abstinence syndrome will become manifest. If it does, it must be treated promptly so that serious complications (e.g., fits) are prevented. Thus the possibility that the patient is dependent on sedatives must be borne in mind so that he/she can be questioned about drug-taking habits when consciousness is regained. In addition, patients should be monitored carefully after recovery, so that the important, early signs of the abstinence syndrome are not missed. If these signs are present, a suitable sedative drug should be given – e.g., phenobarbitone 120 mg or diazepam 20 mg – and the procedure for stabilization and gradual detoxification described on p. 225 should be adopted. Drugs should not be prescribed in the absence of objective signs of withdrawal, even if the patient claims to be suffering from this and asks for drugs.

Another problem, seen most often in those who are dependent on barbiturates and/or methaqualone, is that the patient becomes very restless on recovery from a period of unconsciousness. Such patients may be hostile and aggressive and refuse to stay in bed, staggering around and generally being very difficult to manage. As they are still in an intoxicated condition it is undesirable to prescribe a sedative drug which may precipitate a further episode of unconsciousness. If absolutely necessary, a small dose of chlorpromazine can be administered.

Phencyclidine overdose

Large doses of phencyclidine cause stupor or coma, in which the eyes usually remain open, although the patient only responds to deep pain. The pupils are constricted and there may be roving eye movements, dysconjugate gaze and nystagmus. There is often severe muscle rigidity and episodes of jerky, tonic–clonic movements and facial grimacing. Repeated episodes of vomiting can occur and hypersalivation is common. Life-threatening complications include convulsions, severe hypertension and cardiac arrhythmias (cardiac arrest). Respiratory depression is more likely to develop if opiates, sedatives or alcohol have been taken too.

Gastric lavage can remove large quantities of phencyclidine from the stomach and should be attempted. However, endotracheal intubation is often very difficult because of intense laryngeal spasm and, if intubation is essential for the purpose of ventilation, large (anaesthetic) doses of muscle relaxant may be required.

Severe hypertension should be treated promptly to prevent cerebral haemorrhage. Diazoxide 100–150 mg should be administered as an intravenous bolus and repeated after 10–15 minutes if necessary. Convulsions should be treated with diazepam which is administered slowly and intravenously. The usual dose is 5–10 mg, repeated if required at 10–15 minute intervals.

Convulsions

Convulsions arising in the course of drug abuse and/or dependence usually occur in one of two situations.

1 During withdrawal from a high dose of sedatives in a dependent individual.

2 During severe intoxication with certain drugs – usually stimulants (such as amphetamine or cocaine) or phencyclidine or, more rarely, after very high doses of opiate drugs (such as morphine, pethidine or dextropropoxyphene), or LSD or methaqualone. Convulsions may also develop if prolonged hypotension has led to cerebral anoxia, or if the drug user has a low 'epileptic threshold' so that fits are precipitated by any one of a number of reasons.

Single, short-lived convulsions do not necessarily require treatment. If they occur repeatedly or are prolonged, they should be treated with intravenous diazepam (preferably in emulsion form) injected at the rate of 5 mg/min until the fits are controlled. A dose of 10–20 mg is usually sufficient and can be repeated, if necessary, after 30–60 minutes. If convulsions recur, diazepam can be administered by slow intravenous infusion. Because of the risk of respiratory depression when diazepam is given intravenously, equipment should be available for intubation and ventilation if necessary.

Once the emergency treatment of convulsions has been carried out, their cause should be assessed. Patients suffering from the sedative abstinence syndrome should be stablized on an appropriate drug (diazepam or phenobarbitone) and should undergo supervized detoxification (see p. 225).

Further reading

Advisory Council on the Misuse of Drugs (1988). *AIDS and Drug Misuse. Part 1.* HMSO, London.

Advisory Council on the Misuse of Drugs (1989). *AIDS and Drug Misuse. Part 2.* HMSO, London.

Advisory Council on the Misuse of Drugs (1993). *AIDS and Drug Misuse Update.* HMSO, London.

Ashton H (1987). Cannabis: dangers and possible users. *British Medical Journal,* **294,** 141–142.

Besson JAO (1993). Structural and functional brain imaging in alcoholism and drug misuse. *Current Opinion in Psychiatry,* **6,** 403–410.

Bourne PG (ed.) (1976). *Acute Drug Abuse Emergencies: A Treatment Manual.* Academic Press, New York.

Cremers L & Matot J-P (1994). Dimensions of drug and alcohol use and misuse in HIV-risk behaviour. *Current Opinion in Psychiatry,* **7, No. 3,** 285–291.

Connell PH (1958). *Amphetamine Psychosis.* Maudsley Monograph No. 5. Oxford University Press, London.

Dackis CA & Gold MS (1983). Opiate addiction and depression – cause or effect. *Drug and Alcohol Dependence,* **11,** 105–109.

Edeh J (1990). Clinical complications of substance abuse. In: Ghodse AH & Maxwell D (eds). *Substance Abuse and Dependence,* 204–215. Macmillan Press, London.

Ferrara SD (1994). Psychoactive substances: impairment and accidents. *Current Opinion in Psychiatry,* **7, No. 3,** 278–285.

Ghodse AH (1981). Morbidity and mortality. In Edwards G & Busch C (eds). *Drug Problems in Britain: A Review of Ten Years,* 171–215. Academic Press, London.

Ghodse AH & Creighton FJ (1984). Opioid analgesics and narcotic antagonists. In: Dukes MNG (ed.). *Meyler's Side Effects of Drugs,* 11th edn., 137–155. Elsevier, Amsterdam.

Maxwell D (1990). Clinical complications of substance abuse. In: Ghodse AH & Maxwell D (eds). *Substance Abuse and Dependence,* 176–203. Macmillan Press, London.

McLellan AT, Woody GG & O'Brien CP (1979). Development of psychiatric illness in drug abusers. *New England Journal of Medicine,* **301,** 1310–1314.

Ron MA (1986). Volatile substance abuse: a review of possible long-term neurological, intellectual and psychiatric sequelae. *British Journal of Psychiatry,* **148,** 235–246.

Sapira JD & Cherubin CE (1975). *Drug Abuse. A Guide for the Clinican.* Excerpta Medica, Amsterdam.

Strang J & Stimson GV (eds) (1990). *AIDS and Drug Misuse: the Challenge for Policy and Practice in the 1990s.* Routledge, London.

Strang J & Stimson GV (eds) (1992). AIDS and drug misuse and the research agenda. *British Journal of Addiction, Special Issue,* **87,** 343–498.

8

Special problems

The pregnant addict

Pregnancy

The antenatal care of the pregnant drug addict or drug abuser has exactly the same aims as for the non-drug-abuser – to keep the woman in good health for her own sake, and to give her the best chance of delivering a healthy child. Achieving these aims is often complicated not only by the pharmacological effects of the drugs the mother uses but also by her lifestyle.

To start with, the diagnosis of pregnancy and hence the initiation of antenatal care may be delayed because there is a high incidence of abnormal menstrual cycles and amenorrhoea during opiate administration, that often resolves when drug use is interrupted. Thus, it may happen that a woman who has become pregnant while temporarily abstinent assumes that her subsequent amenorrhoea is due to a resumption of drug-taking, and does not present to an antenatal clinic until well into her pregnancy, when her increasing weight and enlarging abdomen become apparent. This late presentation may be particularly disadvantageous for those living in poor environmental conditions and with poor nutrition who need the vitamin and mineral supplementation routinely provided during pregnancy. Others may attend antenatal clinics, but are frightened to admit their dependence and conceal it from obstetricians and others.

However, once aware of their pregnant condition, many drug addicts do approach their general practitioner or another agency for advice. Their motivation to come off drugs may be high at this time because they are afraid that their newborn child will be taken from them, or at least placed on the Child Protection Register, if they are still taking drugs at the time of birth. It is very important that these women, with all the normal emotional sensitivity and vulnerability of pregnancy, plus their additional anxieties and feelings of guilt, should be handled with tact and sensitivity, so that they are attracted into and are retained in treatment and that nothing deters them from seeking further help.

The majority of pregnant drug addicts are dependent on opiates that cross the placenta and affect the fetus directly. Constantly exposed to these drugs, the fetus also becomes dependent on them and suffers from withdrawal if the mother is deprived of her drugs. This may precipitate fetal distress or death or induce premature labour. On the other hand, an opiate overdose may also affect the fetus adversely. A similar situation arises with those dependent on sedative hypnotics, but this type of drug dependence may be particularly hazardous for the fetus because it is often associated with a chaotic lifestyle, alternating episodes of intoxication and withdrawal, with rapidly fluctuating blood levels of the drug. Obviously, if the mother injects drugs, the fetus is constantly exposed to the risk of infection and the effects of unidentified adulterants.

Whenever possible, pregnant women should be encouraged to come into hospital at least for the initial assessment period and, in an effort to engage all patients in treatment, clinic and in-patient units should be more flexible than usual and ready to make exceptions to their usual policies. The ideal management is to assist the pregnant woman to come off drugs as comfortably and as early in pregnancy as possible. Ideally, the patient should be drug free for at least 2 months before the expected date of delivery as this will ensure a non-addicted infant, even if there is some uncertainty about dates.

For opiate-dependent patients, methadone withdrawal should be achieved gradually, to avoid precipitating fetal distress or premature labour, and the withdrawal programme should be individually tailored according to the severity of dependence, the stage of pregnancy and the general level of cooperation and motivation. When a pregnant patient is unable to cope with being drug free or has presented too late in pregnancy for complete withdrawal to be feasible, then maintenance on the lowest possible dose of oral methadone is an acceptable alternative to the ideal. Generally, and empirically, a dose of 25–30 mg or less methadone daily is acceptable. It is essential that pregnant barbiturate addicts should be weaned off their drugs and should adopt a more stable lifestyle.

Liaison with the obstetrician and with local social services is essential during the treatment of pregnant patients. In many cases it can be anticipated that a case conference will be arranged after the birth to consider the degree of risk to which the baby is exposed and to plan appropriate action. This should be explained to the mother who should be reassured that each situation is assessed individually. It may then be a powerful inducement to her to cooperate fully with the treatment regime and to withdraw from drugs, if she knows that being drug free at delivery and achieving stability substantially improves her chances of keeping her child. On the other hand, if she believes that the child will automatically be removed or placed on the Child Protection Register, she may retreat from any source of professional help only to reappear near term, or even in labour. By this time the baby is genuinely at risk and the opportunity for positive action has been lost.

HIV and AIDS in pregnancy

Antenatal HIV screening

All pregnant addicts (and those planning to have a child) should be encouraged to be tested for HIV antibodies. The woman will then be able to make an informed choice about whether or not she wishes to continue with the pregnancy (or whether or not she wishes to become pregnant). Secondly, if she is found to be HIV-positive, she can be offered appropriate medical treatment, as can the baby, if she continues with the pregnancy.

Effect of pregnancy on HIV and AIDS

Because pregnancy causes suppression of the immune system, there is a theoretical risk that HIV and related infections may progress more rapidly in a pregnant addict. The evidence on this point is conflicting. In the early stages of HIV infection, the woman's health appears to be unaffected by pregnancy. However, if she has stage IV infection (see Chapter 7), with clear evidence of damage to the immune system, then her health may be adversely affected if she becomes pregnant. If the child is infected, the outcome for him/her may be worse. Despite this, a 3-year follow-up of age-matched, HIV-positive pregnant women compared with HIV-positive, non-pregnant women showed no difference between the two groups in terms of the clinical stage of the disease, T4 lymphocyte counts and other laboratory tests. Other studies, however, have shown greater falls in T4 cells in HIV-positive women in pregnancy than in those who were HIV-negative.

Labour

Pain relief in labour

The management of pain relief in labour for women who have been using opiates during pregnancy can be more difficult than usual because the dose of opiate required to achieve adequate analgesia for the mother may be too high as far as the baby is concerned. An epidural anaesthetic may therefore be indicated and this, as well as other approaches to pain control, should be discussed with the mother beforehand, so that her anxieties can be acknowledged and discussed and so that her wishes can be taken into account.

Infection control in the labour room

Although drug abusers who self-inject are more likely to be HIV-positive and more likely to be carriers of hepatitis B virus, no special precautions need be taken for them in the labour room, over and above those taken for any other woman. This of course assumes that all delivery units maintain a high standard of care, with adequate precautions being taken for every delivery, so that there is then no reason to single out and alienate women who are positive for these infections, and staff are not at risk when dealing with undiagnosed cases.

The neonate

Congenital abnormalities

A major concern for the pregnant drug abuser is the fear that her baby will have a congenital abnormality attributable to drug-taking in pregnancy. In fact, there is little evidence that any of the common drugs of abuse are teratogenic. Although LSD produces chromosomal damage in human leucocytes in culture, and can cause congenital malformations in rats and mice, there is no firm evidence of its teratogenicity in humans. Similarly, although cannabis has been suspected of causing limb deformities, this is a fairly common abnormality, so that anecdotal acccounts of such abnormalities in babies born to cannabis abusers do not prove causality. There have been similar stories about the effects of cocaine abuse on the fetus, but again little in the way of proof of teratogenicity.

When interpreting reports of teratogenicity, it should be remembered that a high proportion of drug abusers are poly-drug abusers and may not remember which drugs they took during the critical period of teratogen sensitivity in the early weeks of pregnancy. Furthermore, even if they do remember, illicit drugs are usually impure and may be contaminated with unknown adulterants that may, themselves, be teratogenic. This serves to emphasize the point that, although none of the common drugs of abuse have definitely been implicated as teratogens, their consumption along with unknown contaminants is a violation of the general principle that no unnecessary drugs should be taken during pregnancy.

Low birthweight

Numerically, a far greater problem than the potential risk of teratogenicity appears to be that of low birthweight, which has frequently been reported in babies born to mothers dependent on opiates. Indeed, in one study, 31% of such babies were light for gestational age. The significance of low birthweight is its association with increased infant morbidity and mortality, but it is not clear to what extent these adverse effects are attributable directly to the drug of abuse or to the pregnant addict's lifestyle. There may, for example, have been repeated episodes of drug withdrawal during pregnancy, affecting bloodflow to the placenta and impairing fetal growth. Repeated episodes of infection and maternal undernutrition may also have undesirable effects. It has been suggested that cannabis and cocaine, by impairing fetal oxygenation, may contribute to poor growth. Both drugs increase maternal blood pressure and heart rate, and cocaine causes uterine vasoconstriction; cannabis, like cigarette-smoking, impairs oxygenation by substantially increasing blood carboxyhaemoglobin levels.

A final point worth noting in relation to low birthweight is that the majority of drug abusers smoke and drink alcohol too. Both of these drugs are known to be associated with low birthweight, so that identifying the additional effects of specific drugs of abuse is very difficult.

Neonatal abstinence syndrome

There have been many reports of a neonatal abstinence syndrome developing in babies born to opiate-dependent mothers. It arises because the blood-borne supply of opiates on which the baby has become dependent during its intra-uterine life is abruptly cut off. The infants are described as hyperactive, irritable and restless, with tremors and sometimes convulsions; some may have gastrointestinal disturbance with vomiting. The onset of the neonatal abstinence syndrome depends very much on the duration of action of the opiate on which the mother is dependent. In an infant born to a heroin-dependent mother, signs are usually apparent within 24 hours, but may be delayed to the 2nd or 3rd day, whereas in infants born to methadone-dependent mothers, the withdrawal syndrome does not usually start until 48–72 hours after birth and may be delayed even later.

It should be emphasized that the neonatal abstinence syndrome does not always occur, but depends on the dose of opiate taken by the mother, the duration of her dependence and the timing of the last dose in relation to the time of delivery. When illicit opiates continue to be abused during pregnancy, the adulterants may also affect the manifestations of the abstinence syndrome.

Treatment should be initiated if withdrawal signs are observed. A number of treatments have been tried over the years, including the inhalation of opium smoke and a variety of sedatives, such as paregoric (camphorated tincture of opium), barbiturates and chlorpromazine. Breast-feeding has been advocated if the mother continues to take opiates on the grounds that they are believed to be secreted into breast milk and can thus ameliorate the abstinence syndrome. On theoretical grounds, however, the administration of opiates to the infant after delivery is contraindicated, as any metabolic changes induced by exposure to them *in utero* are likely to be accentuated by their continued use. Chlorpromazine is generally recommended as the drug of choice, but it should be started only if there is evidence of progression in the number or severity of the signs of withdrawal. The dose should subsequently be reduced in a stepwise fashion every 2 or 3 days. Prophylactic treatment, with chlorpromazine or any other drug, is not recommended, because it is unjustifiable to expose those who are not going to manifest the withdrawal syndrome, or those who will do so only mildly, to yet more unnecessary drugs. Instead, an alert watch should be kept so that signs can be treated promptly, if and when necessary. Problems may arise when the mother's drug use is neither known nor suspected, so that diagnosis of the infant's physical condition is delayed.

With the increasing use of psychotropic drugs, many of which have a dependence-producing capacity, other withdrawal syndromes have been described in neonates. The signs of barbiturate withdrawal in the newborn are similar to those of opiate withdrawal although their onset is often delayed, sometimes for up to 4–7 days after birth. This delay can itself be hazardous as mother and baby may be discharged before the withdrawal syndrome manifests itself. Cases of benzodiazepine withdrawal (similar to barbiturate withdrawal) in infants have also been described. Experience in managing neonatal sedative hypnotic withdrawal is limited, but phenobarbitone is a logical choice of drug treatment to minimize the risk of convulsions.

The effects of maternal amphetamine abuse on the neonate are not clear. Although withdrawal signs have been described occasionally, it is not apparent whether these are really due to amphetamine or to concomitant use of opiates.

HIV and the neonate

It is very important that babies born to HIV-positive mothers should be tested for the presence of antibodies and maternal consent for this should be sought. Ideally, this will have been discussed with the mother at some time during her pregnancy, rather than being left until after delivery, when the new mother is likely to be emotionally labile.

Currently, it appears that there is a 13% risk of transmission from mother to baby. Of those that are infected, 83% show laboratory or clinical signs of infection by the age of 6 months; by 1 year, 26% will have AIDS and 17% will die of HIV-related disease. However, these figures undergo frequent revision as the results of longitudinal studies of greater duration become available. It should be noted that a positive HIV test at birth does not necessarily mean that the baby has been infected, because babies are born with the mother's antibodies, which persist for up to 18 months. An antibody test at this later date will give more reliable information, but as this is a long time to wait, other blood tests may be carried out in the interim that may help to determine whether or not the child has been infected. The reliability and sensitivity of these tests (e.g., antigen test, blood culture, immunoglobulin test, polymerase chain reaction) are still being evaluated, and some are difficult to perform on young babies.

Hepatitis and the neonate

Babies born to mothers who are hepatitis B carriers should be immunized as soon as possible after birth, or at least within 12 hours of birth, because this significantly reduces the chance of the baby developing the persistent carrier state. Infants of mothers who are HBV–DNA-positive (indicating active viral replication) are most at risk and active immunization with the vaccine should be combined with simultaneous passive immunization (administration of hepatitis B immunoglobulin) at a different site. This has been shown to have a success rate of over 80% in keeping infants HBsAg-negative at 1-year follow-up. Infants born to mothers who are HBsAg-positive, but HBV–DNA-negative have a low risk of becoming HBsAg-positive and immunization may not be necessary for these children.

Breast-feeding

Although breast milk is acknowledged to be the best food for the newborn baby, other factors must be taken into account when advising drug abusers about breast-feeding.

Firstly, the mother's HIV status is an important consideration. HIV has been found in breast milk and it is thought that transmission to the baby via breastfeeding can occur. For this reason, HIV-positive women in the UK have been advised not to breast-feed. However, in countries where adequate substitutes are not available, the advantages of breast-feeding may outweigh the potential risk that, some would claim, is unproven.

Secondly, it must be remembered that many drugs that may cause toxicity in the infant enter breast milk in pharmacologically significant quantities. Barbiturates and benzodiazepines, for example, do enter breast milk and can cause lethargy and drowsiness in the infant. Therefore, if the mother is still receiving these drugs because detoxification before delivery was not possible, it is not advisable for her to breast-feed her baby. The same advice applies to those maintained on opiates (heroin or methadone) and to those who are likely to abuse illicit drugs after discharge from hospital. As a general principle, breast-feeding is no longer considered the best method of alleviating the neonatal abstinence syndrome (from any drug) and in some cases the mother should be advised to bottlefeed.

The child at risk

Once the hazards of the neonatal period have passed, the question remains of whether there is any longer-term effect of the baby's prolonged exposure to drugs *in utero*. Various studies of children born to opiate-dependent mothers have reported abnormal behaviour patterns in these children as they grow older, and developmental delays are said to occur. Later, impaired concentration, hyperactivity and aggression have also been noted. It is, however, impossible to know if these patterns of behaviour and development are more likely to occur in children born to opiate-dependent mothers than to non-drug-dependent mothers and, if they do, whether they are due to intra-uterine exposure to opiates or to their childhood environment, particularly if parental drug abuse continues.

Drug use by parents does not always indicate that they are bad parents. Nevertheless, there is a natural and often severe anxiety about the well-being of children in such a family. This is partly because the harsh facts of child abuse have become apparent to all, through wide exposure in the media, so that the prevention of any more horrifying instances is now of overriding importance. This has led to some local authorities automatically putting the children of addicts on the Child Protection Register, sometimes at birth. Indeed, a legal precedent (in the UK) was set in 1985 when a care order was made on a baby born to a drug-addicted mother on the grounds that its intra-uterine development was being impaired and neglected, and the baby was then removed from its mother at birth. One should note, in passing, that this is routine in some countries, where every child of a drug-using parent is perceived to be at risk of abuse or neglect by reason of their parents' drug-taking. The opposite point of view is that children of drug abusers are no more or no less at risk than children born to any other group of parents, but undoubtedly the reality lies somewhere between these two opinions – some children are at risk and some are not. Preliminary research suggests that abuse is no more common by drug-using parents than by the rest of the population, but that there is an increased incidence of injury as a result of accidents associated with drug use.

It is clearly of the utmost importance that whenever a drug abuser who is also a parent approaches a treatment agency for help, that the child is not overlooked and that their welfare receives specific and deliberate attention during the assessment procedure. It is essential to identify their physical and emotional needs and to make an accurate assessment of the risks to which they are exposed because of parental drug abuse. This assessment must be made in a systematic fashion so that a complete picture is built up of that child's lifestyle. Then, and only then, should a decision be made about his or her future care. The specific questions to be answered by the assessment procedure are shown below.

1 Provision of basic necessities.
   (a) Is the accommodation adequate for children and are rent and bills being paid? (How much do drugs cost and how is the money raised?)
   (b) Does the family remain in one area or do they move frequently? If so, why?
   (c) Is there adequate food, clothing and heating?
   (d) Does the child attend school regularly and how are they achieving at school?
   (e) Are the child's emotional needs being met adequately?
   (f) Has the quality of childcare changed since drug abuse began? Does it improve during periods of abstinence?
2 Home environment.
   (a) Do other drug abusers share the accommodation; is the family living in a drug-using community?
   (b) Is the accommodation used for selling drugs?
   (c) Is the child left alone while parents are procuring drugs?
   (d) Does the child have to assume parental responsibilities?
   (e) Is the child taken by the parents to places where they may be at risk?
   (f) Is the child engaged in age-appropriate activities?

3   Pattern of parental drug use.
   (a) Type, quantity and method of administration of drug?
   (b) Are drugs used in the child's presence?
   (c) Is drug use stable or chaotic?
   (d) Is there polydrug abuse?
   (e) Is alcohol abused?
   (f) Does the drug-abusing parent swing between periods of intoxication and periods of withdrawal?
   (g) How does this affect childcare?

4   Health risks to child.
   (a) Where are drugs kept?
   (b) Can the child gain access to them?
   (c) If drugs are used by injection, where are syringes and needles kept?
   (d) Are they shared?
   (e) How are syringes and needles disposed of?

5   Family's support and social network.
   (a) Is there a drug-free parent (or supportive partner)?
   (b) Do parents and children associate primarily with drug-abusers, non-abusers or both?
   (c) Are relatives aware of drug use? Are they supportive?
   (d) Will parents accept help from relatives or friends and/or other agencies?

6   Parents' perception of the situation.
   (a) Do parents see their drug use as harmful (or potentially harmful) to themselves or their children? Are they aware of the health risks of their drug-taking practices to the children?
   (b) Do parents place their own needs before those of their children?
   (c) Are parents willing to cooperate with monitoring of the situation by nurseries, schools, health visitor, social worker, etc?

When all this information is elicited, it gives a very good idea of what life is like for the child in that household and, in particular, of the degree to which the child's life is affected by parental drug use, or indeed revolves around that drug use. It will be established, for example, whether there are times when the parent is unconscious from a drug overdose when an unsupervised child might play with a dirty syringe, or take tablets that have been left lying around. If the quality of parenting changes little during episodes of abstinence, there may be scant grounds for optimism that things will improve after detoxification. Many such factors must be taken into account, but from the point of view of the child, the single most important factor that may make home-life possible is the presence of a non-drug-using, supportive parent or partner.

This type of assessment procedure should be carried out regardless of whether it is the father or mother who is abusing drugs. It is of course more important if it is the main care provider (or the only care provider in a single-parent family), usually the mother, who is dependent on drugs, but clearly many of the risk factors are independent of which parent is involved; bottles of tablets or dirty syringes left lying around where an unsupervised toddler can reach them are always dangerous. In some families, both parents abuse drugs and this exposes the child to even greater risk. The age(s) of the child(ren) concerned is also relevant. Younger children are at greater physical risk of neglect and accidental injury and there may be clear evidence of failure to thrive. Older children, although better able to fend for themselves physically, are more likely to recognize drug taking and to understand its significance and so may be more emotionally vulnerable.

When all the information about the child and his/her lifestyle has been gathered, a management plan must be formulated. Where a team approach is adopted for the care of drug abusers, it is essential that a keyworker should be nominated who will maintain contact with the family and who will assume special responsibility for the welfare of the child. It is all too easy, in the midst of dealing with the multidimensional problems of drug abuse, to forget, or at least to overlook, the most vulnerable and least articulate members of the family. It is crucial to have one member of the team whose responsibility it is to remind others of the existence of the children and to safeguard their interests.

The management plan should then identify the existing and potential risks to the children and define the particular circumstances that would, if they arose, give rise to special concern. The name and telephone number of the responsible social worker to be contacted on such an occasion should be recorded and accessible. The way in which the family's situation will be monitored and the children will be visited must be decided, and a date set when the childcare aspects of the case will be reviewed. The particular needs and difficulties of the children should be discussed and the ways of dealing with them decided. Many families with a drug-abusing parent are already known to other agencies (social services, probation service, general practitioner) and it is essential that close liaison is maintained with them. They may be able to play a valuable role in monitoring the situation, but feel unable to complete the total assessment without specialized aid. Again, it is the responsibility of the keyworker from the drug-dependence treatment team to liaise with other involved professionals, so that the situation does not arise in which a child's problems are known to many agencies, but appear to be the responsibility of none. Where there are pre-school age children, the family's health visitor will usually be contacted as he/she is in an excellent position to observe the children for any evidence of failure to thrive, neglect or physical abuse. For older children it may be appropriate to contact the school, where teachers who see the children every day are well-placed to monitor their well-being. Parental consent must, of course, be obtained before schools or other agencies are contacted and confidential information disclosed, but in some situations concern about the child may make it necessary to override the wishes of the family. Satisfactory resolution of a conflict between the needs of the child and the rights of the parent requires good judgement and a high degree of professionalism. In rare cases, under the Children's Act of 1989, if the parents refuse to cooperate in a full assessment of the child's situation, even though the professionals involved believe that there is a risk of significant harm to the child, a Child Assessment Order can be made. This allows a full enquiry to be made into the state of the child's health and development and the way in which he/she has been treated, to decide what further action, if any, is required.

If it appears that there is immediate risk to the child – for example, if drug abuse is chaotic with periods of intoxication, when the parent becomes aggressive, or if a young baby is suffering physical neglect – clearly the child must be removed promptly from the family home. This may be done by means of an Emergency Protection Order, followed by a court case, which may lead to permanent removal of the child or plans for his/her rehabilitation; sometimes wardship proceedings are initiated in the High Court. Such actions are fortunately uncommon. It is more likely that although there is no immediate risk to the child, there is some concern and anxiety about his/her welfare that cannot be adequately monitored and protected. In this situation, a case conference should be called to which all the involved and relevant professionals are invited, as well as the family. The outcome will depend on the individual circumstances, but it is likely that either the child will be removed from the family (by one of the proceedings outlined above), or that the child's name will be placed on the Child Protection Register. This means that there will be active involvement of a social worker with the family and further case conferences to monitor the progress of the child will be held. Liaison and communication between the different professions are formalized and every possible supportive service for parents and child is utilized.

It must be emphasized, however, that it is the exception rather than the rule for a formal case conference to be necessary. While recognizing the potential hazards for children growing up in a drug-abusing household, there is no need to exaggerate their problems, which can usually be adequately managed in a less formal manner by the team of professionals caring for the family. A policy of automatically putting all these children on the Child Protection Register may not substantially improve their management, and risks alienating their parents from all professional help. The rehabilitation of the drug abuser and the family, on which the child's welfare ultimately depends, may thus be adversely affected. A far better approach is to assess each family separately, in the way suggested here, and to respond to the children's needs in an individually appropriate manner.

The drug-abusing doctor – the 'professional' addict

The problems of doctors who abuse drugs have long been recognized and there has always been a tacit understanding that they are a 'special' case. In part, this is one consequence of a medical rather than a criminal approach to addiction, with the medical profession responding with empathy to the problems of one of their own kind, but in some ways the 'professional' addicts (doctors, dentists, veterinary surgeons, pharmacists and nurses), are genuinely different from street addicts. They have access to, and usually take, pharmaceutical preparations of drugs which they obtain by a variety of deceptions. The most commonly abused drugs (after alcohol) are the manufactured opiates, particularly pethidine, but also dextromoramide and dipipanone, morphine and sedative hypnotics such as the benzodiazepines. Self-medication for pain and occupational stress are often cited as reasons for the initiation of drug abuse. Professional addicts suffer fewer complications of drug abuse because they use pure, unadulterated drugs and, if they inject, because they have sterile injection equipment and employ sterile techniques. However, the purity of their drugs means that they can have high levels of intake more easily than street addicts and many may become severely dependent. Their drug-taking is nearly always a solitary activity: doctors, unlike those with no profession, or with a job they do not value, have invested a lot in their career and have much to lose financially and in status and self-respect if their drug-taking is discovered. Many doctors successfully conceal their drug dependence for long periods of time and carry on working with apparently little, if any, impairment of their clinical activities. It has even been reported that doctors on high doses of opiates have been able to become suddenly abstinent with no evidence of the withdrawal syndrome, and it was suggested that it was the overwhelming fear of detection that effectively suppressed the expected manifestations.

Eventually, of course, drug abuse and dependence is likely to come to light because of problems with family, personal health or work. There may be a deterioration in personal appearance, frequent emotional crises, admissions to hospital for illness or as a result of accidents, and so on. Abnormal behaviour with staff or patients may be noticed and there may be inappropriate clinical responses. The 'locked door' syndrome has been described – when the doctor has a drink or takes drugs in privacy. There may also be frequent job changes, with many drug-abusing doctors ending up in temporary positions as locums or in deputizing services.

The identification of doctors with drug problems is usually difficult because they commonly deny that any problem exists – they may deny any use of drugs at all, or if they do admit taking drugs, rationalize this as a consequence of certain recent problems (rather than their cause). They usually minimize the dose of drug taken, the frequency of administration and the duration of this practice. Their denial and rationalization is compounded by the behaviour of friends, colleagues and family, who often have a shrewd suspicion of what is happening, but who are usually reluctant to discuss it openly. Eventually, their conspiracy of silence becomes a covert collusion, so that they cover up deficiencies and avoid any action that might publicly expose the drug-taking behaviour. This protective behaviour enables the continuation of the drug abuse and helps the doctor to avoid or minimize its consequences. In the long term such protection, however well intended, is unhelpful. It delays the initiation of treatment because affected doctors are unlikely to seek help on their own initiative, and it completely ignores the well-being of their patients and the hazards that this drug abuse exposes them to. It should be clearly understood, therefore, that doctors and other health professionals have an ethical responsibility to take action if they feel that a colleague has a drug problem that impairs (however slightly) his/her ability to practise medicine.

The best approach, in this situation, is to discuss the problem with other senior colleagues who are in close working relationship with the affected doctor, so that they can exert their influence in a positive and beneficial way, encouraging him/her to admit to the problem and to seek help for it. This confrontation, clearly not a comfortable situation for anyone, must be carefully planned so that it achieves the desired response. It is often better if two doctors approach their drug-abusing colleague together, one perhaps from the same speciality to offer support and friendship, the other a specialist in drug abuse, or perhaps a doctor recovering from drug abuse, to give expert practical advice on treatment. The affected doctor must not be allowed to rationalize the drug taking and deny the problem, but must face up to the fact that he/she has a problem of which others are also aware. It should be understood that the intervention, which is probably resented as an intrusion into private affairs, is prompted by a genuine concern for the health and well-being of the doctor and that the colleagues, far from trying to stop him/her practising, are looking for a way towards recovery so that medical practice can be continued. At the same time, there should be no doubt that a refusal to seek help will have very serious implications for his/her future career. The doctors confronting the drug abuser should have a plan of action ready, so that they can offer positive suggestions about where and how to seek help. This will reduce the sense of despair that may ensue when the problem, with all its implications, has to be faced for the first time. The intensity of this despair should not be underestimated: it may, in some doctors, lead to attempted suicide. Prompt access to treatment facilities is therefore essential and it may be helpful to emphasize that this can be arranged outside the immediate sphere of work and contacts so that confidentiality is, as far as possible, maintained and damage to self-respect minimized.

Once this hurdle – of confronting the doctor and of forcing him/her to confront the problem and do something about it – has been overcome, the outlook improves considerably. Doctors who have been persuaded by a sympathetic, non-judgemental approach to enter a treatment programme are likely to complete it, and probably have a better than average chance of making a complete recovery. Some, however, having taken very high doses of pure drugs for many years, have a severe degree of dependence and their prognosis is poorer – itself a very good reason for colleagues to practise early rather than late intervention. For all, detoxification is just the first stage of treatment and, like all other addicts, they require long-term help and support during their rehabilitation. Regular attendance at a doctor's self-help group may be of value and long-term treatment with the opiate antagonist naltrexone has been reported to be particularly effective in preventing relapse amongst highly-motivated, abstinent 'doctor addicts'. Those who do become abstinent should be given every opportunity to resume medical practice, although continued supervision, including urine tests, will be necessary for some time. They may need to retrain to enter a field of medical practice that gives less easy access to drugs, and it may be necessary, with their consent, to inform a senior colleague of their previous history so that effective monitoring in the workplace is possible should a relapse occur.

It should be mentioned that some doctors enter treatment, not after friendly persuasion by their colleagues, but by routes in which coercion is more overt. For those doctors who come to the attention of their professional disciplinary organization because of their drug abuse, resumption of medical practice will only be permitted when there is clear evidence of successful treatment and subsequent supervision. In the UK, for example, the General Medical Council (GMC) may receive information about a doctor's drug taking from members of the public or the profession, from health authorities or the police. Rather than initiating disciplinary procedures, this information is referred to the Preliminary Screener who decides whether action by the GMC under its health procedures is required. If it is decided that a doctor's fitness to practise does require investigation, the doctor is invited to undergo medical examination. After this, and if the doctor agrees to abide by the recommendations made about his/her treatment, supervision and professional practice, no further proceedings are taken, except to continue to monitor the case. If, however, the doctor refuses the medical examination or refuses to undergo treatment and continues to abuse drugs, then the case will be referred to the Health Committee, which may suspend the doctor's registration or impose conditions upon it.

Drug-dependent patients on general medical and surgical wards

Drug-dependent patients may require admission to hospital for the treatment of a problem unrelated to their drug dependence, or for one of its many complications. Their admission to a general ward, where the staff are unused to drug-dependent patients, may induce considerable anxiety, because they are often perceived as a potential source of unspecified 'trouble'. It may be helpful in this situation to regard drug-dependent patients, like diabetic patients, as having an underlying condition that requires careful, on-going management, while they simultaneously receive specific treatment for a superimposed problem. Specialist help and advice can be obtained about the underlying drug dependence, and the admission to hospital may thus prove to be a valuable opportunity to engage the patient in long-term treatment for the drug dependence.

The question of prescribing maintenance doses of the drugs of dependence only arises for those who are dependent on opiates and/or sedative hypnotic drugs who will become physically distressed if their drugs are suddenly withdrawn. Patients admitted urgently for the treatment of acute medical or surgical conditions can rarely tolerate the additional physical and mental stress of drug withdrawal, so that this is not an appropriate time to consider detoxification programmes. If the patient is receiving a regular prescription for opiates from a clinic or elsewhere, statements about the daily dosage requirement can and should be checked with the prescribing doctor, and the maintenance prescription can then be continued in hospital.

If no such information is available because the patient uses illicit drugs, it is wiser not to accept his/her demands unquestioningly, but to give nothing at first, observe the patient carefully and prescribe only if and when the manifestations of the opiate abstinence syndrome begin (p. 74). Some patients may have only a slight degree of physical dependence and minimal tolerance, and if their uncorroborated claims about the necessary dose are met in full, the greater purity of the pharmaceutical preparation may result in unexpectedly large doses being given, with the risk of ensuing intoxication. It may also cause more severe physical dependence, so that by the time of discharge the patient is taking higher doses than on admission. On the other hand, patients who are given insufficient drugs to control the abstinence syndrome are more likely to discharge themselves prematurely or to persuade friends to bring extra drugs in for them. It is therefore necessary to titrate the dose of prescribed opiate according to the individual's need, using the method of stabilization outlined on p. 213. Methadone, which can be prescribed to addicts by any doctor, without the requirement of a licence, is a suitable choice of opiate.

The same principles of management apply to those who are dependent on sedative hypnotic drugs. They should be stabilized on a sedative drug of the same class as that on which they are dependent as soon as they show any signs of the potentially dangerous abstinence syndrome (see p. 185).

Because drug-dependent individuals often abuse a range of different drugs, they may unwittingly become physically dependent on more than one. Medical staff should be aware of the possibility that someone diagnosed and treated as opiate dependent may also be at risk of developing the sedative abstinence syndrome and should be alert to the need to treat it promptly with the appropriate drug, should it arise unexpectedly. Because long-term maintenance on sedative drugs is not a feasible treatment option, a decision must be made according to the individual needs of the patient about when drug withdrawal should be initiated and how it should be coordinated with other aspects of treatment.

Although it is common for drug-dependent patients to inject their drugs, this should not be permitted in hospital. Their admission can thus be used to show them that drugs taken orally can adequately control and prevent the abstinence syndrome, and to encourage them to adopt this much safer method of drug administration. If medical reasons preclude oral administration, the drugs should be administered intramuscularly.

Opiate-dependent individuals who require analgesics pre-operatively or for severe pain can be given opiates if these are indicated, but they will require higher than usual doses because of acquired tolerance. As a rough guide, they will need the usual analgesic dose in addition to their usual maintenance dose. If heroin is required for the relief of pain due to organic disease or injury, it can be prescribed for an addict by any doctor, without the need for a special licence. In practice, this situation arises only rarely, as there is a natural reluctance to prescribe heroin to those who are dependent on opiates.

The problem of visitors bringing in illicit drugs has already been mentioned. Staff should be aware of this possibility and may, on occasion, have to refuse admission to undesirable visitors. Similarly, routine procedures for the security of drugs on the ward must be strictly implemented, so that no opportunities for abusing drugs are offered to individuals who, because of the severity of their dependence, may not be able to resist them. Medical staff should also remember their statutory obligation to notify the Home Office of any patient who is dependent, or whom they suspect of being dependent, on notifiable drugs; they should not assume that another doctor will already have done this.

Drug-dependent patients in accident and emergency departments

Drug-dependent individuals present frequently to accident and emergency (A & E) departments, either following an overdose or with some other drug-related problem. It is rare for them to attend for a medical problem that is not directly or indirectly caused by their drug taking. Some patients of no fixed abode, or with no general practitioner (GP), use one or more A & E departments as their source of primary health-care and attend frequently for one thing or another, becoming well-known to all the staff. Others are brought in unconscious, with depressing regularity, following repeated overdoses.

Such recidivism is one reason why drug-dependent individuals are unpopular in A & E departments, where non-specialist doctors can feel deskilled and ill-equipped to deal with them. However, the basic tools of history-taking, observation, physical and mental state examination and investigation are all that is required. The doctor needs to be informed of the statutory aspects of addiction and to be aware of local specialist services that are available for onward referral. A written, departmental policy or guidelines for the management of intoxication and drug prescribing for drug abusers is helpful.

Drug withdrawal and drug-seeking attendance

Some drug-dependent individuals attend A & E departments asking for and sometimes demanding drugs, on the basis that their prescribed supplies have been lost or stolen. Commonly, elaborate stories are told to account for this, or they may present themselves as temporary residents who are unexpectedly 'stranded' and unable to return to their treatment unit for their routine prescription. Attendance at night, when verification is impossible, is common. Others may complain of severe symptoms of withdrawal.

In these situations, the golden rule must always be that nothing should be prescribed unless there are clear physical signs of the appropriate abstinence syndrome, that should be carefully documented. In particular, it may be necessary to resist manipulative statements: that the refusal to prescribe will force the individual to resort to illegal activity. Any deviation from this principle may mean that non-dependent, casual users are provided with pharmaceutically pure preparations of dependence-producing drugs, or that the hospital is used deliberately by drug-dependent individuals as a supplementary source of supply; this will increase the severity of their dependence and may contribute to a drug overdose. It is imperative, therefore, that a careful history should be taken to corroborate the account of dependence, and that a thorough physical examination is carried out to establish the nature and severity of the claimed abstinence syndrome.

Of course, if there is any evidence of the sedative abstinence syndrome, treatment should be prompt to prevent the onset of withdrawal fits. Nowadays, barbiturate withdrawal is rare, but can be managed initially by giving phenobarbitone 120 mg orally. It has largely been replaced by benzodiazepine dependence, often as one component of polydrug abuse. Those dependent on benzodiazepines should be given diazepam 20 mg orally; those with a mixed sedative abuse (that often includes alcohol), should receive two capsules of chlormethiazole orally. Their condition should be reviewed after 1 hour, when the intense agitation and distress associated with sedative withdrawal should be at least partially relieved. At this stage, when patients are calmer and more receptive to advice, every effort should be made to encourage them to be admitted to hospital for stabilization and detoxification. The risks of unsupervised sedative withdrawal should be fully explained, and patients should understand that if they come into hospital, they will be given medication to prevent the recurrence of the previous distressing symptoms. Some patients consistently refuse to be admitted to hospital; unless their mental state warrants compulsory admission to hospital under the 1983 Mental Health Act, they cannot be detained, and should be allowed to leave. In other cases, there may be a lack of availability of beds. In such cases, urgent referral should be made to psychiatric or drug-treatment services, or patients should be strongly advised to consult their GP as soon as possible. In the meantime, they can be provided with an adequate dose of their sedative drug to prevent the onset of the abstinence syndrome before they contact their GP. For example, they may need 20 mg diazepam 6-hourly, as takeaway medication for a minimum period, i.e., overnight They should not be given supplies for a longer period because of the likelihood that they will take an overdose, inject it or supply it to someone else.

The clinical situation of opiate-dependent individuals experiencing the abstinence syndrome, although equally distressing, represents no serious danger. If symptoms are mild, consideration should be given to prescribing for symptomatic relief only, perhaps using a combination of a low dose of a phenothiazine (e.g., thioridazine 25 mg qds) and an antispasmodic, anti-diarrhoeal drug (e.g., co-phenotrope, one to two tablets qds) More severe cases may be given methadone mixture 20 mg orally and should then be observed for 1 hour, by which time they should be feeling much better. They should be advised to seek treatment for their opiate dependence and, if possible, referred for specialist advice. A urine specimen taken before methadone administration may be helpful in any future assessment. The opiate abstinence syndrome is not, on its own, an indication for urgent admission to hospital, nor is there any need to prescribe methadone for the patient to take home.

Milder analgesic drugs, i.e., codeine, dihydrocodeine and dextro-propoxyphene preparations are dependence forming. Although the patient may, originally, have been prescribed them during treatment for a gen-uinely painful condition, those who then become dependent on them often obtain supplies by attending several general practitioners and A & E depart-ments with plausible symptoms such as back pain. Physical examination and investigations may be unhelpful in distinguishing between simulated and actual pain and the doctor should be particularly cautious if the patient requests an opiate painkiller or has attended previously in similar circumstances. Prescribing a non-steroidal anti-inflammatory drug would be preferable. Patients who present with more extravagant simulations of very painful conditions such as renal colic may suggest Munchausen's syn-drome, in which dependence on opiates is only one component of the disor-der. Buprenorphine and pentazocine are also abused and may be sought by attenders at A & E departments claiming to have chronic, painful condi-tions. In assessing these patients, the doctor needs to achieve a balance between prescribing to relieve suffering and withholding addictive medica-tion from those who are using it inappropriately. The general principle remains that, if in doubt, only small quantities should be prescribed and the patient referred to their general practitioner, who should be informed of their attendance at hospital.

Drug overdose

It is also common for drug-dependent patients to attend the A & E depart-ment after a drug overdose and the management of such cases is described in Chapter 7. Many of these patients are likely to be unconscious and, unless there is evidence of self-injection, or they are known to the staff of the department, their dependent status may not be suspected. Those who are dependent on sedative hypnotic drugs are likely to present in a state of chronic intoxication when they may be verbally and sometimes physically aggressive towards staff and other patients. Although in this condition they may be extremely disruptive to the functioning of a busy department, so that most staff would prefer them to leave, they should not be discharged in this abnormal mental state. Specifically, they should not be removed by the police to be held in police cells. There is always a risk that these patients may lapse into unconsciousness and that skilled medical care may be urgently required. Hospitals that have to cope regularly with these patients sometimes designate a special area of the A & E department where they can be contained and subsequently sleep off their overdose under medical supervision. When they have recovered a more normal mental state, they should be persuaded to seek help for their underlying dependence.

It is worth emphasizing that A & E staff have a key role to play in the diagnosis of drug dependence, and particularly in identifying drug-dependent individuals among the vast numbers involved in incidents of deliberate self-poisoning. There is clear evidence that many of those who take a drug overdose apparently accidentally, or in a suicidal attempt or gesture, are in fact dependent on these drugs. This may be established if a careful and detailed history is taken with attention paid to points such as the past history of drug overdose, the number of drugs taken, the duration of drug taking and so on, rather than concentrating only on the management of the presenting incident of overdose. Awareness of the possibility of drug dependence will lead to earlier diagnosis and earlier intervention and probably to a better prognosis.

Engagement in treatment

Drug-dependent patients present to A & E departments with a whole range of other problems, of course. The management of many problems has been described elsewhere in this book, but in some ways, the treatment of the immediate complications of drug dependence is only a minor component of the total management of these patients in A & E departments. What is far more important is that these departments are often the only point of contact between drug-dependent individuals and health-care professionals, and are therefore their only route into treatment for their drug dependence. It is therefore essential that the staff who treat them for the complications of their dependence try wholeheartedly to engage them in long-term treatment, rather than adopting the 'sticking-plaster' approach of dealing with the immediate problem and sending the patient away as quickly as possible. It is, of course, completely understandable if they feel like doing just that. As a group, these patients are demanding, difficult and unpopular. Staff who are unaware of the nature of drug dependence do not fully under-stand the overwhelming compulsion to take drugs and perceive the atten-dant complications as self-induced and unworthy of much sympathy. In addition, many drug-dependent patients are very uncooperative, particu-larly when intoxicated, and they rarely express any appreciation for what has been done for them. In other words, they are ungratifying patients to whom the staff are likely to have hostile attitudes.

It requires a high degree of training and professionalism for staff to overcome these attitudes and to respond to drug-dependent patients in a more constructive way. For example, the continual re-attendance of a patient can be used to establish a relationship that may eventually be instrumental in persuading that patient to accept a referral to a drug-dependence treatment unit (DDTU). Such help should be offered whenever a drug-dependent patient attends for treatment because there is evidence that at a time of crisis – when recovering from an overdose, or after experi-encing the effects of drug withdrawal – the patient may be particularly receptive to intervention, and this opportunity to engage the patient should not be lost.

To facilitate the referral process, staff need to have ready access to and knowledge of local advice and treatment agencies, preferably in the form of a comprehensive directory of local services. If the A & E department is in a hospital with a drug unit on site, it is mutually beneficial to establish liaison and referral procedures.

Data collection and statutory requirements

The strategic response to drug-abuse problems depends on information and knowledge of the scale and nature of these, both locally and nationally. It is therefore essential that A & E staff are aware of, and fulfil, their statutory obligation to notify the Home Office of the drug-dependent individuals whom they see (p. 343). In addition, in the UK, many Regional Health Authorities have now established Substance Use Databases (SUD). For these, information is collected on anonymized forms, covering any drug abuse problem, and is not restricted to addiction to notifiable drugs. Clearly, this new database offers the potential for much more comprehensive monitoring of drug-abuse problems, provided that all agencies involved with drug abusers participate by completing the forms. For convenience, combined SUD and Home Office Notification forms are available in some regions.

With the enlarging scope of recreational and experimental drug use, and the development of designer drugs, the A & E department is in the frontline of coping with the adverse effects, and there may be few sources of detailed knowledge of the pharmacological and physiological actions of these new drugs. Good record-keeping will assist in increasing knowledge and, at all times, a urine sample should be collected for toxicological analysis of any attender who is suspected of having a drug-abuse problem. Although the result of analysis is unlikely to be immediately available to influence the management of the patient at that time, it can prove extremely useful in the follow-up and continuing care of the patient.

Drug-dependent patients in the GP's surgery

With the growing number of drug abusers and drug-dependent individuals in the population, GPs are likely to see them more often and have an important role to play in their treatment and management. Although some individuals with drug-related problems recognize that they have a problem and seek help for it, others may approach their GP about an apparently unrelated complaint. An alert doctor, aware of the dependence-producing liability of many of the newer psychoactive drugs, may be able to recognize drug dependence in its early stages and to intervene before it becomes severe and difficult to treat. In particular, it is now recognized that although symptoms such as anxiety, tremor, insomnia and depression, as well as many somatic symptoms, may indicate underlying psychiatric illness or other personal problems, they may also be the early manifestations of the benzodiazepine withdrawal syndrome, and a clear indication of physical dependence upon these drugs. Sometimes the drugs may have been prescribed by the GP, but such is their widespread availability nowadays that the patient may have 'borrowed' them and/or have used up an old supply, and the doctor may well be unaware of this self-medication with prescription-only drugs.

Another common way for GPs to come into contact with a drug-dependent individual is to be approached by someone seeking treatment as a temporary or private patient for a chronic, painful condition requiring potent analgesics, or for insomnia, requiring a prescription for hypnotics. The history is often very plausible, but it transpires later that it is a total fabrication and that the patient has approached a number of doctors, sometimes under an assumed name, in a deliberate attempt to obtain a prescription for drugs on which he/she is dependent. It is, of course, an offence for a patient who is already receiving controlled drugs on prescription from one doctor not to disclose this fact to another doctor who is also going to prescribe them. However, there are many who are not deterred by this and who have a 'collecting round' of several doctors. This is particularly likely to occur with those who are dependent on opiates, and is an excellent reason for the GP approached to check the Home Office Index to find out if the patient has been notified. If the patient is found to be dependent on opiates (or sedatives), drugs should only be prescribed if there is clear objective evidence of the appropriate withdrawal syndrome, and then only as a single dose, preferably to be consumed on the premises. Doctors who prescribe more liberally are likely to find that, as word gets round, they are visited by many more such patients, eager to benefit from a 'soft touch'. Because these patients may be quite prepared to break the law in order to obtain their drugs, it is essential that drugs, syringes, needles and prescription forms are not left unattended.

If it becomes apparent that a patient is abusing drugs or is dependent upon them, or if the GP suspects that this may be the case, the first step must be a thorough assessment of the patient's drug problem. This should include a full drug history and examination of the patient's physical and mental state (see Chapter 4). It is essential to establish whether or not the patient is physically dependent on any drug. If the doctor has had long contact with the patient (and often the family), he/she is likely to be familiar with the patient's social situation, but if not, this is an area that requires clarification. Observed specimens of urine should be taken for drug screening as the findings may provide helpful corroboration of the patient's history.

GPs, like all other doctors, have a statutory obligation to notify the Home Office of an addict who attends their surgery or of any individual whom they suspect of being addicted to a notifiable drug. Notification should be made even if the GP does not treat or prescribe for the patient (p. 343).

The problems of drug abuse and drug dependence are now so great that it is not possible for every case to be referred for specialist treatment, nor is it desirable that this should be done. Indeed, many patients, and particularly those who have become dependent on sedative hypnotic drugs, in the course of medical treatment, may deeply resent referral to a special clinic that they perceive to be the last resort of treatment for 'junkies' and the like. For others in an early stage of a drug-taking career and with only a mild degree of dependence, it may be positively disadvantageous to introduce them to a clinic where they are likely to meet more experienced drug takers and be introduced to the drug sub-culture. Finally, and perhaps most important of all, the GP is likely to have a longstanding acquaintance with the patient, that can be used to enhance psychotherapeutic counselling.

However, some patients have such severe and complex problems that they need all the multidisciplinary resources and expertise of a specialist drug-treatment clinic. Opiate abusers, for example, using other drugs as well; sedative abusers taking large doses of these drugs and who are therefore at risk of withdrawal convulsions; and those chaotic drug abusers whose life has become wholly centred on drugs and drug taking, cannot be satisfactorily treated in a general practice setting, and should be referred to a specialist treatment facility.

When the GP decides to treat the patient him/herself, the goal of treatment is always to help the patient come off drugs, rather than to offer any maintenance treatment. If the patient is physically dependent on opiates/sedatives, a contract should be agreed between doctor and patient specifying the drug to be prescribed, the total duration of treatment and the rate of dose-reduction. If methadone is indicated, prescription must be on a daily basis and six handwritten prescriptions will be required each week (see Chapter 11). Pharmacological treatment is only appropriate for those who are dependent on opiates or sedative hypnotics (e.g., benzodiazepines, barbiturates). No drugs should be prescribed for those who are dependent on stimulants such as amphetamine. During detoxification it is best to avoid prescribing any other psychoactive substances. Apart from the obvious risk of causing dependence on yet another type of drug, it is very important that the patient should learn non-pharmacological responses to symptoms and problematical situations. Counselling, psychotherapy and instruction in simple techniques of relaxation may all be helpful and will also convey this important message. However, if symptoms of insomnia, anxiety and craving are severe and distressing in a patient who is otherwise doing well, a phenothiazine such as thioridazine 25 mg bd can be prescribed – it has few or no addictive properties and the patient is very unlikely to escalate the dose. Drug-dependent patients should be seen at least weekly and there should be frequent, preferably random, urine tests. Every effort should be made to involve the patient (and their family) in local self-help groups and other activities conducive to a drug-free lifestyle.

Patients who have been referred to a specialist DDTU may continue to consult their GP for other apparently unrelated conditions. On no account should any psychoactive drugs be prescribed for these patients without prior consultation with the responsible doctor at the DDTU. For example, if the patient is complaining of severe symptoms of drug withdrawal it is very important that the clinic doctor should be aware of this, so that treatment can be adjusted accordingly rather than the picture being clouded by the patient obtaining drugs from another source. In addition, there is also the risk that some patients may try, quite deliberately, to obtain extra drugs from their GP, and the clinic should be informed of this drug-seeking behaviour.

Substance abusers detained in police custody

Substance abusers are frequently detained in police custody and the advice of forensic physicians (police surgeons) is often requested in these circumstances. These doctors are experienced in dealing with issues such as the individual's fitness to be detained, the need for treatment and fitness for interview. However, if the detainee needs to be transferred to hospital, other doctors and other health-care professionals become involved in their care too, and it is important that they also are aware of particular issues that are relevant to detainees.

The rights and clinical safety of the detainee

Individuals detained in police custody are entitled to the same standard of clinical care as any other member of the public and transfer to hospital may be indicated if, for example, there is an allegation that the detainee has taken drugs prior to their arrest and there is concern about the level of consciousness.

It must be emphasized that consent should be sought for any examination that is undertaken. Also, detainees have the right to have prescribed treatment continued while they are in custody, as long as it is clinically safe to do so. Thus, if the detainee has medication prescribed for him/her in his/her possession, its continued use can be authorized. Sometimes it may be necessary and possible to contact the pharmacist or prescribing doctor to verify details of the prescribed drug. However, on occasion, and particularly if the detainee claims to be suffering from withdrawal symptoms from drugs obtained illegally, treatment will be prescribed at the discretion of the forensic physician. In this situation, a careful and well-documented history and examination is essential; it should be remembered that substance abusers may not be frank and that inconsistent information may be given for some perceived secondary gain. However, an honest history is more likely if the detainee has confidence in the forensic physician and in his/her independence of the police.

Prescribing and drug administration

If a decision is taken that medication is necessary to alleviate symptoms and signs of opiate withdrawal, for example, the doctor may prescribe a drug, such as codeine, that he/she carries with him/her. National Health

Service prescriptions must not be issued for persons detained in custody, for whom drugs should be prescribed on a private prescription. Although all medication in the police station is usually held by the custody officer, on behalf of the detainee, no police officer may administer controlled drugs. Thus if a detainee requires opioid drugs, he/she administers them to him/herself under the supervision of the forensic physician. This does not necessarily require the forensic physician to be present at the time, only that he/she has authorized this treatment. Injectable preparations are utilized only in exceptional circumstances, and in such cases the forensic physician would administer or personally supervise drug administration.

Discharge from hospital

An individual who is well enough to be discharged from hospital may not be fit enough for detention in a police cell. The hospital doctor should take this into account before discharge and, if necessary, recommend reassessment by the forensic physician when the detainee returns to the police station, because this does not happen automatically.

Intimate searches

The authorization of a police officer of the rank of Superintendent or above is required before an intimate seach can be carried out. It must be carried out at a hospital or other medical premises (not a police station) by a registered medical practitioner or registered nurse, and the responsibility for performing the examination lies with the forensic physician and not the hospital doctor. The forensic physician must have obtained informed consent from the detainee and permission from senior medical/nursing staff at the hospital or other medical premises concerned.

Fitness for interview

Forensic physicians and other doctors may be asked for their opinion about a detainee's fitness for interview. Before offering this opinion they should be aware of the proposed time and likely duration of the interview. They will then need to establish whether there is evidence of substance abuse; if the patient is currently under the influence of drugs and/or alcohol; whether there is evidence of the abstinence syndrome; and whether the detainee is fully aware of his/her surroundings, is well enough to cope with a stressful interview, can understand the questions put to him/her and can instruct solicitors.

Particular problems arise if the individual concerned is suffering from drug withdrawal because of the risk of giving a false confession, which is later retracted. This may occur because detainees believe that compliance will result in early release with charges being dropped or altered, while stubborn denial leads to further detention and difficulty in obtaining necessary drugs. In particular, the physical and mental distress caused by drug withdrawal, may make it difficult for the individual concerned to retain coherence of his/her story and to maintain his/her defence, when questioning is carried out by skilled interrogators. If drugs are prescribed to alleviate the abstinence syndrome, it may be argued, later, that the treatment itself impaired the individual's fitness for interview and this may affect the admissibility of any confession.

Where a detainee is obviously intoxicated, it is customary to wait until the effects of the drug(s) wear off before the interview begins. However, when hallucinogenic drugs have been taken, the mental state may fluctuate markedly in the recovery stages and it may not be apparent that the detainee is not fit to be interviewed immediately.

Driving licences

In the UK, holders of driving licences or those applying for a licence are obliged by law to notify the Driver and Vehicle Licensing Agency (DVLA) as soon as they become aware that they are suffering from a 'prescribed disability' (as set out in the regulations of the Road Traffic Act) or any other condition likely to make the driving of a vehicle a source of danger for the general public. Addiction/use of or dependency on illicit drugs are prescribed disabilities and patients should be told of their obligation to inform the DVLA. If they fail to do so, their driving licence and insurance may be considered invalid.

The current UK regulations are in line with the requirements for medical standards of driver licensing set out in the second EC directive. If there is evidence of cannabis abuse, the consequence is a 6 month driving ban; this period is doubled for other drugs (amphetamines, heroin, morphine, methadone, cocaine, LSD/hallucinogens, including the abuse of Ecstasy and other psychoactive substances that are currently fashionable) if evidence of abuse or dependence is confirmed by urine screening. A 'Till 70' licence will be restored only after satisfactory independent medical examination, and urine tests negative for drug abuse The patient is recommended to seek help from medical or other agencies during the period off driving. It should be noted that patients on consultant-supervised oral methadone replacement can have a driving licence, subject to annual review: however, if patients are receiving methadone-maintenance treatment intravenously, it is recommended that their driving licence should be refused or revoked.

The above rules apply to those with an 'ordinary', Group 1 licence for cars and motorbikes. Those holding vocational, Group 2 licences, for vehicles such as lorries and buses, can expect to have their licence refused or revoked for 3 years, during which time there should be no evidence of dependency or continuing misuse. On application for a licence, a specialist medical examination is required with a negative urine screen for drugs of abuse.

Persistent solvent abuse also requires driving to cease and the DVLA to be informed. The licence would be restored after medical enquiries confirm no continuing abuse.

Epileptic fits or seizures may occur in conjunction with drug abuse, and there is an obligation to notify the DVLA of this. In this situation, the licence would be revoked for 1 year after a single seizure or for 2 years if more than one seizure has occurred.

If a doctor believes that a particular patient, when driving, is a grave risk to the public at large (perhaps because of a chronic state of intoxication due to sedative hypnotic dependence), he/she may consider overriding normal standards of medical confidentiality and informing the DVLA. This is a matter for the clinical judgement of the individual doctor who should be prepared to justify the decision if it is questioned.

Travelling abroad

Drugs such as amphetamines, barbiturates and the opiates in Schedules 1–3 of the Misuse of Drugs Regulations (Chapter 11) are subject to legal restrictions on their import- and exportation. However, ordinary travellers are allowed to import/export and possess limited quantities of medically necessary controlled drugs, by virtue of an 'open general licence' held at the Home Office. This is intended to cover an average prescription for 15 days, and up to 500 mg methadone would be reasonable. Larger quantities, even if the drugs have been legally prescribed, require an individual export licence which is issued by the Home Office (drugs branch). This facilitates passage through British customs but, like the 'open general licence', has no legal status outside the UK. Details of the import licence required by the country of destination (if importation is permitted at all), can be obtained from that country's embassy.

The question of an addict taking drugs abroad is most likely to arise for stable opiate addicts on methadone maintenance who want to go abroad on holiday. If the doctor in charge of the patient's treatment has personal contact with colleagues in DDTUs in other countries, it may occasionally be possible to arrange for methadone to be prescribed by them for the period of the holiday. Generally, however, it must be accepted that opiate dependence significantly curtails an individual's freedom to travel – and this may be used as an additional incentive for coming off drugs.

References and further reading

Brewster JM (1986). Prevalence of alcohol and other drug problems among physicians. *Journal of the American Medical Association*, **255**, 1913–1920.

Ghodse AH, Reed JL & Mack JW (1977). The effect of maternal narcotic addiction on the newborn infant. *Psychological Medicine*, **7**, 667–675.

Ghodse AH (1990). Clinical complications of substance abuse. In: A H Ghodse & D Maxwell (eds). *Substance Abuse and Dependence*, 16–231. Macmillan Press, London.

Guidelines for the Clinical Management of Substance Misuse Detainees in Police Custody (1994). HMSO, London.

Richmond RL & Anderson P (1994). Research in general practice for smokers and excessive drinkers in Australia and the UK. *Addiction*, **89**, 35–62.

Riley D (1987). Management of the pregnant drug addict. *Bulletin of the Royal College of Psychiatrists*, **11**, 362–365.

Robertson JR (1985). Drug users in contact with general practice. *British Medical Journal*, 290, 34–35.

Stimson GV, Oppenheimer E & Stimson CA (1984). Drug abuse in the medical profession: addict doctors and the Home Office. *British Journal of Addiction*, **79**, 395–402.

Willette RE & Walsh JM (eds) (1983). *Drugs, Driving and Traffic Safety*. WHO Offset Publication No 78. WHO, Geneva.

9

Follow-up and treatment outcome

Introduction

Those who have read the earlier sections of this book will appreciate that there is no quick solution, no 'cure' for drug abuse, and anyone who has come into contact with drug abusers will know, from personal experience, that they can be one of the most difficult groups of patients to treat.

So what does happen to them? What is the outcome for drug abusers and drug-dependent individuals? Do they get off drugs or are they always addicted? Do they carry on taking drugs until they kill themselves or are they likely to die from an unrelated illness? If they become abstinent, what brings about this fundamental change, and when is it likely to occur? Does treatment 'work'? If so, which treatment is 'best'?

There are no simple answers to any of these questions. Drug abusers are a heterogeneous population, and the individuals who make up that population have different personality attributes and exist in different life situations. They suffer from one or more of a range of drug-related problems, of variable severity, and the eventual outcome of their drug abuse, like its initiation, depends on the unique interaction between drug, individual and society. To this already complex formula must be added yet another variable – the effect (if any) of treatment intervention. Thus, while one heroin-dependent individual may successfully achieve and maintain abstinence, another attending the same clinic may die from an overdose, while a third may attain stability when provided with a regular prescription for methadone. Similarly, among a group of adolescents experimenting with glue sniffing, most will 'grow out of it', but an occasional youngster will persist in abusing solvent for many years and may, in the process, seriously damage his/her liver and kidneys.

Endless anecdotal examples could be given of patterns of drug abuse and of the different outcomes that ensue. Most research, however, has concentrated on what happens to those who abuse opiates, sometimes with a tacit assumption that all opiate abusers are necessarily dependent on their

drug and are therefore 'addicts'. In contrast, there is a striking paucity of
information about what happens to those who abuse other drugs and/or
are dependent upon them, and this yawning gap in our knowledge base is
usually papered over by extrapolations from studies of opiate 'addicts'.

In addition, there is often a lack of clarity and little agreement about
what exactly is meant by 'outcome'. Drug-taking status is an obvious component of any assessment procedure, but it must be precisely defined. For
example, an individual who has successfully become abstinent from opiates
may then abuse a whole range of other drugs such as cannabis, alcohol
and sedatives, and may become dependent upon one or more of them. How
should this person be described as far as outcome is concerned? In a multidimensional approach to drug abuse, detoxification and abstinence are
rarely the only goals of treatment. Elimination or reduction of criminal
activity, cessation of all illicit drug use and the establishment of socially
acceptable behaviour, such as obtaining employment, maintaining a basic
standard of living by legitimate means and maintaining stable relations
with family and friends, are all considered important and may be included
as outcome criteria in the evaluation of treatment. In a methadone
maintenance treatment programme, they are of course the most important
indicators of the success of the treatment.

Another question that needs to be addressed is the timing of assessment
procedures. Exactly when should 'outcome' be assessed? For those undergoing detoxification, completion of the detoxification programme is a major
landmark of their treatment, and the proportion who manage to reach it is
an indication of the acceptability of the treatment programme to patients –
an important factor when patient motivation is crucial to recovery. In a
chronic and relapsing illness, however, evaluation at a single point in time
is not enough; to be meaningful it must extend over months and years and
this in itself raises further problems, particularly when different treatment
modalities are being composed and different goals of treatment are
included. For example, those individuals who are imprisoned, or go into
hospital, or decide to enter a therapeutic community, have limited opportunity to use illegal drugs, commit crimes or become employed, and this may
affect the result of outcome assessment. Sophisticated analysis of data can
control for time at risk in outcome studies, but the important point to be
grasped here is that bland statements of success of different treatment
strategies should never be taken at face value. Claims of '75% cure rates'
for drug dependence require further clarification. When are 75% of patients
considered 'cured'? At the end of a course of treatment? If so, what has
happened after 6 months, or 1 year? If 75% of patients are abstinent from
their original drug of abuse, how many are taking a substitute drug from
the same class; how many are using alcohol or other drugs? When these

points are clarified and taken into account, the figures for 'successful' treatment are usually much lower – and more meaningful. On the other hand, beneficial consequences of intervention and treatment may not be manifest immediately, and may not therefore be recognized as a consequence of treatment. For example, even if relapse to drug taking occurs within days of completion of a detoxification programme, the experience of abstinence, albeit temporary, may be instrumental in a later decision to enter a therapeutic community or to engage in other long-term treatment programmes.

The difficulties of assessing the outcome of treatment for drug abuse are compounded by a basic ignorance of what might be termed the 'natural history' of the condition. It is by no means clear what happens if there is no treatment and no intervention by any health-care worker, and it is therefore impossible to know whether any changes following the intervention are causally related to it or might have occurred anyway. Many studies evaluating treatment compare illicit drug taking, employment status etc. in the year following the treatment intervention with what was happening the year before. Any differences are attributed to the effectiveness or ineffectiveness of the treatment process.

It is important to remember, however, that professional intervention is only one factor in a complex and ever-changing situation, and it is arrogant to assume that it lies at the root of all subsequent change. For example, an opiate addict undergoes detoxification in an in-patient unit and, after being discharged, continues to attend a non-user's group regularly; after vocational rehabilitation he is able to gain regular employment and never abuses opiates, or indeed any illicit drug, again. Is this happy ending due to the effectiveness of in-patient detoxification, or could the fact that his wife is pregnant and has said that she will leave with the baby unless he comes off drugs and gets a job, explain why treatment on this occasion was successful? Or could it be that he has attained sufficient maturation of personality that he can now cope without drugs? Undoubtedly, all of these may be important factors independently and their interaction may account for the patient eventually achieving abstinence. The statistical evaluation of outcome can never unravel such complexity.

Natural history of drug dependence

One of the reasons why it is impossible to be definite about the outcome of drug dependence and to evaluate accurately the effect of treatment intervention is because of our ignorance of the natural history of the condition. Indeed, the very term 'natural history' is somewhat misleading because it assumes the existence of a predictable pathological process with an inevitable course, whereas in any discussion of drug abuse and dependence there is constant awareness of the way in which external factors interact to affect the course of events. In the absence of a 'typical' natural history, it may be more helpful to consider drug dependence in terms of different drug-taking 'careers'. Examination of a large number of these careers may permit the extraction of certain commonalities that tell us something about the nature of drug dependence and its eventual outcome.

First and foremost, it is clear that although there are many routes into drug abuse and thence to drug dependence, once the dependent state has been reached it is generally a chronic condition lasting for years rather than months, and one that is difficult, but not impossible, to overcome. Within this long-term perspective, it is also clear that it is a condition of relapse and remission. Very few drug-dependent individuals achieve permanent abstinence the first time that they try, and of those who eventually achieve it, the majority have had several, often numerous, attempts. They may have tried to become abstinent, but only managed a temporary reduction in dose, or they may have become abstinent but resumed drug taking within days, weeks or months. It is sometimes assumed that this cycle of abstinence and drug taking is a consequence of treatment and its subsequent failure, but a similar pattern of behaviour is reported by addicts attending drug-dependence treatment units for the first time. A careful history usually elicits an account of at least one, and often several, episodes of abstinence achieved on the individual's personal initiative and with no professional intervention.

It is very important that all who work with or who have contact with drug-dependent individuals understand the fluctuating nature of the condition. Resumption of drug taking after a period of abstinence is then not perceived as failure, but as an indication of the severity of the underlying addiction, and it becomes the cue not for recrimination but for a more energetic attempt to induce another remission. Furthermore, the natural cycle of relapse and remission must be borne in mind in any assessment of treatment outcome, just as it is in the evaluation of other fluctuating conditions such as multiple sclerosis.

In the absence of information about what happens to drug-dependent individuals who remain aloof from all professional intervention, it may be possible to gain some understanding of the natural history of the condition by following the fortunes of cohorts of addicts over a number of years, accepting that any 'treatment' or contact with health-care professionals is just one component of the totality of a drug-taking career. A particularly interesting study along these lines was initiated in 1969 of a representative sample of subjects being prescribed heroin at London drug clinics. The initial survey of the drug use and behaviour of 128 people revealed considerable heterogeneity, but it was possible to classify them into four groups:

1   the 'stables' suffered from fewest complications of drug abuse, avoided other users and usually had regular employment;

2   the 'junkies' did not work, had a high rate of complications and were deeply involved in criminal behaviour and the drug sub-culture;

3   the 'two-worlders' tended to be employed and to avoid complications, but were involved in the drug sub-culture;

4   the 'loners' were not involved in criminal activity or the drug sub-culture, nor were they involved in the conventional world of work. They were often unconventional in appearance and living arrangements.

In the absence of a modern study, it is not clear how far this classification might be reproducible today (26 years later), but it emphasizes the variety of behaviour that exists within just one group of drug-dependent individuals. These people were followed up by record searches and personal contact for 10 years. At the end of this time, 19 (15%) had died, 49 (38%) were still attending the clinic and 60 (47%) were not. The mortality of drug dependence will be discussed later in this chapter, but what of those who had not died, but had survived for 10 years?

Of the 49 individuals still attending the clinic in 1979, all were receiving prescriptions for opiates (methadone and/or heroin) and the majority had received prescriptions continuously for the 10-year period. On the whole, other aspects of their lives were unproblematical and the majority were employed. It appears that they had settled down into a life of fairly safe but chronic addiction and it seems unlikely that this would have changed in the future. It is interesting that the group identified as 'stables' in 1969 had indeed proved stable: they were more likely than any other group to be still receiving prescriptions for heroin and to have received such prescriptions continuously between 1969 and 1979. In contrast, no 'junkies' were still receiving heroin in 1979.

It is often assumed that when addicts stop attending the clinic and are lost to follow-up, that they have probably resumed drug taking. This study, which made energetic and thorough attempts to trace addicts and to confirm their drug-taking status, suggests otherwise; over the years the number of people remaining addicted declined, and after 10 years 38% (estimated) had stopped using heroin and other opiates. Having become abstinent, they did not generally abuse other drugs or alcohol. By 1979 their average period of abstinence was more than 6 years and it seemed unlikely that drug taking would be resumed thereafter.

In another study, a cohort of all 83 addicts attending a London drug clinic in July 1971 was followed up 11 years later by a search of medical notes and Home Office records. At that time, 29 (24%) were known to be still using drugs, the majority receiving injectable methadone on prescription despite an 'official' clinic policy of weaning addicts off injectable drugs. Once again, as in the study described earlier, this group showed a definite move towards stability, with a marked fall in the number having complications of drug use or being involved in criminality, and a slight increase in the attainment of stable relationships and regular employment. Whether this increased stability is a result of continued and often uninterrupted prescription of opiate drugs, or the cause of their prescription is not clear. It may be argued, for example, that it was the provision of a regular supply of opiates that kept addicts out of trouble and permitted the development of a stable and uncomplicated lifestyle – but it could also be true that continued prescribing was a consequence of the addicts' underlying stability because a chaotic lifestyle (abuse of other drugs, excess side-effects, etc), would probably have led to cessation of prescription.

Whatever the reason, in two long-term studies of British opiate addicts attending drug clinics, about 30% settled down to a state of chronic but uncomplicated addiction. It is interesting that a third, somewhat different, study reported a similar result: 86 injecting drug users, most of whom used opiates, attended a clinic that did not prescribe opiates at all. After a follow-up period of up to 6 years, 30% were continuing to inject regularly, many of them having subsequently attended clinics which did prescribe for them.

Another finding to emerge from many studies carried out in drug clinics is that if abstinence is going to occur, it is more likely to happen early in a drug user's career. For example, when 40 patients who became drug free were compared with 40 patients at the same clinic who did not become drug free, the mean time between claimed first use of opiate and first attendance was 3.9 years for the group who became abstinent, but was 8.7 years for the others. The message is clear from many sources that it is the less chronic addicts who are likely to become abstinent in the short term, and that short-term or early improvement is more likely to lead to long-term improvement. This phenomenon has been described as the 'rush' in the numbers becoming abstinent early in their drug-taking career, followed by a much slower 'trickle' of addicts coming off over subsequent years. The slow but steady decline over the years in the numbers continuing to be dependent may be evidence of the effect of maturation – that, eventually, many addicts will 'grow out of' drug taking.

Mortality

It is widely believed that to be an 'addict' (i.e., an opiate addict) is to dice with death. Indeed, many people believe that early death is the inevitable outcome of addiction. Mortality statistics refute the latter belief while confirming the hazards of the condition. For example, an oft-quoted study of addict deaths between 1947 and 1966 estimates their mortality rate to be 28 times that expected for a population with similar demographic characteristics. Since then, there have been many studies of addict deaths, but their differing research methodologies make interpretation and comparisons difficult. In general, however, most of these studies report that 2–3% of addicts are dead within 1 year of making contact with a clinic or helping agency.

However, as has been remarked before, addiction is a chronic condition and it is important to find out what happens to those who survive the first year. Do more and more addicts die as time goes by, or is mortality concentrated in the early years of an addiction career, with 'stable' addicts, who have learned to live with their addiction, surviving comfortably into old age? The answers to questions such as these are relevant to an understanding of the natural history of addiction, but they are difficult questions to resolve because of the difficulties of following cohorts of addicts over long periods and of knowing when and why they died. It may be labouring the obvious to point out that the eventual outcome for any cohort (addict or not) followed for a sufficiently long period of time will be a 100% mortality rate, but this emphasizes the statistical problems surrounding the study of chronic conditions with an increased mortality rate.

Despite these pitfalls, mortality studies are useful investigative tools both for indicating trends in drug addiction and for providing data about the most serious forms of addiction – that is, those from which the addict has died. One source of information in the UK is the Home Office list of those addicts, previously notified, who have been removed from the current index by reason of death. During the 15-year period, 1967–81, 1499 notified addicts died, and when they were divided into annual cohorts, according to the calendar year in which they were first notified, it was found that approximately 1.6% died within that calendar year and that 3.3% died by the end of the subsequent calendar year (Fig. 9.1). These percentages were fairly constant over the whole of the study period, that encompassed a range of different enthusiasms and policies for treating addiction: in the early years, clinics opened and started to prescribe heroin; then injectable methadone was substituted and then oral methadone. Clinics became more reluctant to prescribe opiates and now usually do so only as part of a

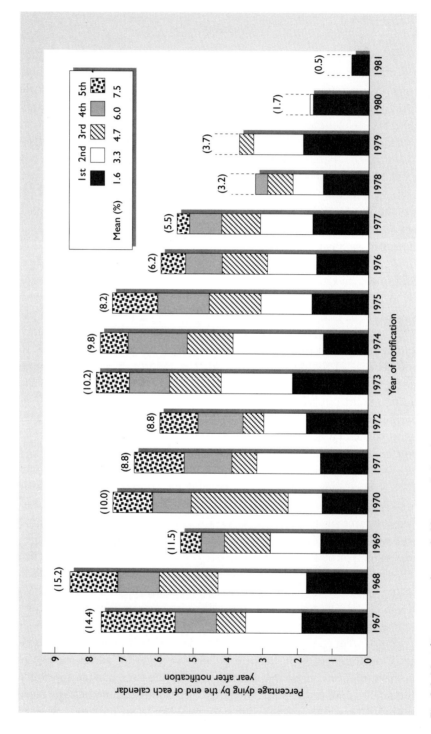

Fig. 9.1 Mortality among cohorts of addicts notified each year. Figures in parentheses are percentages of each annual cohort dead at follow-up (1982). (Source: Ghodse et al., 1985.)

therapeutic contract. None of these measures seem to have had any impact on early mortality and the uniformity of the results over the 15 years suggests that these death rates perhaps represent the elusive 'natural history' of addiction. When the results are corrected to reflect annual mortality, rather than death within a specific calendar year, the true death rate for the first year approaches 3%, for the second year 1.9%, and for the third 0.7%.

When the older, 'therapeutic' addicts were excluded from the calculations, mortality due to recreational opiate addiction was found to be approximately 16 times that expected for a similar population of non-addicts.

Other studies have also described this high mortality rate – 15% of a representative sample of heroin addicts attending London clinics in 1969 were dead 10 years later, and 20% were dead in another 11-year follow-up study (described in the previous section). Many studies have been undertaken, often with noticeable differences in the mortality rates discovered, but these probably reflect differing research methodologies rather than true differences in outcome.

When the 15-year study described above was updated to 1990, it was found that out of 63 571 addicts newly notified during the 24-year period from 1967 to 1990, 3668 (5.8%) were dead by the end of 1990. The number of deaths has tended to increase each year, with occasional reversals, from 51 in 1967 to 125 in 1979 and to 333 in 1990. However, when these deaths are expressed in terms of an annual mortality rate (number of deaths each year expressed as the rate per thousand of the population at risk), this has showed a steady decline from 25.4/1000 per year in 1968–70, the first 3 years after the opening of the clinics, to 10.9/1000 per year in 1978–80 and to 5.9/1000 per year in 1988–90. The majority (3248, 88.5%) of these deaths were of non-therapeutic addicts (p. 23), with a male: female ratio of about 4:1. The mean age at death for this group over the whole period was 30.2 years, although within the last 3 years of the study this increased to 31 years.

What do these young addicts die of? Even with long periods of administration, pure opiates do not cause direct tissue damage, and it is evident from the chronic, stable addicts described above that a substantial proportion can and do survive comparatively unscathed. Those who die often do so because of the effects of other drugs, such as sedative hypnotics. This point is illustrated by several studies. For example, in the 24-year study of deaths of notified addicts, drugs caused or were implicated in 1779 deaths (48.5%). Heroin accounted for the lowest proportion of deaths (4%), while methadone accounted for 6.5% and barbiturates were implicated in about

8%; other opiates (e.g., dipipanone, dextromoramide) accounted for the largest percentage (12.7%), closely followed by other drugs (12.3%) Fig. 9.2 shows the percentage of deaths caused each year by the main drug classes and it is clear that during the last 25 years, different drugs have been of different significance. It shows, for example, the importance of barbiturates in the 1970s and their subsequent decline; the significance of other opiates throughout the 1980s; and the increasing percentage of deaths caused by 'other drugs' in recent years.

These mortality findings are not confined to notified addicts. A study carried out in the coroners' courts of Greater London identified 134 deaths due to drug addiction in the period 1970–74, of which only 79 (59%) were addicts who in life had been notified to the Home Office. Once again, many (71) deaths were primarily due to barbiturate overdose, and only 44 of the addicts were known to the Home Office. It is worth noting in passing that even those whose drug problem is so severe that it ends in death may escape 'official' attention and notification.

Several further observations may be made from these and other studies. Addicts usually die as a result of a drug overdose that causes respiratory failure, and consequent cerebral anoxia and unconsciousness; this in turn may lead to asphyxia, due to postural causes or inhalation of vomit. Bronchopneumonia following respiratory depression is also common. Infectious complications, such as hepatitis and endocarditis, can be and sometimes are fatal, but these are less common causes of addict deaths. A fatal drug overdose is frequently a polydrug overdose with at least two central nervous system depressants being taken together and sometimes more, so that their effects on respiration are potentiated.

It was striking (during the 1970s, at any rate) that addicts known to the Home Office because of their addiction to a notifiable drug were more likely to die from the effect of a supposedly less dangerous, non-notifiable drug. In other words, the high mortality of opiate dependence at that time was largely, but not wholly due to non-opiate drugs – an indication and a reflection of the complexity of drug-taking behaviour and clear evidence that drug abuse is rarely confined to a single substance. As the hazards of barbiturates became more apparent, and as safer alternatives (benzodiazepines) became available, barbiturates were prescribed less frequently and addict deaths due to these drugs declined correspondingly. Indeed, the evidence from the Home Office study of an overall reduction in mortality rates over the last 24 years may be directly attributable to the reduced availability of barbiturates. However, the basic behaviour of taking a drug overdose has not changed and other drugs are taken instead of barbiturates – usually opiate drugs such as dipipanone and dextromoramide or other unspecified opiates.

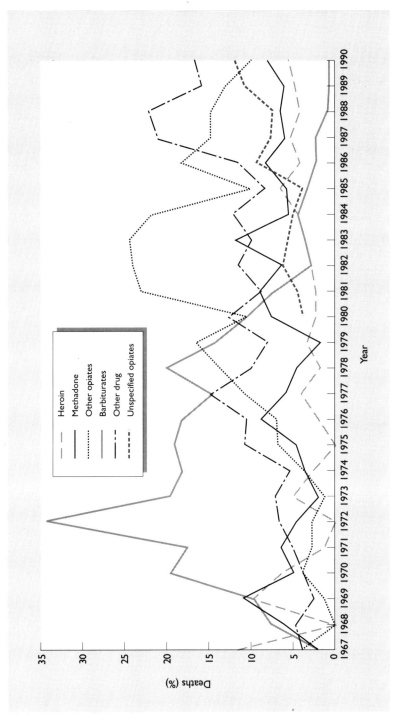

Fig. 9.2 Percentage of drug-related deaths per year.

In summary, therefore, although opiate dependence is not invariably
fatal, many – predominantly young – people die from it. The mortality rate
in the earlier years of dependence appears to have remained fairly constant
over a number of years, suggesting that this is perhaps an unvarying component of the 'natural history' of the condition. In other words, just as x%
of patients with carcinoma of the stomach die within 2 years of diagnosis,
so 4.9% of opiate-dependent individuals die within 2 years of notification to
the Home Office. Subsequent mortality may be affected more markedly by
'external' factors. In the UK, addicts' deaths are usually due to drug overdoses and prescribed drugs are at the core of this aspect of the problem. Far
from being a new phenomenon, prescribed drugs have always played a
large part in addiction in Britain and this may be the inevitable consequence of a medical, rather than a criminalizing, response to addiction.
These findings emphasize how, even in death, addiction is intimately
involved with and influenced by apparently peripheral issues. Mortality
rates are decided not only by the severity of the dependence syndrome, but
also by the availability of drugs to the general population, which in turn
depends in part on doctors' prescribing practices. In the months and years
to come, it is likely that addict mortality will be profoundly affected by yet
another external factor – the HIV virus – which will make future interpretation of scanty statistics even more difficult.

Outcome of treatment

The high mortality rate of opiate dependence emphasizes the severity of the
condition for some individuals and, on a wider scale, drug abuse and
dependence have far-reaching implications for society as a whole. The need
for effective treatment is clear and becomes daily more important as the
numbers involved increase steadily. It is no longer sufficient to offer treatment on an *ad hoc* basis; its usefulness must be assessed. In this context, it
is important to be precise about the goals of specific treatment modalities.
For example, if treatment is aimed at reducing criminality and illicit drug
abuse, it is necessary to know if it actually has this effect and for what proportion of patients. Similarly, if the purpose of a treatment programme is
detoxification, it is useful to know what proportion of patients actually
achieve abstinence and whether other methods of detoxification are better
or worse at achieving this. If an out-patient programme is aimed at preventing relapse, how many people stay drug free and for how long?

The answers to these questions are important, primarily for the sake of
the individual, but they also have important financial implications. When
large numbers of patients are involved, resources (staff, time, money)

should not be wasted on ineffective treatment, and if comparable treatment programmes yield similar results, it is common sense to adopt the most economical. Cost-effectiveness may be further improved if patient characteristics can be identified that permit patients to be assigned to the treatment that is most likely to help them attain achievable goals.

Despite the obvious difficulties of treatment evaluation, many research studies are addressing this problem – or at least some aspect of it. None can give a complete answer about the 'best' treatment, but separate studies, focussing on specific answerable questions, are providing worthwhile information. Gradually, a picture is emerging, as yet far from complete, that shows some of the effects and consequences of different treatment interventions.

As always, vast studies have been carried out in the US on a scale unknown elsewhere. The Drug Abuse Reporting Programme (DARP), for example, described 44 000 patients attending 52 different agencies from 1969 to 1974. Follow-up research strategies and patient characteristics of 6402 patients were selected for follow-up. The treatment modalities studied included methadone maintenance (MM), therapeutic communities (TC), out-patient drug-free programmes (mostly non-opiate drug users) and short-term detoxification (DT). Outcome was defined as 'highly favourable' if there was no use of illicit drugs (except less than daily use of cannabis) and no arrests or imprisonments during the year, and as 'moderately favourable' if there was no daily use of illicit drugs and no major criminality (i.e., 30 days in prison; no crimes against the person or crimes of profit). Sophisticated statistical analysis, with 'time at risk' adjustments, demonstrated that the most favourable outcomes were associated with MM, TC and DT and that patients on these three programmes did about equally well. Those on short-term detoxification programmes and those who registered with one of the treatment agencies, but never actually engaged in treatment, had significantly poorer outcomes. It was found that the amount of time spent in treatment was reasonably well-correlated with outcome and, more specifically, that if the patient was engaged in treatment for less than 90 days, the outcomes of MM, TC and DT were no different from those of DT patients. This finding is of interest because it confirms clinical experience and common-sense expectation that in a chronic illness, change is unlikely to be effected by fleeting contact with treatment. It also suggests that it is the amount of treatment contact rather than the type of therapeutic approach that is important in achieving the particular outcome they were measuring (which for some patients included drug abstinence, but for MM patients did not). In the UK, a study of addicts who had spent time in a therapeutic community found that those who stayed more than 6 months were less likely to have subsequent criminal convictions and less likely to resume self-injection.

The DARP findings stress the importance of understanding that retention in treatment is a phenomenon in its own right. If drug abusers are going to be helped, they must stay in contact with the helping agency. We need to know who the drop-outs are and why they leave treatment. Some studies have already suggested that retention in treatment (or outcome) can be predicted from psychobiological testing or from typologies derived from cluster analyses of patients' characteristics. Thus personality traits, once studied from the point of view of the aetiology of dependence, may come to be of more interest as predictors of outcome. One finding has been that patients with fewest and least severe psychological problems did 'well' (according to several outcome criteria), regardless of which treatment programme they were assigned to. Those with more severe psychological problems did poorly in all treatment programmes, although they did rather better with methadone maintenance than in the more confrontational situation of a therapeutic community. Further information on these and similar factors will become available from another large-scale US study – the Treatment Outcome Prospective Study (TOPS), which is a longitudinal investigation of drug abusers, during and after treatment.

In the meantime, if some patients benefit equally from all treatment programmes, it makes financial sense to manage them in less expensive out-patient treatment programmes rather than in costly in-patient units. With experience, it may become possible to identify patient characteristics to permit assignment to the most appropriate treatment facility, and some success has already been reported with this strategy. It was found, for example, that if patients with low severity of psychological problems also had significant family and/or employment problems, they fared much better if treated in an in-patient setting. Overall, the effectiveness of treatment could be improved by matching patients to what seemed on clinical grounds to be the most appropriate programme, although once again, patients with severe psychological problems did badly.

The different methodologies and criteria of outcome used in American and British studies make any comparison difficult. Nevertheless, it is interesting that in the survey of British addicts being prescribed heroin in 1969, there were very few differences between those who were going to continue taking opiates and those who were going to stop. They could not, for example, be differentiated on characteristics such as social class, sex, employment, crime, drug use or income, so that prediction about prognosis and treatment would have been very difficult. In fact, the main difference seemed to be that those who subsequently stopped taking opiates were younger, had a shorter history of addiction and were prescribed smaller doses of opiates.

Of course, the prescription of opiates to addicts when they present for treatment is an important, often essential, component for retaining them in treatment. The extent to which addicts should get what they want as a way of attracting them to, and keeping them in treatment, is a difficult question to resolve. The point is elegantly illustrated by research carried out in London in the 1970s, when some patients attending a clinic were offered injectable heroin (undoubtedly the drug of choice for most opiate addicts), while the rest had oral methadone. A year later, three-quarters of the heroin group were still attending the clinic compared with less than one-third of the methadone group, most of whom had left treatment early in the year. However, those receiving heroin had changed very little – they continued to take their heroin and most were still involved in the drug sub-culture. In other words, heroin had kept them in contact with the treatment agency, had maintained the status quo of their addiction and had reduced their involvement in criminal activity. In contrast, after a year, the methadone group had polarized into two sub-categories. Some had given up drug use altogether and were not involved in criminal activity, but others were injecting illicit opiates regularly and had a high conviction rate. It seemed, therefore, that the more confrontational approach of not giving the addict the preferred drug 'precipitated' abstinence for some, at the price of effectively driving others away from the treatment agency altogether.

In most countries the choice between heroin and methadone does not exist, because heroin is not even included in the pharmacopoeia, and where it is, it is rarely permissible to prescribe it to addicts. Even in the UK, the choice nowadays is usually whether to prescribe to keep patients in treatment and thereby reduce some of the complications of addiction and the problems that addicts pose to the rest of society, or to deny opiates and at least give some addicts a better chance of becoming abstinent.

Public debate on this issue has become more vigorous since the advent of AIDS, because of concern about protecting the general population from this disease. A body of opinion believes that the general purpose of the treatment of addiction should change from one that emphasizes abstinence for as many addicts as possible, to one of 'harm reduction' – ostensibly the reduction of harm that addicts may do to themselves, but with the clear, ulterior purpose of reducing the harm they may do to society as a whole by spreading AIDS. This debate illustrates how the treatment of addiction and its evaluation can be radically affected by societal factors. It is this ever-shifting background that makes assessment of treatment outcome so difficult.

Discussion

Despite the very patchy nature of our knowledge, it is possible to draw together some of the information that has been gathered and to present the rudiments of an answer to the question posed at the beginning of this chapter, 'What happens to addicts?'.

Firstly, it is apparent that opiate dependence is a serious condition with a high mortality rate. This is particularly worrying because of the youth of those concerned and because of the feeling that they may have stumbled into drug abuse and dependence because of a combination of circumstances, and that death is too high a price to pay for youthful error.

Nevertheless, a diagnosis of opiate dependence is not a death sentence. The majority of opiate abusers do survive – some (perhaps 30%) settling into a state of chronic dependence, with areas of their life, other than drug taking, more or less normal and involving stability of relationships, home and employment. It appears that this group can function normally only if they take an opiate regularly and that their drug is as necessary for them as insulin is for a diabetic, or vitamin B12 injections for someone with pernicious anaemia. Others (perhaps 30–40%) become abstinent. Those who are young and have a shorter history of addiction are the most likely to achieve this outcome – which is undoubtedly the safest and most satisfactory.

It is therefore important to encourage everyone who seeks help to attempt abstinence while their chances of achieving it are highest, and before they become entrenched in a permanent drug-taking lifestyle. Not everyone will achieve abstinence in the early stages of their drugtaking career, and even those who do are likely to need several 'tries'. It is worth pointing out that the prognosis for 'new' addicts, presenting in the 1990s, may be better than that established for addicts who presented for treatment in the late 1960s–70s. 'Modern' drug addicts have a daily dose of opiates that is much lower than their counterparts in the 1960s, so on pharmacological grounds their dependence can be considered less severe.

At present, there is no sure way of predicting at the beginning of a dependence 'career' which route a particular individual is likely to follow. It seems as if the most stable and 'settled' are the most likely to end up as stable, chronic addicts, but in the UK this may be a reflection of a system that permits opiate maintenance. It also appears that those with the most severe psychological problems do less well, often continuing to abuse a variety of drugs in a chaotic fashion. They suffer the medical, legal and social consequences of their drug abuse until such a time as they do eventually 'mature' into abstinence, settle down into a more stable pattern of drug taking, or kill themselves.

It is also not clear what part, if any, treatment can play in tipping the balance towards the desired outcome of abstinence or, failing that, of methadone maintenance, and away from chaotic drug abuse and/or death. There is some (slight) evidence that the British medical 'drug clinic' approach to opiate addiction may slightly increase the early numbers becoming abstinent (the 'rush'), although there is very little effect on the later 'trickle'. Mortality statistics suggest a hard core, apparently unhelped by treatment, who die early in their addiction career, and this bears out clinical experience of a group who do badly whatever measures are attempted.

On the brighter side, both the health-care professionals and the drug-dependent individuals must hang on to the fact that a good proportion can achieve abstinence and be considered 'cured'. This is rarely achieved rapidly – drug dependence is a chronic condition unlikely to be affected by brief encounters with treatment intervention – but if a prolonged period of help is accepted, this offers real hope of drug abstinence. Compulsory 'help', in terms of enforced abstinence during imprisonment, is rarely useful because relapse is more likely to occur upon release.

So far we have concentrated exclusively on the outcome of dependence of those addicts who have come to 'official' attention and who have remained within its range long enough for someone to assess what happens to them. But what of the rest? Undoubtedly, 'out there', beyond any statistics or follow-up studies, are many opiate-dependent individuals who make only fleeting contact with health-care workers and many who make no contact at all during the course of their drug-taking career. Their numbers are unknown, but it is abundantly clear that they exist: drug abusers approaching a clinic for the first time characteristically report a history of many years of drug abuse and long periods of regular self-injection; some make contact only briefly and never return; they describe friends who have injected regularly for years who have never sought help. Sometimes, this is due to a reluctance to become involved with a clinic or any official body, sometimes because they fear they will be prescribed inadequate quantities of opiates. Whatever the reason, and with a covert activity such as illicit drug abuse there may be many, these addicts and their fate remain unknown.

This profound ignorance seriously affects our understanding of the outcome of opiate dependence. It is rather like trying to understand the outcome of a streptococcal infection by studying only those admitted to hospital with the more sinister consequences such as rheumatic heart disease, arthritis or Sydenham's chorea, while ignoring all those with more common manifestations such as tonsillitis and cellulitis. It is therefore worth making a guess at what happens to these unrecognized thousands.

Undoubtedly, some die with their addiction still undetected and unknown to any authority until they die as a consequence of it. Mortality statistics do not, however, suggest that the majority of young unknown addicts perish. Some probably become chronically dependent, obtaining drugs regularly from illicit sources, but it is impossible to believe that they all go on to a state of permanent, covert, chronic dependence. In the 25 years or so since the beginning of the drug-dependence explosion in the UK, such a large population would have developed that it is unlikely that it could remain excluded from all statistics. Presumably, therefore, many become abstinent, probably in a very similar way to those who achieve abstinence by means of professional help – with periods of voluntary abstinence, followed by relapse into drug taking, until eventually some achieve permanent abstinence. Indeed, it may be very common for abstinence to be achieved in this way with no professional intervention, because the individuals concerned are likely to be young and at an early stage of their addiction career – just the group most likely to become successfully abstinent. Those who present for professional treatment, on the other hand, are likely to be the more severely dependent who can no longer afford to support their escalating drug habit.

Obviously, this is all conjecture, but it emphasizes the point that although opiate dependence is a serious and chronic condition, there is cause and room for optimism. Abstinence is an attainable outcome for many, perhaps even the majority, and treatment is a way of propelling more drug-dependent individuals towards that outcome, more rapidly than they might otherwise have reached it. However, the importance of treatment is much greater than any theoretical 'success' rate. The fact that treatment exists is a clear statement that the dependent state need not be permanent, that drug-dependent individuals can be helped and that they are worthy of help. By its very existence, treatment offers hope, sparks motivation, and improves outcome; and these benefits extend beyond those who are in formal receipt of the different treatment interventions.

Although this chapter has concentrated wholly on opiate dependence and its outcome, some of the observations that have been made clearly apply to other forms of substance dependence too. The chronic nature of dependence and the pattern of relapse and remission are common to all types of drug dependence and it is possible to identify similar types of outcome. For example, people attending slimming clinics for years to obtain regular prescriptions of amphetamine, or those taking barbiturates or benzodiazepines regularly for insomnia, equate with chronic, stable opiate addicts on methadone maintenance. Similarly, there are individuals with chaotic patterns of sedative abuse who die as a result of their drug taking. The plethora of self-help groups that have sprung up tell eloquently of the difficulties of achieving abstinence – whatever the underlying drug of dependence. It is these (and other) underlying commonalities that justify different types of drug dependence being treated in similar ways, despite the different pharmacological properties of the drugs involved. There have, however, been few attempts to formally assess the long-term outcome of dependence on drugs other than opiates.

References and further reading

Bewley TH, Ben-Arie O & James IP (1968). Morbidity and mortality from heroin dependence: 1. Survey of heroin addicts known to the Home Office. *British Medical Journal*, **1**, 725–726.

Cottrell D, Childs-Clarke A & Ghodse AH (1985). British opiate addicts: an 11-year follow-up. *British Journal of Psychiatry*, **146**, 448–450.

De Leon G, Wexter H & Jainchill N (1977). The therapeutic community: success and improvement rates 5 years after treatment. *International Journal of Addiction*, **12**, 301–321.

Ghodse AH, Sheehan M, Stevens B, Taylor C & Edwards G (1978). Mortality among addicts in Greater London. *British Medical Journal*, **2**, 1742–1744.

Ghodse AH, Sheehan M, Taylor C & Edwards G (1985). Deaths of drug addicts in the United Kingdom, 1967–1981. *British Medical Journal*, **290**, 425–428.

Hartnoll RL, Mitcheson MC, Battersby A *et al.* (1980). Evaluation of heroin maintenance in controlled trial. *Archives of General Psychiatry*, **37**, 877–884.

Judson BA & Goldstein A (1982). Prediction of long-term outcome for heroin addicts admitted to a methadone maintenance program. *Drug and Alcohol Dependence*, **10**, 383–391.

Marlatt GA & George WH (1984). Relapse prevention: introduction and overview of the model. *British Journal of Addiction*, **79**, 261–273.

Marlatt GA & Gordon JR (eds) (1985). *Relapse Prevention: Maintenance Strategies in the Treatment of Addictive Behaviours*. Guildford Press, New York.

McLellan AT, Woody GE, Luborsky L, O'Brien CP & Druley KA (1982). Increased effectiveness of drug-abuse treatment from patient-program matching. In: Harris LS (ed.) *Problems of Drug Dependence*, 335–341. NIDA Research Monograph 43, Department of Health & Human Services, Rockville.

Rounsaville BJ, Tierney T, Crits-Cristoph K, Weissman MW & Kleber HD (1982). Predictors of out come in treatment of opiate addicts: evidence for the multidimensional nature of addicts' problems. *Comprehensive Psychiatry*, **23**, 462–478.

Simpson DD (1984). National treatment system evaluation based on the Drug Abuse Reporting Program (DARP) follow-up research. In: Tims FM & Ludford JP (eds). *Drug Abuse Treatment Evaluation: Strategies, Progress and Prospects*. NIDA Research Monograph 51. Rockville Department of Health & Human Services, Rockville.

Stimson G & Oppenheimer E (1982). *Heroin addiction. Treatment and Control in Britain.* Tavistock, London.

Strang J, Gossop M & Stimson G (1990). Identifying the problem. In: Ghodse AH & Maxwell D (eds). *Substance Abuse and Dependence,* 80–97. Macmillan Press, London.

Thorley A (1981). Longitudinal studies of drug dependence. In Edwards G & Busch C (eds). *Drug Problems in Britain: A Review of Ten Years,* 117–169. Academic Press, London.

Tims FM & Leukefeld CG (eds) (1984). *Drug Abuse Treatment Evaluation: Strategies, Progress and Prospects.* NIDA Research Monograph 51. Rockville Department of Health & Human Services, Rockville.

Vallant G (1973). A 20-year follow-up of New York narcotic addicts. *Archives of General Psychiatry,* **29,** 237–241.

10

Prevention of drug abuse

Introduction

In the light of our knowledge of the consequences and complications of drug abuse, of the difficulties of treatment, and of the high mortality rate, the old adage, that prevention is better than cure, is beyond dispute. For drug-related problems, the value of prevention goes way beyond the individual benefits it confers, important though these are for the people whose lives are thus preserved. Prevention is also crucial for society as a whole and this is more apparent now than ever before. Drug trafficking, associated as it is with organized crime on an enormous scale, can threaten the very fabric of society by undermining law and order and the economy. In addition, the advent of AIDS, which is probably the most serious threat to the health of the world population since the Black Death, has made the prevention of drug abuse by injection relevant to everyone. No longer can drug dependence and abuse be shrugged off and ignored by those who are not affected; it is now in the immediate interest of everyone in the community that effective preventive measures should be adopted.

Although the need for prevention is clear, the best course of action is not. Because the causes of drug abuse are multiple, interrelated and multidimensional, its prevention is similarly complex. Unlike an infectious disease, there is no single causative factor to be opposed or countered by a single preventive measure, and it has proved very difficult to identify and assess which factors among many might be susceptible to preventive intervention.

It is not surprising, therefore, that different cultures and societies choose and employ quite different preventive measures, that may need to vary in response to new trends in drug abuse.

For example, one approach to preventing dependence on prescribed drugs has been to try to modify the chemical structure of drugs to reduce (eliminate) their dependence-producing liability. Pharmaceutical companies are constantly producing new psychoactive drugs for which they make

extravagant claims in this respect. Usually, however, when more people
start to use the drug, its dependence potential becomes apparent and cases
of abuse and of dependence on it are reported. So far, this approach to preventing dependence has been strikingly unsuccessful, as evidenced by the
barbiturates, which were replaced by non-barbiturate hypnotics such as
methaqualone, which in turn gave way to benzodiazepines. Now that these
too have come under the cloud of dependence, a new anxiolytic has
appeared opportunely on the market, and the same claims are being heard
again.

Although solvents are not prescribed drugs, a similar approach is being
adopted to control their abuse, and new solvents are being developed which
it is hoped lack 'sniffing' appeal.

An interesting example of preventing drug abuse by tackling the drug
itself comes from the US, where there was a serious outbreak of pentazocine
(Fortral, Talwin) abuse. Talwin tablets intended for oral use were crushed
and injected together with tablets of the antihistamine tripelennamine,
resulting in a 'high' said to be similar to that caused by heroin. The pharmacological response was to add naloxone, an opiate antagonist, to the
preparation of pentazocine; if the drug was taken orally, as intended, its
analgesic effect was unimpaired because naloxone is inactive by the oral
route. If the drug were injected, however, the naloxone antagonized the
effect of pentazocine and the drug abuser did not experience any 'high'.

Clearly, measures such as these are peripheral to the main issues of prevention and can only be employed in occasional, circumscribed areas of
the totality of drug abuse. Nevertheless, they may sometimes be of value.

Definitions of prevention

A traditional approach has been to divide preventive measures into
primary, secondary and tertiary prevention. For *primary prevention* the aim
is to prevent the initiation of drug abuse. Limiting the availability of drugs
is an important component of this strategy, usually combined with educational programmes for those perceived to be at risk of starting to experiment with drugs. *Secondary prevention* depends on the early identification of
drug abusers so that they can be treated promptly, to prevent the development of a state of severe dependence and to reduce the total number of
those dependent on drugs. *Tertiary prevention* involves the treatment of
those with a severe drug abuse or dependence problem, with the aim of
mitigating the effects of harmful use. On the principle that most newcomers
to the scene are introduced to drugs by an experienced user, vigorous
efforts at treatment should also have a preventive effect.

A slightly different approach to prevention distinguishes between measures aimed at reducing the risk of engagement in substance abuse, and measures aimed at reducing the harm associated with drug abuse. In the present climate of anxiety about the wider risks of HIV and AIDS, more emphasis is now being placed on harm reduction. This approach acknowledges that, as total eradication of drug abuse is impossible, every effort should be made to minimize its harmful consequences, both for the individual concerned and for society as a whole.

Unfortunately, strategies aimed at harm reduction may oppose more fundamental measures to stem the initiation of drug abuse and, conversely, statutory controls on drugs to reduce their availability may actually increase the likelihood of harm for existing drug abusers who may resort to more dangerous drugs or use drugs with a high adulterant content.

When there is conflict of this type, the overriding concern is to minimize the risk of new people starting to take drugs. It is not surprising, therefore, that the mainpin of any preventive approach is to reduce drug availability by statutory control. At one stage, this was the only way of tackling drug-abuse prevention, but it has gradually become apparent that, on its own, this is never sufficient. Unless total eradication of supply is achieved – an impossible ideal – drug abuse continues. The modern approach therefore is to couple the goal of reducing the supply of drugs with that of reducing demand for them, recognizing that, while neither approach is sufficient on its own, each augments the effectiveness of the other. The importance of demand reduction received international acknowledgement in the 1988 United Nations Convention against Illicit Traffic in Narcotic Drugs and Psychotropic Substances (see Chapter 11)

Reducing the availability of drugs of abuse

The basis of all strategies to control the availability of drugs of abuse and dependence is statutory control and law enforcement. In all countries, laws are passed to control the production, supply, import, export, sale, prescription and possession of these drugs. The underlying principle is that there should be sufficient drugs available for any genuine, medical need, but no surplus, and that these drugs should be 'guarded' (i.e., controlled) to ensure that none are diverted for illicit abuse.

The measures used to control the availability of drugs vary according to the type of drug involved. Different methods of control are used for prescription drugs (e.g., methadone, barbiturates, benzodiazepines, amphetamines) and for illicit street drugs (e.g., LSD, cocaine, cannabis, heroin). In the UK, heroin occupies a unique position: it can be medically prescribed, but because most of the abused heroin is smuggled into the country, many of the measures used to control its availability are the same as those employed for illicit drugs rather than for prescription drugs. Although cocaine can still be prescribed in the UK, this rarely happens.

Illicit drugs

The illicit street drugs currently causing most concern globally are heroin, cocaine and cannabis. Large quantities are smuggled into the major consumer countries – USA, Canada, Western Europe, Australia, New Zealand – from the producing countries, which are mostly in South and Central America and Asia. The main thrust of preventive action in the consumer countries has been to try to keep the drugs out by vigorous customs control at national boundaries, coupled with equally vigorous police activity to detect and prosecute those who buy and sell the drugs. Severe penalties are usually imposed on those who buy and sell large quantities of these drugs. However, it is generally admitted that only a fraction of the total imported is ever detected, and although massive seizures are frequently made, this appears to have little effect on drug availability. Because of their own failure to keep drugs out, the consumer countries have looked further afield and have encouraged attempts to reduce availability by curtailing production abroad. Crop eradication, by burning or spraying with herbicides, financial inducements for crop substitution, destroying illicit factories where drugs are extracted and purified, and destroying air strips to prevent drugs being moved out, have all been tried. Despite immense input in terms of time, money and effort, the plant crops from which the drugs are extracted (opium, cannabis, coca) continue to be grown, apparently in increasing acreage, because they are far more profitable than any other crop. Stopping their cultivation would adversely affect employment, income and standard of living – and not just for those immediately involved in this activity.

Income from these crops may be integral to the producer country's economy and those who control the drug trade are very wealthy and usually have considerable political power. In addition, the producer countries themselves have, so far, had little experience of serious drug problems because there the drugs are consumed in a socially controlled way, as they have been for centuries, by smoking or chewing the vegetable matter rather than in a highly purified and potent form. The drug problems of the rich, importing countries, have up to now caused little concern and have seemed an inadequate reason for tackling a difficult and politically unpopular problem. Recently, however, the picture has changed and several of the producer countries have begun to experience the real impact of a serious drug problem. A more determined effort to eradicate excessive crops may thus become more acceptable to their population.

An additional impetus for action in these countries is that there is serious concern about the environmental impact of illicit cultivation of narcotic drugs, which now accounts for an increasing proportion of tropical deforestation. Land-clearing techniques such as 'slash and burn' in the depths of the rain forest, often in steep-sloped mountain environments, lead to a high degree of soil erosion and nutrient depletion. Problems are compounded by high levels of chemical use, in the form of herbicides, fungicides and fertilizers. Furthermore, it is now common for drug extraction and purification to take place in clandestine refineries close to the site of cultivation, and toxic by-products are dumped indiscriminately, polluting water supplies that are used to irrigate food crops, and causing significant public-health risks.

Whatever the measures taken by individual countries, there is little cause for optimism. If crops of cocaine, opium and cannabis are forced out of one geographical area, there is every likelihood that they will be grown, equally successfully, elsewhere in the world, and for the same reason. The potential profit is so enormous that even large increases in the cost of production have only minimal impact on the final profit margin. Even if there were total crop eradication worldwide, chemists, spurred on by the promise of those profits, could undoubtedly synthesize any of these drugs in illicit factories, just as LSD, amphetamines and many designer drugs are synthesized today.

Prescription drugs

Because drugs such as barbiturates, benzodiazepines and amphetamines are (or should be) available only on prescription, the doctor who prescribes them, and who therefore acts as the 'barrier' between the drugs and the general population, is the key figure in any attempt to reduce their availability. Improving doctors' prescribing practices may therefore be an important preventive strategy, both in terms of reducing the likelihood of an individual becoming dependent on drugs in the course of treatment and in terms of reducing 'overspill' of prescribed drugs to the black market.

In the course of their training, doctors learn about psychiatric illnesses and the psychoactive drugs available for their treatment. Once qualified, however, they see many patients with symptoms suggestive of psychiatric illness, but who are not suffering from an identifiable disease state. They complain of non-specific symptoms such as depression, anxiety, sleeplessness, inability to cope and headache, that reflect life's stresses but do not necessarily indicate psychiatric illness. They are normal responses, experienced by most people at some time or another, to a difficult situation, and if the situation is very difficult, the symptoms too may be very severe. The point at which they are felt to be sufficiently severe to seek medical help varies from one individual to another, and the point at which drug treatment is judged to be necessary is similarly arbitrary. Because the symptoms are often very distressing, and because modern psychoactive drugs can provide almost immediate relief, it is a natural and humane response to offer symptomatic treatment by prescribing these drugs. The doctor is well aware that in many cases the treatment is not curative but the principle of symptomatic treatment is, after all, a well established component of clinical care. For these patients the underlying problem, whether personal, interpersonal or social, is usually beyond the doctor's power of intervention.

Although well intentioned, the lax prescribing of psychoactive drugs often has unintended effects on the individual concerned and has become so widespread that it has far reaching consequences for society as a whole. For the individual, the rush to provide symptomatic relief may mean that the underlying condition is not investigated and is never identified. To make matters worse, the drugs themselves may further impair the patient's ability to cope with the problems. The drugs are potentially harmful, with a variety of side-effects. They are liable to abuse and may be taken in overdose, giving rise to considerable problems of diagnosis, treatment and rehabilitation. There is always a risk of dependence, even when taken under controlled medical conditions. Most important of all, however, is that inappropriate prescription to individuals contributes to a vast pool of these drugs within the community as a whole. How many households, one wonders, do not have a supply of psychoactive drugs, often the remnants of earlier courses of treatment? It is these medicines, legitimately obtained on prescription and now as easily available as any 'over the counter' medication, that provide a never-ending source of drugs for abuse and dependence, just as surely as do the fields of opium poppies and the plantations of coca bushes and cannabis.

The education of doctors in the rational prescription of psychoactive drugs is therefore crucial to reducing their present, very liberal availability. Doctors should learn from a very early stage of their training the full implications of their prescribing habits. Their training should prepare them adequately to cope with the many patients who will present complaining of the non-specific symptoms outlined above. A scientific approach to the prescription of psychoactive drugs must be inculcated from the beginning, before casual and unthinking habits become entrenched. For example, the specific condition or symptom to be treated must be clearly identified, and the decision to prescribe a psychoactive drug must be made on the positive grounds of its effectiveness, rather than for negative reasons, such as the patient's expectations or the doctor's need to be seen to be responding. The drug with the least potential for abuse should be prescribed, although alleged differences between drugs of the same class should be treated with scepticism. The dose and the appropriate duration of treatment must be decided. Prescription of the optimum dosage is very important: too small a dose is pointless, exposing the patient to many of the risks of treatment for little or no therapeutic benefit; too large a dose increases the risk of toxicity and dependence and means that more of the drug is available to spill over into the communal 'pool'. Patients should understand at the outset that treatment with any of these drugs will be for a limited period, usually only for a few weeks. This period depends, in part, on the pharmacological properties of the drug and, in particular, on the time taken for tolerance to develop to the effects of the drug. Once this occurs, the prescribed dose is no longer effective and to continue the drug at that dose is of little or no use. Side-effects should be monitored throughout and patients thought to be at risk of developing dependence on the drug should be identified at the start. All of these decisions and observations are usually made automatically when non-psychoactive drugs are prescribed, but the usual clinical approach is often abandoned when psychoactive drugs are involved, perhaps because it seems less appropriate if the underlying problems are social rather than medical.

Once the stage has been reached when prescribing becomes a positive, therapeutic decision rather than a semi-automatic response, there are likely to be many more occasions when the prescription of psychoactive drugs is seen to be wholly inappropriate. For example, if the real cause of the patient's anxiety is a long-standing social problem, there is little point in prescribing benzodiazepines for a month, which is the maximum advisable duration of treatment with these drugs for anxiety.

Similarly, chronic insomnia is rarely benefited in the long term by treatment with hypnotics. In these or similar situations, when a pharmacological solution is seen to be inappropriate, it may still be very difficult for the doctor to withhold symptomatic relief when confronted by a patient suffering real and distressing symptoms. It is therefore very important that doctors become familiar with practical and effective alternative treatment strategies, such as behaviour therapy, psychotherapy, counselling etc. Some of these methods may appear technical and difficult when described in scientific jargon, but they are often no more than the application of common sense principles to patient management. In practice, most doctors employ them unconsciously as part of their total therapeutic relationship with their patients. If any attempt to reduce the availability of psychoactive drugs is to be successful, these non-pharmacological responses will have to receive far more attention in medical education than at present, so that they become a recognized and a respectable component of the therapeutic response, rather than merely second-rate 'alternatives' or 'afterthoughts' to prescribing. Behavioural approaches have the additional advantage of helping people to take responsibility for their own problems, rather than expecting a pharmacological solution, and in the long term may help to reverse the trend towards the medicalization of psychosocial problems.

Medical education, therefore, has a crucial role to play in reducing the availability of prescribed drugs for abuse. This begins with undergraduate education, where basic information about psychoactive drugs and the consequences of their abuse should be formally taught and should receive the attention merited by a condition that can cause widespread public health and social problems. Because there is a constant stream of new psychoactive drugs coming into the market all the time, it is essential that during their undergraduate education, doctors also acquire the skills necessary to evaluate information about new drugs, so that extravagant claims for effectiveness and lack of dependence liability can be assessed critically. Undergraduate education, however, is only the starting point. The practising doctor, as well as keeping abreast of new drugs and treatments, is also exposed to a variety of influences. Continuing education is essential, and it is important that all the institutions and organizations that are in a position to train and influence the doctor exert their influence in the direction of the rational use of psychoactive drugs. Their involvement may take the form of seminars, conferences, articles in journals, etc., and they also play an important role in liaising with other bodies such as government and pharmaceutical industries.

The role of pharmaceutical companies in training doctors is often ignored because it is felt that their ultimate goal, of increasing the sale of their products, opposes the aims of rational prescribing and of reducing the availability of psychoactive drugs that might be abused. However, because governments can and do impose strict control on drugs that are widely abused, the optimal prescribing of their products is ultimately in the best interest of the pharmaceutical companies too and their role in research and information dissemination is too important to be discounted.

The risks of certain drugs, such as cocaine, heroin and other opiates, are seen to be so great that special legal restrictions are imposed upon their prescription. The degree of restriction and the drugs involved vary from country to country, but the basic principle is that clinical freedom to prescribe as the doctor wishes is sacrificed for the sake of control, because the drugs concerned are being widely abused. Such measures are usually imposed in response to an upsurge in abuse and are intended to prevent the situation worsening. Their effectiveness may be reduced by a shift in the pattern of abuse to another less restricted and therefore more easily available preparation. In other words, the problem is not eliminated but transferred to new areas. It is for this reason that imposing restrictions, although sometimes necessary as an immediate response, is far less significant as a long-term preventive measure than genuine improvements in prescribing practices. Some countries have carried this restriction a stage further and have adopted a national drug policy with only a very limited number of drugs available for prescription. The psychoactive drugs included in this list have been well tried out in practice and the information necessary to ensure their proper use is available. New drugs are added to the list only if they have clear-cut advantages over existing drugs.

Other health-care professionals, apart from doctors, are also involved in controlling the availability of psychoactive drugs. In some countries, for example, many of these drugs can be obtained 'over the counter', without the need for any prescription, and the pharmacists who sell them and who have a vested financial interest in their sale must be included in any educational initiatives. Even in countries where prescriptions are always required, pharmacists may be important in detecting abuse and may be able to exert a beneficial influence on patients who seek their advice about taking psychoactive drugs. In some parts of the world, community nurses too may have supplies of these drugs under their control.

Reducing the demand for drugs of abuse

The great difficulties of reducing the availability of drugs for abuse emphasize the need to reduce public demand for them: if no-one wanted heroin or cocaine, the illicit market for them would collapse; if there were no longer the expectation that the doctor can and therefore should relieve all discomfort, far fewer prescriptions for psychoactive drugs would be required. Demand reduction, however, is a preventive approach that attracts comparatively little attention because it depends heavily on worthwhile, but unnewsworthy educational campaigns to influence society's attitude towards drugs and drug taking. Unfortunately, one need look no further than the next cigarette smoker to know that there is no straightforward relationship between education – teaching people about drugs and the dangers of drug abuse – and actually changing their drug-taking behaviour. Spelling out the risks of a particular type of drug abuse does not necessarily mean that those who indulge in it will actually stop doing so and there is evidence that ill-chosen material, intended to scare people away from drug abuse, may instead arouse an interest in the topic and stimulate some individuals, who would not otherwise have become involved, to try drug taking for themselves.

The content of any educational effort is therefore of the greatest importance. Broadly-based health campaigns that encourage healthy lifestyles are generally agreed to be the best approach. Within this framework, healthy eating, participation in sport and physical activities and the appropriate use of medicines are emphasized.

In other words, the message is positive – what should be done to achieve and maintain a healthy lifestyle, rather than emphasizing what is forbidden or dangerous. The individual is encouraged to assume personal responsibility for his/her own health, that would clearly be damaged if drugs were abused. The advantage of this sort of approach is that with appropriate modification of presentation and detail, it is suitable in its broad outline for all ages and all groups. From primary school onwards, the emphasis is on a positive attitude towards health, and within this framework the safe use of medicines can be emphasized – that they should be taken only when necessary for the treatment of illness, that medicines should always be stored safely, that one person must never take another's medicine, and so on.

From this baseline position it is possible to move on quite naturally to non-pharmacological responses for coping with both physical and psychological symptoms. It is very important that people learn that there is not always a 'pill for every ill' and that for many conditions for which there is no cure, symptomatic relief, using traditional, homely remedies is appropriate. A child given lemon and honey for a sore throat, rather than a medicated lozenge, or a hot-water bottle for a stomach ache, rather than a spoonful of medicine, is being taught by practical experience that the first response to discomfort is not necessarily a pill, a medicine, or a drug, but commonsense self-help. Such lessons carried on into adulthood teach that psychological symptoms too may be managed by non-pharmacological methods. In this context, one can question whether it is wise for indiscriminate pill taking of any sort to be positively promoted in any way. Should 'over the counter', non-prescription medicine be widely advertised on television, for example? Should children take daily vitamin pills, when a good diet can supply their needs? Practices such as these run contrary to the basic message of only taking medicines when absolutely necessary, to treat recognized disease states, and they invest medicine taking with an undesirable ordinariness.

Although it is very important that the trend of recent years to medicalize social problems should be reversed, it is equally important that the proper use of medicines should not be discouraged. Amid all the concern about psychoactive drugs and the catalogue of problems consequent on their use, it should not be forgotten that it is this group of drugs that has revolutionized the care of the mentally ill during the last 30 years or so. The drugs have permitted many who would otherwise have been confined to institutions to live within the community and have removed much of the stigma of mental illness. It is essential, therefore, that efforts to limit inappropriate use of drugs in general and of psychoactive drugs in particular, do not develop into a general condemnation of all drug taking. There are many people for whom it is absolutely essential to take drugs regularly, perhaps on a daily basis, perhaps for life, for the treatment of physical or mental illness. Those with a genuine requirement for such treatment should not be discouraged from this wholly appropriate use of drugs, nor made to feel guilty about it.

Once again, doctors have an important role to play in this long-term, public education programme. Their attitudes towards prescribing and their prescribing practices may significantly affect their patients' attitudes too. Doctors who prescribe rationally and who explain their decisions to their patients can make a medical consultation a genuinely educational experience and can contribute regularly to the prevention of drug abuse.

In addition to the education of the community as a whole, specific target groups can be identified for whom more specialized campaigns may be appropriate. Young people are usually perceived as a group for whom preventive education is most important, perhaps because much drug abuse starts at this age, when it is intimately related to peer-group pressure and youthful curiosity. It is also a time for rebellious attitudes and behaviour, when campaigns against drug abuse may have exactly the opposite effect, stimulating an interest in drugs just because they are 'anti-authority'.

Many other target groups can also be identified. Pregnant women, for example, aware that the health of their unborn child is dependent on their own good health, may be particularly receptive to health education. Young professionals, who may be tempted to take cocaine as a symbol of their success; old people who sleep poorly and who would like regular prescriptions for hypnotics; doctors, with their prescription pads always in front of them – all can be recognized as being at special risk, and worthy of special preventive efforts.

For these more specialized preventive campaigns it may seem appropriate to focus the anti-drug message on the particular drug that is the current cause of concern. This permits a simple and direct communication to get the immediate message across, but by stressing the hazards of a particular drug, it is out of tune with modern thinking about the much bigger problem of substance abuse as a whole. Instead, where possible, it should be integrated within existing frameworks and health-care programmes. For example, older adolescents may be approached through programmes in youth-training or work-experience schemes, while the health-promotion clinics established by primary health-care teams for specific patient groups can play an important preventive role in which active patient participation is encouraged.

Harm reduction

Syringe-exchange schemes

Recently, attitudes towards prevention have changed considerably and there is now much greater emphasis on the need to prevent or at least to reduce the harm associated with drug abuse and dependence. This is not a new response. For years, some professionals have advocated that opiate addicts should be prescribed injectable heroin, which they prefer, rather than theoretically safer oral methadone, to prevent them resorting to black market sources with all the attendant hazards. They point out that the harmful consequences of drug abuse are rarely due to the effect of the drug itself, but are more often due to the method of its administration and the presence of adulterants. The arrival of AIDS has reinforced these arguments and, ever since it became apparent that intravenous drug users are a high-risk group for contracting HIV and AIDS, there has been a body of opinion advocating the provision of sterile injection equipment to addicts who inject drugs. It is argued that this will be a genuine public-health measure and good preventive medicine because, theoretically, if sufficient syringes were provided, there would be no need to share injection equipment at all, and the transmission of the HIV virus between addicts and from them to the non-drug-using population would be reduced.

The simplicity of this approach is appealing, but it has certain inbuilt disadvantages. There is a very real risk, for example, that the easy availability of sterile syringes and needles may make the transition to injecting easier and more acceptable and might encourage more young drug abusers to start injecting and to do so sooner; equally there may be less incentive for others to give up injecting. Such a policy could therefore lead to an increased number of injectors within the population, which would undoubtedly mean an increased number of severely dependent individuals. Furthermore, it would not completely eliminate the sharing of injection equipment, which is associated with socializing and communal feeling in the drug sub-culture and not just with the shortage of needles, so there are bound to be some individuals who would carry on sharing regardless of the hazards. In addition, there will always be occasions when the drug user forgets to carry his/her own syringe or has attempted to have a fix when he/she did not intend to.

There are certain practical problems associated with the policy too, such as the number of syringes to be issued per day, and restrictions on those who may receive them. Should they, for example, be given to anyone who asks for them, even before they inject for the first time? Logically, to prevent AIDS and hepatitis they should be freely available, but many professionals caring for drug abusers feel very uncomfortable in a situation in which they seem to be condoning, if not positively encouraging self-injection, which inevitably leads on to a more severe dependent state. A common policy is to provide syringes on a 'new for old' basis only. This prevents the accumulation of large stocks of injection equipment outside the 'system' and ensures the safe, ultimate disposal of potentially contaminated syringes and needles. However, it cannot control, or even estimate, how many times or by how many people a returned syringe and needle has been used. In practice, in some areas where syringe-exchange schemes have been introduced, local communities complain bitterly that used syringes and needles are left lying around and are a serious hazard to young children.

Although the provision of sterile injection equipment is not as simple as it seems at first, syringe-exchange schemes have proliferated rapidly. Research into their effectiveness is difficult because of the long-time lag between infection with HIV and seroconversion (presence of detectable antibody) and because HIV is not exclusively transmitted by sharing contaminated injection equipment. However, it appears that providing sterile injection equipment can contribute to the adoption of safer drug-use behaviour amongst injecting drug users and will therefore reduce the incidence of AIDS among addicts. However, it should be noted that even without providing free syringes, fear of AIDS may bring about beneficial changes in techniques of drug administration, with a reduction in all complications due to injection.

Perhaps the best way forward is to judge each case on its merits, rather than to adopt a stereotyped response. Where it is clear that a stable addict does inject regularly and will continue to do so, and if one can be confident that the injection equipment will not be shared, it may be sensible to provide syringes and needles. On the other hand, it is foolish to pretend that the chaotic polydrug abuser, who is frequently intoxicated and for whom sharing injection equipment is an integral part of drug-taking behaviour, is a safe person to entrust with a supply of syringes and needles.

The provision of syringes and needles to addicts has been discussed in some detail because it is of considerable topical interest. It is not, however, the only aspect of harm reduction. Another similarly controversial question has risen about whether young solvent abusers, at risk of fatal accidents while intoxicated, should be instructed in safer techniques of solvent sniffing – such as not putting a plastic bag right over the head, not sniffing alone, not sniffing in dangerous places (e.g., roof tops, canal banks). Preventive education of this type, although potentially life saving, at best conveys a very ambivalent message about drug taking and at worst seems to encourage the practice.

These examples emphasize the unpalatable fact that the laudable aim of harm reduction may sometimes conflict with the much more important aim of preventing and reducing the underlying problems of drug abuse and dependence. It is worth noting that the harmful consequences of drug abuse were largely ignored by the general population until one of these consequences, AIDS, became a serious threat to themselves as well. The vociferous support for harm reduction since then suggests that it is motivated more in unthinking self-interest than in a genuine concern for the well-being of drug abusers. For the latter group, the best approach is undoubtedly to encourage them vigorously to become abstinent from drugs. This is achieved more easily if it is attempted early in a drug-taking career, and ideally it should be attempted before self-injection becomes established and causes severe physical and psychological dependence. Easy access to treatment facilities is therefore a very important factor in harm reduction. Only if treatment and persuasion fail should measures that may reinforce dependence be considered.

Substitute prescribing

The use of methadone for the stabilization, detoxification or maintenance of opiate-dependent individuals has been described in some detail in Chapter 6. One of the reasons for adopting this type of substitute prescribing is to attract more drug users to services, so that treatment, in its broader sense, can be initiated as soon as possible. It may have very positive benefits in terms of harm reduction, in that the patient may cease to use illicit drugs, may stop injecting, or at least use a sterile injection technique. However, while substitute prescribing may be a helpful tool in helping the drug-dependent individual to move towards abstinence or towards intermediate goals, there is a very real risk that this progress may be unacceptably slow and that the patient may be maintained indefinitely in an opiate-dependent state, without any clear decision having been taken that this is the right course of action for this particular patient. It follows that if the potential benefits of substitute prescribing are to be fully realized, it is essential that treatment interventions should have a clearly defined aim, and that there are well-established routes into detoxification.

Outreach services

Despite general acknowledgement of the importance of easy access to treatment and the consequent growth in drug services in recent years, the majority of drug users are not in touch with these services. Indeed, there may be a period of several years between starting illicit drug use and making contact with a helping agency. Reducing this time lag early in a drug-taking career, when intervention is most likely to be successful, is essential for effective prevention. Because waiting for drug users to attend established services is clearly an inadequate response, outreach services have been developed that are proactive in making contact with drug users to offer them short-term help and to refer them on to appropriate helping agencies.

If outreach services are to be effective, some type of needs assessment is essential. For example, the reasons why existing services are not being used will have to be established and, if necessary, these services will be reviewed and modified so that they are acceptable and attractive to those who need them. In particular, outreach can aid the development of effective liaison and referral mechanisms between a wide range of agencies, including voluntary services and statutory health and social services.

However, outreach workers will never be able to achieve contact with all drug users, nor will they be able to achieve onward referral to an appropriate agency for all those with whom they do come into contact. Therefore, an important aspect of their work is to achieve change at community level and to achieve harm reduction by a cascading educational process. Thus, when working with a certain number of individuals, they also try to ensure that their message reaches other drug users with whom their client comes into contact. Because outreach developed as an attempt to reduce the spread of HIV and AIDS, much of the work is focused in this area, with an emphasis on advice on safer sexual practices and safer injecting practices and on practical measures such as the provision of condoms and sterile injection equipment. Effective harm reduction, however, encompasses far more than this, and outreach workers should not lose opportunities to discourage regular drug use among experimental users, to discourage injection by potential injectors, to encourage established injectors to switch to safer, oral administration of drugs and to encourage drug injectors and their sexual partners to be immunized against hepatitis B.

Conclusion

The prevention of drug abuse and drug dependence, like the treatment and the conditions themselves, is a chronic process. Once again, we see that there are no quick and easy solutions but a number of measures, none effective alone, but each making some contribution to the totality of a comprehensive programme. The preventive measures that seem likely to be most effective include reducing the availability of drugs by effective law enforcement, including the application of penalties severe enough to deter those who make huge profits by dealing in illicit drugs. Reduction of the availability of prescription drugs, however, relies less on law enforcement and much more on the education of doctors in rational prescribing. This is closely related to the problem of changing public attitudes towards medicine in general and psychoactive drugs in particular. Educating the public to reduce the demand for psychoactive drugs is a very long-term project. It probably offers the best hope for the prevention of drug abuse in years to come, but it will undoubtedly take a long time to reverse the trends of recent decades.

In addition, this approach emphasizes the fact that effective prevention will never be brought about, or imposed on the community, by the actions of professionals and experts alone. On the contrary, it is absolutely essential that the whole community has a strong commitment to prevention. Already there are clear signs of this happening, usually where a particular type of drug abuse has become so prevalent that local people have made a determined effort to overcome it. For example, in some places heroin abuse is so rife that parents have got together in very powerful self-help groups, not just for mutual support, but also to work actively to eliminate drug-taking from their community. Unfortunately, it seems that the problem has to be severe before this kind of response is initiated, but it is reassuring that when a community is genuinely under threat it can and often does respond energetically.

Parallels can be drawn with what has happened and what is happening with cigarette smoking: community attitudes and responses to smoking now permit far more coercive and draconian measures to be taken than could have been contemplated 20 years ago, and the prevalence of cigarette smoking in the UK has declined steadily. In China, too, after liberation, fervent support on the part of the community enabled the total eradication of problems related to the use of opium. Continuing commitment to prevention has resulted in China remaining comparatively free of drug-related problems, at least until fairly recently.

It is to be hoped that the long-term, educational approaches outlined in this chapter will bear fruit in years to come and that pharmacological solutions to personal problems will cease to be the norm. In the meantime, the importance of indirect factors, such as improved housing, education, leisure opportunities and employment, that can all influence drug taking significantly, should not be ignored.

Most of these preventive measures are neither dramatic nor newsworthy and it is difficult to evaluate their effectiveness. It is understandable that when governments are faced with an upsurge of drug abuse of one type or another, they require a more obvious response than a dogged perseverance with long-term programmes, however sound in principle they may be. In this situation, where they need to be seen to be responding to a crisis with some urgency, changes in the law or a strident advertising programme are often thought to be appropriate. However, the effectiveness of these responses and of the other approaches outlined here must not be taken for granted. They should be carefully evaluated by means of ongoing epidemiological programmes, that can detect changes in drug abuse and monitor the effects of preventive approaches.

References and further reading

Advisory Council on the Misuse of Drugs (1984). *Prevention*. Home Office, London.

Advisory Council on the Misuse of Drugs (1988). *Aids and Drug Misuse: Part 1*. HMSO, London.

Advisory Council on the Misuse of Drugs (1989). *Aids and Drug Misuse: Part 2*. HMSO, London.

Advisory Council on the Misuse of Drugs (1993). *Aids and Drug Misuse Update*. HMSO, London.

Bandy P & President PA (1983). Recent literature on drug-abuse prevention and the mass media: focussing on youth, parents, women and the elderly. *Journal of Drug Education*, **13**, 255–271.

Bell CS & Battjes R (eds) (1985). *Prevention Research: Deterring Drug Abuse Among Children and Adolescents*. NIDA Research Monograph 63. Department of Health & Human Services, Rockville.

Dorn N (1981). Social analyses of drugs in health education and the media. In: Edwards G & Busch C (eds). *Drug Problems in Britain: A Review of Ten Years*, 281–304. Academic Press, London.

Dorn N (1990). Preventive issues and legal aspects. In: Ghodse AH & Maxwell D (eds). *Substance Abuse and Dependence*, 232–243. Macmillan Press, London.

Ghodse H & Khan I (1988). *Psychoactive Drugs: Improving Prescribing Practices*. WHO, Geneva.

Glynn TJ, Leukenfeld CG & Ludford JP (1983). *Preventing Adolescent Drug Abuse: Intervention Strategies*. NIDA Research Monograph 47. National Institute of Drug Abuse, Washington DC.

International Narcotics Control Board (1992). *Report of the INCB for 1992. (E/INCB/1992/1)*. United Nations Publication, New York.

International Narcotics Control Board (1993). *Report of the INCB for 1993. (E/INCB/1993/1)*. United Nations Publication, New York.

Pittman DJ (1994). Substance misuse prevention, health promotion, and health education. *Current Opinion in Psychiatry,* **7, No 3**, 269–273.

Schaps E, di Bartolo R, Moskowitz J *et al.* (1981). A review of 127 drug abuse prevention program evaluations. *Journal of Drug Issues,* **1, 11**, 17–43.

Schuster CR (1992). Drug abuse research and HIV/AIDS: a national perspective from the US. *British Journal of Addiction,* **87**, 355–361.

Strang J, Heathcote S & Watson P (1987). Habit-moderation in injecting drug addicts. *Health Trends,* **19**, 16–18.

Tyrer P & Murphy S (1987). The place of benzodiazepines in psychiatric practice. *British Journal of Psychiatry,* **151**, 719–723.

World Health Organization (1983). *The Use of Essential Drugs*. Report of a WHO Expert Committee, Technical Report Series 685. WHO, Geneva.

World Health Organization (1993). *Health Promotion in the Work Place: Alcohol and Drug Abuse*. Report of a WHO Expert Committee, Technical Report Series 833. WHO, Geneva.

11

The law and drug-control policy

International controls

The need for international measures to control drug abuse and dependence has long been recognized. They were initiated at the beginning of the century and continue today. A number of multilateral treaties were signed over the years and the international system of control became complicated and cumbersome. It was revised and modernized by the Single Convention on Narcotic Drugs, which was adopted in 1961 and was subsequently widened and strengthened by the 1972 protocol. Additional problems arose due to the introduction of new, synthetic, psychoactive drugs, that were widely used for the effective treatment of mental illness, but which were often accompanied by the development of dependence and abuse. The Convention on Psychotropic Substances (1971) extended the international drug-control system to cover some of these new drugs, while the 1988 Convention against Illicit Traffic in Narcotic Drugs and Psychotropic Substance was introduced to hamper the activities of drug traffickers by depriving them of their ill-gotten gains and freedom of movement.

These three Conventions aim to ensure the safe use of potentially dangerous psychoactive substances. They recognize that these substances often have legitimate scientific and medicinal uses that must be protected, but that their abuse gives rise to public-health, social and economic problems. Vigorous measures, involving close international cooperation, are required to restrict their use to legitimate purposes.

The Conventions list the controlled substances in different schedules with different levels of control, depending on the balance between therapeutic usefulness and the risk of abuse. Countries that ratify the Conventions are obliged to adopt appropriate legislation, introduce necessary administrative and enforcement measures and cooperate with international drug-control agencies and with other parties to the Conventions. Internationally devised measures are thus translated into national controls by individual states within their own legal systems.

The Single Convention on Narcotic Drugs

The Single Convention puts strict controls on the cultivation of the opium poppy, coca bush and cannabis plant and their products, which for the purpose of the Convention are described as 'narcotics' (although cocaine is a stimulant drug rather than one which induces sleep). The Convention lists these substances in four schedules and a considerable number of opiate-like, dependence-producing drugs that are synthesized by scientific methods and manufactured industrially thereby come under varying degrees of control, according to their potential harmfulness and therapeutic usefulness.

Schedule I is the major schedule, roughly corresponding (except for heroin and cannabis) to Class A drugs of the UK Misuse of Drugs Act 1971 (see p. 340). It includes the raw, plant materials, such as opium, coca leaf and cannabis and many of their derivatives. These drugs are subject to all of the controls specified by the Convention.

Schedule II includes the drugs more commonly used for medical purposes that require less strict trade and distribution controls because there is a smaller risk of their abuse.

Schedule III drugs are the same as those in Schedule II, but in lower concentrations and controlled proportions so that they are not liable to abuse.

Schedule IV includes a very few drugs that are subjected to extra controls because they have particularly dangerous properties and/or are of limited therapeutic use. Cannabis and heroin are both included in Schedule IV of the Single Convention.

Parties to the Single Convention undertake to limit the production, manufacture, export, import, distribution, stocks of, trade in, and use and possession of the controlled drugs so that they are used exclusively for medical and scientific purposes. The production and distribution of the drugs is licensed and supervised so that annual estimates and statistical returns can be made to the International Narcotics Control Board (INCB) of the quantities of drugs required, manufactured and utilized, and the quantities seized by police and customs officials. The accumulation of returns from many countries provides global information about the movement – licit and illicit – of these drugs.

The Psychotropic Convention

The Psychotropic Convention extends the same principles of control as the Single Convention to cover drugs such as central nervous system stimulants, sedative hypnotics and hallucinogens. As of 1995, 105 substances are covered by the Psychotropic Convention, but this number is likely to increase as new drugs are introduced to the market. The drugs are listed in four schedules with different degrees of control.

Schedule I includes hallucinogens such as LSD which are dangerous drugs, causing serious risks to public health and with little, if any, therapeutic use. They are therefore controlled very strictly to limit their use chiefly to research.

Schedule II contains the stimulant sympathomimetic drugs (e.g., amphetamine) which are of very limited therapeutic value. They are highly addictive drugs and are strictly controlled, although the special provisions of Schedule I, limiting use to authorized individuals only, are omitted.

Schedule III covers fast and medium-acting barbiturates that have been widely abused, but which are therapeutically useful.

Schedule IV includes a variety of hypnotics, tranquillizers and analgesic drugs that are widely used therapeutically (in some countries), but which have a marked dependence-producing liability.

All of these drugs are available only on medical prescription and parties to the Convention undertake to ensure that prescriptions are issued in accordance with sound medical practice and that labelling, packaging and advertising conform to certain rules.

1988 United Nations Convention against Illicit Traffic in Narcotic Drugs and Psychotropic substances

This Convention defines drug-trafficking activities, which now include money laundering and illicit activities related to precursors, in a comprehensive and innovative manner. Countries are required to establish these activities as criminal offences and create penalties adequate to their serious nature. To facilitate the tracing, freezing and confiscation of proceeds and property derived from drug trafficking, courts are empowered to make available or to seize bank, financial or commercial records, and bank secrecy cannot be invoked in such cases. Furthermore, the Convention bars all havens to drug traffickers, particularly through its provisions for extradition of major drug traffickers, mutual legal assistance between states on drug-related investigations, and the transfer of proceedings for criminal prosecution. Another significant landmark is the commitment of parties to eliminate or reduce illicit demand for narcotic drugs and psychotropic substances. Over 60 states are now party to the 1988 Convention which came into force in 1990.

United Nations drug abuse control organs

The United Nations General Assembly is ultimately responsible for the control and supervision of international efforts to restrict the use of drugs to their proper medical purposes. It operates in this field through the Secretary-General and the Economic and Social Council (ECOSOC) which is assisted and advised by the Commission on Narcotic Drugs.

Recognizing the central role that must be played by the United Nations in fostering concerted international activity in this field, a special session of the General Assembly was convened in 1990 to consider, as a matter of urgency, the question of international cooperation against illicit production, supply, demand, trafficking and distribution of narcotic drugs, with a view to expanding the scope and increasing the effectiveness of such cooperation. The General Assembly adopted a Global Programme of Action to achieve the goal of an international society free of illicit drugs and drug abuse, and created the United Nations International Drug Control Programme, which integrated the structures and functions of the former United Nations drug units (i.e., the Division of Narcotic Drugs (DND), the United Nations Fund for Drug Control (UNFDAC)) as well as the secretariat of the International Narcotics Control Board (INCB)

Commission on Narcotic Drugs

The Commission on Narcotic Drugs (CND) was established in 1946 and is the central policy-making body within the United Nations system for dealing with all questions related to the global effort of drug abuse control. It consists of representatives of 53 Member States, elected by the Economic and Social Council, and its annual meetings are also attended by observers from other governments, other United Nations organs and from agencies and organizations with an interest in drug control.

As well as planning and developing general strategies against drug abuse, a central function of the Commission is to advise on changes in the current system of international drug control, making proposals for new conventions and drug-control instruments. More specifically, the Commission makes decisions on bringing new substances under the control of the Conventions and decides what level of control is required. To this end, it receives information and recommendations from the World Health Organization (WHO), which it may accept or reject (or sometimes amend) in the light of economic, social, legal and administrative factors that are considered relevant.

Subsidiary bodies of CND coordinate the Commission's work at regional level. There are regional groupings of the operational Heads of National Drug Law Enforcement Agencies (HONLEA) in Asia and the Pacific, as well as in Africa, Latin America, the Caribbean and Europe, and inter-regional meetings of HONLEA strengthen international cooperation further.

The International Narcotics Control Board *economy*

The International Narcotics Control Board (INCB) is an independent body created by the Single Convention. It reports to the Economic and Social Council through the Commission on Narcotic Drugs. There are 13 members of the Board who are proposed by the member states of the United Nations and elected by the Economic and Social Council. Once on the Board, however, they serve impartially in their personal capacities for periods of 5 years at a time. Three members, nominated by WHO, have medical, pharmacological or pharmaceutical experience.

The major responsibility of the INCB is to limit the cultivation, production, manufacture and utilization of the drugs that are controlled by the Conventions to the amounts that are necessary for medical and scientific purposes. Parties to the Conventions undertake to keep records of the flow and handling of the controlled substances so that they can provide the INCB with estimates of the total annual requirements of each controlled substance, and later with statistics about actual manufacture, international trade and consumption. The Board can then compare estimates with actual total use, to establish that the drugs available in each country for medical purposes are accounted for at the main stages of production, manufacture and trade. If there are discrepancies between consumption and statistically calculated available quantities, or between estimates and actual use, these can be investigated and the causes clarified. In this way the Board can assist governments to achieve the correct balance between supply and demand for controlled drugs. Under the 1988 Convention, traffic in precursor substances that are important for the illicit manufacture of narcotic drugs and psychotropic substances is also monitored, and this too is the responsibility of the INCB.

The INCB also receives information about illicit drug activity within national borders and uses this information, together with that about all aspects of the licit drug trade, to determine whether the aims of the Conventions are being endangered by any country. If they are, it can make recommendations on remedial measures or, as a last resort, propose sanctions against defaulting countries. The INCB maintains dialogues with governments, both through regular consultations and by special missions, arranged in agreement with the governments concerned. This type of 'quiet diplomacy' has brought about the strengthening of legislation in several countries which have acknowledged the need for coordination of national drug-control efforts.

The INCB's other activities include training programmes for drug-control administrators and producing an annual report on the global situation of the working of the Conventions and on illicit production and traffic of drugs. This report, which is submitted to the Economic and Social Council through the CND, contains recommendations to governments and is supplemented by technical reports on the licit movement of narcotic drugs and psychotropic substances.

United Nations International Drug Control Programme

Created in 1990, the United Nations International Drug Control Programme (UNDCP) has continued with the work of the Division of Narcotic Drugs and of the United Nations Fund for Drug Abuse Control, performing a variety of functions deriving from the international drug-control treaties and specific mandates of the General Assembly, ECOSOC and CND. It is therefore responsible for coordinating UN drug-control activities, for promoting the implementation of the international Conventions and for providing effective leadership in international drug control. In particular, it carries out the Secretary-General's functions under the international Conventions, assisting CND and INCB in implementing their treaty-based functions and promoting new instruments as necessary.

UNDCP plays a very important role in providing technical assistance, through expertise and training, to help governments to set up adequate drug-control structures and to define comprehensive national plans. These may encompass a wide range of activities such as integrated rural development and crop substitution, enforcement of drug-related laws, prevention, treatment and rehabilitation of drug addicts, as well as legislative and institutional reforms so that governments are better able to fight drug abuse. New areas of concern for UNDCP include the damaging environmental effects of illicit cultivation and processing of drugs and the fight against 'money laundering'. Its 16 national and subregional field offices assist governments in the development of initiatives to enhance the concept of joint operations between different countries. Its important work in these areas is dependent on voluntary contributions to the Programme's budget, which in 1992 amounted to 93% of all resources available to UNDCP (about

$US 100 million); the remainder of its funding comes from the regular budget of the United Nations.

World Health Organization

Because drug abuse constitutes a serious health hazard of steadily growing proportions in many countries, the WHO, which is the competent international health authority, is closely involved on many fronts in the fight against it. Within the field of control, for example, WHO is involved and concerned with regulations about the prescription of controlled drugs and their advertising. In addition, it has developed reporting programmes to monitor the adverse side-effects of psychoactive drugs in relation to their risk of abuse and dependence potential, and programmes to establish the epidemiology of drug dependence.

The Conventions assign specific responsibilities to WHO in respect of changes in the control of substances and of placing them in appropriate schedules. WHO studies the medical and scientific characteristics of drugs in order to assess their therapeutic usefulness and dependence liability, and then evaluates the public health and social problems related to their abuse. To make these assessments, WHO relies on collaboration with member states. The fundamental research, whether biological, medical or epidemiological, is carried out in national universities and industrial laboratories which provide a steady flow of information to WHO, which in turn provides resources for research. Once the assessment is completed (by a group of experts), WHO communicates its findings to CND together with recommendations on control measures. The final decision about control is taken by the Commission which also takes into account economic, social, legal and administrative factors which have been communicated to it from the UNDCP and the INCB. Research of this kind is always important, but its value is magnified many times over if standardized methodology is adopted by several countries. International comparisons then become possible and a truly global picture of patterns of drug abuse and dependence emerges, which permits appropriate international responses to be made.

Other WHO activities related to drug control include the promotion of the rational use of psychoactive substances, not just through regulations but through education. To this end, guidelines for rational use are being compiled, together with a list of essential drugs for basic health needs, which serves as a guide for countries in identifying their own needs and priorities concerning drug availability. WHO is also involved in inter-regional training courses for health-care professionals on prevention and treatment of drug dependence.

Other United Nations organizations

Although drug-abuse control is not their main function, a number of other United Nations organizations are actively involved in this area. They include the following.

United Nations Educational, Scientific and Cultural Organization (UNESCO) focuses on the prevention of drug abuse through public education and awareness and works to integrate preventive education concerning drug use into school curricula and out-of-school activities.

United Nations Children's Fund (UNICEF) is involved particularly in relation to the estimated 100 million 'street children' who are often drug abusers and drug sellers.

The *International Maritime Organization*, the *International Civil Aviation Organization* and the *International Postal Union* have all introduced measures aimed at combating the illicit transport of drugs, while the *Food and Agriculture Organization* is involved in raising the income level of farmers so that the incentive to cultivate prohibited crops is reduced.

Although it is not an agency of the United Nations, the *International Criminal Police Organization (ICPO/Interpol)*, which is composed of national law enforcement agencies, works with the United Nations to improve information about the flow of illicit drugs and illegally acquired assets across international borders.

Control in the UK

Misuse of Drugs Act 1971

The Misuse of Drugs Act 1971, which became fully operational in 1973, replaced earlier laws and is the principal legislation in the UK for controlling drug use and preventing misuse. It deals with nearly all drugs with abuse and/or dependence liability, laying down specific requirements for their prescription, safe custody and record-keeping and defining the offences related to their production, cultivation, supply and possession.

The Act lists the drugs that are subject to control and classifies them in three categories according to their relative harm when misused.

Class A includes alfentanil, carfentanil, cocaine, dextromoramide, dipipanone, heroin, lofentanil, LSD, methadone, morphine, opium, pethidine phencyclidine (and injectable forms of Class B drugs).

Class B includes oral preparations of amphetamines, barbiturates, cannabis, cannabis resin, codeine, glutethimide, pentazocine, phenmetrazine and pholcodine.

Class C includes certain appetite suppressants such as phentermine, diethylpropion and mazindol, and sedatives such as meprobamate, methyprylone and most benzodiazepines.

The penalties for offences involving controlled drugs depend on the classification of the drug: penalties for misuse of Class A drugs are more severe than for Class B drugs, which in turn are more severe than for Class C drugs. The Act also distinguishes, in terms of the penalties that may be imposed, between the crimes of possession and drug trafficking, with the latter receiving much more severe punishment.

An important part of the Misuse of Drugs Act is that the Home Secretary is empowered to make regulations to supplement the control of drugs. Many of these regulations have a direct effect on doctors and their work, although their clinical freedom to prescribe whatever drugs they consider necessary is largely unimpeded.

Misuse of Drugs Regulations 1985

These regulations define the classes of people (e.g., midwife, doctor, public laboratory analyst) who are authorized to possess or supply controlled drugs and the situations in which they are permitted to do so.

As far as doctors are concerned, the regulations provide a more practical classification of controlled drugs than that described earlier which was primarily for crimino-legal purposes. The regulations divide the drugs into five schedules, with different requirements and rules governing prescribing, safe custody and record-keeping for each schedule.

Schedule 1 includes drugs such as LSD, cannabis, raw opium and coca leaf, for which there are no therapeutic indications. Special authorization is required from the Home Office for their possession and supply (which is usually for the purpose of research).

Schedule 2 includes drugs which are, on the whole, widely used in clinical medicine, but which have a high dependence liability, e.g., heroin, morphine, pethidine, dextromoramide, dipipanone, methadone, fentanyl, cocaine and amphetamine.

The regulations give specific instructions for the safe custody of these drugs, which are usually kept in locked safes, cabinets or rooms which have to comply with precise specifications. Doctors (and others) should note that it is not considered safe to leave Schedule 2 drugs in a locked car (e.g., when visiting a patient). A register must be kept to record the use of these drugs.

Prescriptions for Schedule 2 drugs must conform to precise legal requirements. They must be hand-written by the prescriber who must sign and date them and whose address must be stated (i.e., they cannot be produced by a printer from a computer or be typed). The prescription must state:

1   the name and address of the patient;
2   the drug and the form in which it is to be dispensed (e.g., tablets, mixture) and, if appropriate, the strength of the preparation (e.g., methadone mixture x mg/ml);
3   the dose;
4   the total quantity or the number of dose units to be dispensed. This must be written in both words and figures.

All of this information is required by law. It is an offence for a doctor to issue an incomplete prescription for a drug controlled under Schedule 2, and it is an offence for a pharmacist to dispense the prescription if it is incomplete. 'Repeat' prescriptions for these drugs are not permitted, nor can they be issued as an 'emergency supply' by a pharmacist at the patient's request. Special arrangements exist when these drugs are prescribed to addicts in the course of treating their dependence.

Schedule 3 includes barbiturates, diethylpropion, mazindol, phentermine, meprobamate, methyprylone and pentazocine. These are all drugs that are known to cause dependence and that have been extensively abused. Prescriptions for Schedule 3 drugs must conform to the same legal requirements as those outlined above for Schedule 2 drugs, but there are no requirements for safe custody (except for diethylpropion), and there is no need to keep a register.

The term 'controlled drugs' is widely, although imprecisely, used as a collective description of the drugs in Schedules 2 and 3 of the Misuse of Drugs Regulations 1985, and has come to mean those drugs that are subject to the prescription requirements of the regulations. Strictly speaking, all drugs listed in the Act (or Regulations) are 'controlled' drugs.

If phenobarbitone is the only drug from Schedule 2 or 3 on the prescription form, the requirement for a hand-written prescription does not apply. This exemption is a recognition of the role of phenobarbitone in the treatment of epilepsy, when there is little risk of the development of drug abuse.

Schedule 4 includes benzodiazepine drugs which were brought under control of the Misuse of Drugs Act by the 1985 Regulations. They are, however, subject to only minimal control, and although they are 'prescription-only medicine', their prescriptions do not have to fulfil the requirements applicable to Schedule 2 and 3 drugs, nor are there any safe custody requirements.

Schedule 5 drugs are preparations which contain drugs listed in Schedules 2 or 3, but in such small quantities that they are harmless, or compounded in such a way that recovery of the drug in quantities that might be harmful is impossible or unlikely. For example, diphenoxylate is a Schedule 2 drug, but as Lomotil (2.5 mg diphenoxylate with atropine sulphate 25 μg) it is a Schedule 5 drug and exempt from all controlled drug requirements except that of retaining invoices for a 2-year period.

Obligation to notify

Under the Misuse of Drugs (Notification of and Supply to Addicts) Regulations 1973, a doctor is required to notify the Chief Medical Officer at the Home Office, in writing, of the personal particulars of any patient whom he/she considers (or has reasonable grounds to suspect) is addicted to certain controlled drugs. According to these regulations, a person is regarded as being addicted 'if, and only if, he/she has, as a result of repeated administration, become so dependent on the drug that he/she has an overpowering desire for the administration of it to be continued'.

These are the controlled drugs to which the regulations apply.

1   Cocaine.
2   Dextromoramide (Palfium).
3   Diamorphine (Heroin).
4   Dipipanone (available as Diconal).
5   Hydrocodone (Dimotane DC).
6   Hydromorphone.
7   Levorphanol (Dromoran).
8   Methadone (Physeptone).
9   Morphine.
10   Opium.
11   Oxycodone.
12   Pethidine.
13   Phenazocine (Narphen.
14   Piritramide (Dipidolor).

Addiction to papaveretum (Omnopon) which contains morphine should also be notified.

It is not necessary to notify the Chief Medical Officer if continued, long-term administration of any of these drugs is necessary for the treatment of organic disease. In other words, patients receiving opiates to relieve severe pain – often those who are terminally ill – need not and should not be notified.

The information provided to the Chief Medical Officer should include:

1   name and address of patient;
2   sex;

3   date of birth;
4   National Health Service number;
5   date of attendance;
6   drug(s) of addiction.

There is also space on the form to record where the patient was seen (e.g., hospital out-patient department, general practice, etc.), the patient's nationality and what drugs, if any, have been prescribed by the reporting doctor. Since September 1987, when a new form was introduced (HS2A/1 Rev), there is also a question about whether the patient injects any drugs (including those which are not notifiable, but which are commonly abused, such as amphetamine). It is hoped that the answers to this question will help the authorities to obtain a more complete picture about patterns of drug abuse in general and about injection practices in particular. This database may be of great importance when planning preventive strategies against HIV and AIDS.

It is important to emphasize that notification is a statutory obligation of all doctors and that failure to notify is a contravention of the Misuse of Drugs Act that can result in disciplinary action against the doctor. The completed form should be sent to the Home Office within 7 days of attending the patient (regardless of whether drugs were prescribed or not). If a doctor does not know all the necessary particulars, the available information should be given and the remainder notified as soon as possible.

Notification is not necessary if the doctor, or another doctor in the same general practice, has notified the Home Office of that patient within the previous 12 months. Similarly, a hospital doctor need not notify if he/she or another doctor from the same hospital has sent in a notification form for that patient within the previous year. In practice, of course, a hospital doctor may not know and indeed is very unlikely to know if a colleague has notified a particular patient, but as many doctors remain unaware of their obligation to notify, it is wiser to assume that it has not been done and to complete the necessary form oneself. No harm is done by repeated (unnecessary) notification. Only if the patient is currently attending a drug-dependence treatment unit (DDTU) at the hospital, which sends in regular returns to the Home Office, is it safe to assume that the patient has already been notified.

Prescribing controlled drugs to addicts

If a decision is made to prescribe opiates or other drugs regularly to someone who is dependent upon them, either in the short term for detoxification, or in the long term for maintenance treatment, it is essential that the prescriptions be dispensed on a daily basis. This is because it would be very unwise to give several days' supply of drugs to an addict all at once. As the prescription forms FP10 and FP10 HP are valid for supply on one occasion only, it follows that if these forms are used, six prescriptions must be written each week, with 2 days' prescription being dispensed on Saturday.

To facilitate prescribing for addicts, a new prescription form, FP10 (MDA), has been introduced to enable GPs to write a prescription for several days' treatment on a single form, to be dispensed in instalments. Not more than 14 days' supply should be ordered on one form, and the number of instalments to be dispensed and the interval between each instalment should be specified. Form FP10 (MDA) may only be used to prescribe Schedule 2 drugs to addicts and all other prescription-writing requirements for these drugs must be complied with.

Whenever possible, the patient should be introduced to the particular pharmacist who has agreed to dispense the prescription, so that there is no confusion about the identity of the patient. It should be made clear to the patient that the prescription will not be dispensed in advance and cannot be collected 'in arrears'. The pharmacist should be encouraged to report back to the prescribing doctor if drugs are not collected, and always to check with the doctor if the patient requests any alteration in the dispensing arrangements. Prescriptions are often posted directly to the pharmacist.

Special arrangements have also been made for doctors working in specialist DDTUs, when they prescribe controlled drugs to addicts, to save them from having to write six prescriptions per week for each patient on maintenance or detoxification treatment. They are provided with a different prescription form (FP10HP(ad)) which can only be used for prescribing cocaine, dextromoramide, diamorphine, dipipanone, methadone, morphine or pethidine and which permits these drugs to be dispensed in instalments so that only one prescription is needed each week. The quantity to be dispensed on each occasion and the interval between instalments must be stated. These doctors may also obtain exemption from the handwriting requirement for Schedule 2 and 3 drugs, so that prescriptions can be typed ready for them to sign. This exemption applies only to the named institutions in which they work.

Prescribing heroin, cocaine and dipipanone to addicts

Under the Misuse of Drugs (Notification of and Supply to Addicts) Regulations 1973, only doctors who hold a special licence, issued by the Home Secretary, are permitted to prescribe heroin, dipipanone or cocaine for addicts for the purpose of treating their addiction. In practice, most doctors holding this licence work in the specialist clinics for treating drug dependence, where the prescription of these highly addictive (and therefore highly sought-after) drugs is under scrutiny and discussion by members of a multidisciplinary team. It is hoped in this way to control and restrict the prescription of these drugs to those cases for whom it is justified and necessary, and to prevent the re-emergence of a 1960s-type situation when some doctors prescribed unnecessarily large doses that contributed to the black market in drugs.

However, any doctor may prescribe heroin, dipipanone or cocaine to any patient (including addicts) if the drug is required for the treatment of organic disease. Thus an addict who needs heroin or morphine, for example, to provide analgesia after an abdominal operation, may be prescribed the necessary dose by the responsible doctor without recourse to a DDTU. The statutory obligation to notify the Home Office is not affected.

Medicines Act 1968

It has been noted previously (see p. 115) that some drugs with a potential for misuse are available without a prescription 'over the counter'. Under the Medicines Act there are two classes of such drugs.

1 *Pharmacy Only Medicines* which can only be sold in a registered pharmacy.

2 *General Sales List Medicines (GSL)* which can also, under certain conditions, be sold in other shops – usually only in strictly limited quantities.

Medications with a potential for misuse (codeine, antihistamines, stimulant-like drugs) come within the former group.

Intoxicating Substances Supply Act 1985

Solvents, which are commercially available substances with a variety of uses, are not covered by the Misuse of Drugs Act, and the Intoxicating Substances Supply Act was therefore introduced in an attempt to deal with solvent sniffing. This act makes it an offence for a person to supply or offer to supply to someone under the age of 18 years, substances that the supplier knows, or has reason to believe, will be used 'to achieve intoxication'. The law is directed primarily at irresponsible shopkeepers, to deter them from selling solvents or volatile substances to youngsters who are going to sniff them. However, it is difficult to prove that a shopkeeper knows what the substance will be used for and there have been few prosecutions under this act. Nevertheless, the threat of legal action probably acts as a deterrent.

Health and Safety at Work Act 1974

Under this act, employers are required to ensure, as far as reasonably practicable, the health, safety and welfare of all their employees, and employees are required to take reasonable care of the health and safety of themselves and others who may be affected by their acts or omissions at work. This clearly has implications for substance abusers but, in addition, an employer who knowingly allows a drug abuser to continue working without doing anything either to help the abuser or protect other employees may also be liable to charges.

Advisory Council on Misuse of Drugs

The Advisory Council on Misuse of Drugs (ACMD) was set up under the Misuse of Drugs Act 1971. It is made up of at least 20 members who are appointed by the Home Secretary and who include representatives of the medical, veterinary, dental and pharmacy professions and of the pharmaceutical industry. Individuals with wide and recent experience of the social problems connected with drug misuse are also included.

The ACMD is responsible for advising the government about appropriate measures to educate the public about the dangers of drug misuse, about the best ways of treating drug misusers and helping their rehabilitation and about promoting research into drug misuse.

A particular and very important function of the ACMD is to review drugs which are being misused or which appear likely to be misused and to advise the government on measures to prevent this. Often this involves a drug being brought under control of the Misuse of Drugs Act, or being put under stricter control because there is evidence that its misuse is increasing. Thus new controls can be initiated in response to changes in the drug scene without the need for a new Act of Parliament if a different drug becomes problematical. The potential for a (comparatively) swift response to changing trends of drug abuse is essential if new and perhaps dangerous patterns of drug abuse are to be dealt with effectively before the problem gets out of control.

In practice, of course, even swift responses depend on the gathering of relevant information and are slow in comparison with the rapid changes of the drug scene, so that 'solutions' are always late. Nevertheless, the ACMD reduces the duration of potentially damaging delays.

References and further reading

Bakalar JB & Grinspoon L (1984). *Drug Control in a Free Society.* Cambridge University Press, Cambridge.

Bruun K (ed.) (1983). *Controlling Psychotropic Drugs: The Nordic Experience* Croom Helm, London.

Bruun K, Pan L & Rexed I (1975). *The Gentlemen's Club: International Control of Drugs and Alcohol.* University of Chicago Press, Chicago.

Bucknell P & Ghodse AH (1991). *Misuse of Drugs,* 2nd edn. Waterlow, London; first supplement to the second edition (1993). Sweet & Maxwell, London.

Comparative Analysis of Illicit Drug Strategy (1992). Monograph series No 18. Australian Government Publishing Service, Canberra.

Edmondson K (1987). Government drug agencies and control of drug misuse. *British Journal of Addiction,* **82**, 139–146.

Farmer R (1990). Preventive issues and legal aspects. In: Ghodse AH & Maxwell D (eds). *Substance Abuse and Dependence,* 244–254. Macmillan Press, London.

International Narcotics Control Board (1992). *Report of the INCB for 1992. (E/INCB/1992/1).* United Nations Publication, New York.

International Narcotics Control Board (1993). *Precursors and chemicals frequently used in the illicit manufacture of narcotic drugs and psychotropic substances: Report of the INCB on the Implementation of Article 12 of the United Nations Convention against Illicit Traffic in Narcotic Drugs and Psychotropic Substances of 1988 (E/INCB/1993/4).* United Nations Publication, Vienna.

Oppenheimer T (1988). Strengthening international action of drug abuse: outcomes from a very important meeting. *British Journal of Addiction,* **83**, 605–608.

Porter L, Arif AE & Curren WJ (1986). *The Law and the Treatment of Drug and Alcohol Dependence Persons: A comparative study of existing legislation.* WHO, Geneva.

Rexed B, Edmondson K, Khan I & Samson RJ (1984). *Guidelines for the Control of Narcotic and Psychotropic Substances in the context of the International Treaties.* WHO, Geneva.

United Nations (1987). *Report of the International Conference on Drug Abuse and Illicit Trafficking.* United Nations Publications, New York.

Appendix 1

The European Substance Use Database

The European Substance Use Database (EuroSUD) (see overleaf) is a brief initial assessment instrument collecting basic demographic data about drug users who present to services, as well as information about their current drug using behaviour and the types of treatment intervention offered to them. The information contained on the EuroSUD may be used for either clinical or research purposes. The Database itself is a valuable epidemiological tool at local, national and international levels. EuroSUD computer programmes, written in shareware software, enable data-entry and report-generation at local level at minimal cost. The EuroSUD is currently in use in treatment centres in 10 European countries.

European Substance Use Database

Interviewer's name : _____

Job title : _____

Agency name : _____

BASIC CLIENT DATA

1 CLIENT DATA

Client's initials [ ] [ ] **OR** code [ ] [ ] [ ] [ ]   Female [ ]

Date of birth [/ /] **OR** age [ ] [ ]   Male [ ]

Postcode **OR** postal district [ ] [ ] [ ] [ ] [ ] [ ] [ ]

2 CONTACT DATA:

Date of contact   / /

Type of contact: Face-to-face [ ]
                  Telephone   [ ]
                  Letter   [ ]
                  Indirect   [ ]

3 SUBSTANCE PROFILE: substances used over last 12 months

STATE SUBSTANCE NAME BELOW
Put main substance first.
If alcohol used at all, fill in final slot on table.

	Frequency of use over last 30 days							Most usual route over last 30 days						Source over last 30 days					DURATION OF THIS DRUG EPISODE	AGE OF FIRST USE
	NO USE	LESS THAN ONCE PER WK	ONCE PER WK OR MORE	ONCE DAILY	2/3 TIMES DAILY	4 OR MORE TIMES DAILY	NOT KNOWN	ORAL	SMOKED	INJECTED	SNIFFED/ SNORTED	OTHER ROUTES	NOT KNOWN	ILLICIT	PRIVATE DR	NHS DOCTOR	OTHER	NOT KNOWN		
1.																				
2.																				
3.																				
4.																				
5.																				

ALCOHOL: Units consumed per week

4 Injecting details

Have you ever injected?   Y [ ] N [ ]   Has a HIV test ever been offered to you?   Y [ ] N [ ]

Have you ever shared?   Y [ ] N [ ]   Have you ever completed a Hep. B vaccination course?   Y [ ] N [ ]

How long ago was most recent sharing ...... years ...... months ...... days

REFERRAL DETAILS

5 REFERRED BY:
(tick one only)
Self [ ]
Dr [ ]
Hospital [ ]
Social services [ ]
Voluntary agency [ ]
Legal services [ ]
Police [ ]
Other, specify: [ ]

6 REASON FOR ATTENDANCE:
(tick up to 4)
Financial [ ]
Job [ ]
Family/Relationships [ ]
Medical [ ]
Psychological [ ]
Housing [ ]
Pregnancy [ ]
Casualty [ ]
Needle Exchange [ ]
Other, specify

7 DRUG-RELATED CONTACTS:
(in last 6 months)
(tick up to 3)
Non-statutory agency [ ]
Doctor [ ]
NHS Drug Team [ ]
Legal Services [ ]
Social Services [ ]
Accident & Emergency [ ]
Other, specify: [ ]

CLIENT DETAILS

8 ETHNIC ORIGIN:
(tick one only)
White [ ]   Black Caribbean [ ]
Indian [ ]   Black African [ ]
Mid East [ ]   Black other* [ ]
Far East [ ]   Not Known [ ]
Other* [ ]
*Specify_____

9 EDUCATIONAL ATTAINMENT:
(tick one only)
No qualifications [ ]
High School quals [ ]
Professional quals [ ]
Degree/Diploma [ ]

10 LIVING WITH:
(tick one only)
Alone [ ]
Self & children [ ]
Partner/spouse [ ]
Partner/spouse & children [ ]
Parents [ ]
Friends [ ]
Other, specify: [ ]

Client lives with someone   [Y] [N]
with substance use problems
There is a family history   [Y] [N]
of substance use

11 DEPENDENT CHILDREN:
How many? [ ]
Age of youngest [ ]

12 TYPE OF ACCOMMODATION:
(tick one only)
Parental home [ ]
Owner occupied [ ]
Private rented [ ]
Council rented [ ]
Housing association [ ]
Squat [ ]
Rehab/hostel [ ]
Hospital [ ]
Prison [ ]
No fixed abode [ ]
Other, specify: [ ]

13 OCCUPATIONAL STATUS:
(tick one only)
Unemployed [ ]
Employed [ ]
Self-employed [ ]
Childcare/housewife [ ]
Student [ ]
Armed forces [ ]
National Service [ ]
Retired [ ]
Voluntary work [ ]
Other, specify [ ]

14 CURRENT/USUAL JOB:
(BLOCK LETTERS please)

15 PROPOSED ACTION:
(tick up to 3)
Referred to other agency [ ]
Assessment [ ]
Detoxification [ ]
Long-term prescribing [ ]
Prescribing contract [ ]
Counselling [ ]
Family support [ ]
Rehabilitation [ ]
No action [ ]
Other intervention, specify: [ ]

16 REFERRED TO:
(tick up to 3)
Outpatient drug facility [ ]
Inpatient drug facility [ ]
NHS Doctor [ ]
Private Doctor [ ]
Non-statutory agency [ ]
Accident & Emergency [ ]
Psychiatric services [ ]
Social Services [ ]
Other, specify: [ ]

Appendix 2

Substance Abuse Assessment Questionnaire

Name of interviewer:		
INDEX No.	[ ] [ ] [ ] [ ] [ ]	1–5
STUDY No.	[ ] [ ]	6–7
CARD No.	[0] [1]	8–9

Section I (a):
Initial information (general assessment)

1 Date of interview: [ ] [ ]/[ ] [ ]/[ ] [ ]   10–15

2 Place of interview: [ ]   –16
    1   Treatment centre
    2   Hospital
    3   Home
    4   Other (specify): ....

3 Date of referral: [ ] [ ]/[ ] [ ]/[ ] [ ]   17–22

4 Client's name: ....   [ ] [ ]   23–24

5 Client's address: .... [ ] [ ] [ ] [ ] [ ] [ ]   25–30
    ....
    ....
    Tel No.: ....
    Post code: ....

6 Client's sex: [ ]   –31
    1 Male   2 Female

7 Client's date of birth.   [ ] [ ]/[ ] [ ]/[ ] [ ] 32–37

For example, 1 September, 1963 =   [0] [1]/[0] [9]/[6] [3]

99 99   99 = not known

8 Client's age: [ ] [ ] 38–39

9 Ethnic group: [ ] [ ] 40–41

01 White	06 Black Caribbean
02 Indian	07 Black African
03 Pakistani	08 Black other*
04 Bangladeshi	09 Other*
05 Chinese	99 Not known

* Specify ....

10 Marital status: [ ] –42
1 Single
2 Married/Cohabiting
3 Separated
4 Divorced
5 Widowed
9 Not known

11 Number of children: [ ] [ ] 43–44

12 Ages of children to nearest whole year: [ ] [ ] 45–46
     [ ] [ ] 47–48
     [ ] [ ] 49–50
     [ ] [ ] 51–52
     [ ] [ ] 53–54

Should the client have more than 5 children please place the youngest child's age in the first two boxes and the eldest child's age in the last two boxes.

13 Does client have a ....
1 Yes   2 No   8 Not applicable   9 Not known

Family doctor	[ ]	–55
Social worker	[ ]	–56
Probation officer	[ ]	–57
Other professional care worker	[ ]	–58

(specify): ....

Name and address of key person:

....

....

Tel: ....

14 Source of referral: [ ] [ ] 59–60
    01   Self
    02   Family/friend/cohabitee
    03   Family doctor/community health centre
    04   Accident & Emergency/Hospital
    05   Drug clinic
    06   Psychiatric service
    07   Police
    08   Probation/courts/lawyer
    09   Social services
    10   Voluntary agency/hostel
    11   Other (specify): ....
    99   Not known

15 Current living arrangements: [ ] [ ] 61–62
    01   Alone
    02   With spouse or partner
    03   With spouse/partner and children
    04   Self and children
    05   Friends/hostel
    06   Parents
    07   Other (specify): ....
    99   Not known

16 Type of accommodation at address: [ ] [ ] 63–64
    01   Parental home
    02   Owned by client and/or his/her spouse/partner
    03   Rented house/flat
    04   Squat
    05   Hospital
    06   Therapeutic community
    07   Probation hostel
    08   Prison
    09   No fixed abode
    10   Other (specify): ....
    99   Not known

17 Education – number of years of   [ ] [ ]   65–66
schooling completed:
  88   Still attending
  99   Not known

18 Schooling: [ ]   –67
  1   No formal education
  2   Special educational needs
  3   No qualifications
  4   High school qualifications
  5   Professional qualifications
  6   Degree/diploma

19 Occupational status: [ ] [ ]   68–69
  01   Unemployed
  02   Employed
  03   Self-employed
  04   Child care/housewife
  05   Student
  06   Armed forces
  07   National service
  08   Retired
  09   Voluntary work
  10   Other (specify): ....
  99   Not known

20 Current/usual job: *[ ] [ ]   70–71

  *Local coding system to be used

21 Longest period of unemployment: years   months
                                       [ ] [ ]   [ ] [ ]   72–75
  88   Not applicable (still at school/college)
  99   Not known

22 Longest period in same job: years   months
                                       [ ] [ ]   [ ] [ ]   76–79
  88   Not applicable (still at school/never employed)
  99   Not known

INDEX No.	[ ] [ ] [ ] [ ] [ ]	1–5
STUDY No.	[ ] [ ]	6–7
CARD No.	[0] [2]	8–9

23 How many jobs has Client had since leaving school?

number   [ ] [ ]   10–11

    88   Not applicable (still at school/college)
    99   Not known
    00   Never employed

24 Reason for attendance
    1 Yes   2 No   8 Not applicable   9 Not known

Financial	[ ]	–12
Job	[ ]	–13
Family/relationships	[ ]	–14
Medical	[ ]	–15
Psychological	[ ]	–16
Housing	[ ]	–17
Pregnancy	[ ]	–18
Accident & Emergency	[ ]	–19
Needle exchange	[ ]	–20
Other (specify):	[ ]	–21

25 Are there any other agencies involved with the client?   [ ]   –22
    1 Yes   2 No   8 Not applicable   9 Not known
    If Yes, specify   ....
                       ....
                       ....

26 Has client received treatment for their drug use before?   [ ]   –23
    1 Yes   2 No   8 Not applicable   9 Not known

Section I(b): Drug use assessment
INDEX No.   [ ] [ ] [ ] [ ] [ ] [ ]   1–5
STUDY No.   [ ] [ ]   6–7
CARD No.   [0] [3]   8–9

1 Substance profile (see pp. 358–359):

2 How were you introduced to drug taking?   –52
   1   Partner
   2   Sibling
   3   Friend or acquaintance
   4   Parent or relative
   5   Drug dealer
   6   Doctor (include therapeutic addicts)
   7   Other (please specify): ....
   9   Not Known

3   How long do you consider that you have had a 'drug problem'?
                         years   months
                       [ ] [ ]   [ ] [ ]   53–56
   99   Not known

For example, four and a half years =   [0] [4] [0] [6]

4 Have you experienced any of the following symptoms over
   the last 6 months?
   1 Yes   2 No   9 Not known
   Opiate withdrawals   [ ]   –57
   Sedative withdrawals   [ ]   –58
   Convulsions   [ ]   –59
   Hallucinations   [ ]   –60
   Paranoid state   [ ]   –61
   Depersonalisation   [ ]   –62
   Derealization   [ ]   –63
   Flashbacks   [ ]   –64

5 How soon after you wake up in the morning do
   you use drugs?   [ ]   –65
   1   Immediately
   2   After breakfast/a few hours
   3   After several hours
   4   Not known

1 Substance profile

Substance profile	Ever used 1 Yes 2 No 3 Not known	Age at first used 88 Never used 90 Has used, but age unknown 99 Not known	Duration of use 1 Once or twice 2 < 6 mths 3 7 mths–1 yr 4 2–5 yrs 5 6–10 yrs 6 > 10 yrs 8 N/A 9 Not known	Frequency of use over last 30 days 1 No use 2 Less than once per week 3 Once per week or more 4 2/3 times daily 5 4 or more times daily 8 N/A 9 Not known	Most usual route over last 30 days 1 Oral 2 Smoked 3 Injected 4 Sniffed/ snorted 5 Other routes 8 N/A 9 Not known	Source over last 30 days 1 Illicit 2 Private doctor 3 Family doctor 4 Hospital doctor 5 Other doctor 6 OTC/legal purchase* 8 N/A 9 Not known	Box code
01 Heroin	[ ]	[ ][ ]	[ ]	[ ]	[ ]	[ ]	10–16
02 Methadone	[ ]	[ ][ ]	[ ]	[ ]	[ ]	[ ]	17–23
03 Other opiates (specify):	[ ]	[ ][ ]	[ ]	[ ]	[ ]	[ ]	24–30
04 Barbiturates	[ ]	[ ][ ]	[ ]	[ ]	[ ]	[ ]	31–37

No.	Substance						Column
05	Benzodiazepines	[ ]	[ ] [ ] [ ]	[ ]	[ ]	[ ]	38–44
06	Other sedatives (specify):	[ ]	[ ] [ ] [ ]	[ ]	[ ]	[ ]	45–51
07	Antidepressants Major tranquillizers (specify):	[ ]	[ ] [ ] [ ]	[ ]	[ ]	[ ]	52–58
08	Cocaine	[ ]	[ ] [ ] [ ]	[ ]	[ ]	[ ]	59–65
09	Amphetamines	[ ]	[ ] [ ] [ ]	[ ]	[ ]	[ ]	66–72
10	Other stimulants (specify):	[ ]	[ ] [ ] [ ]	[ ]	[ ]	[ ]	72–78

INDEX No.   [ ] [ ] [ ]   1–5
STUDY No.   [ ] [ ]   6–7
CARD No.   [0] [4]   8–9

No.	Substance						Column
11	Cannabis	[ ]	[ ] [ ] [ ]	[ ]	[ ]	[ ]	10–16
12	Hallucinogens	[ ]	[ ] [ ] [ ]	[ ]	[ ]	[ ]	17–23
13	Solvent inhalants	[ ]	[ ] [ ] [ ]	[ ]	[ ]	[ ]	24–30
14	Alcohol	[ ]	[ ] [ ] [ ]	[ ]	[ ]	[ ]	31–37
15	Tobacco	[ ]	[ ] [ ] [ ]	[ ]	[ ]	[ ]	38–44
16	Other (specify):	[ ]	[ ] [ ] [ ]	[ ]	[ ]	[ ]	45–51

* OTC, over-the-counter medications.

6 How much money do you estimate you spend in an
   average week on drugs?
   Please state currency: ....,........................
                          [ ] [ ] [ ] [ ] [ ] [ ]   66–71

7 Have you been absent from work for more than 2 days
   in the last month because of drug use?   [ ]   –72
   1 Yes   2 No   8 Not applicable   9 Not known

8 In the last 12 months how many weeks have you been totally drug free?
   Insert number of weeks   [ ] [ ]   73–74
   99   Not known

   > For example, seven weeks = [0] [7], No weeks = [0] [0]

   INDEX No.   [ ] [ ] [ ] [ ] [ ]   1–5
   STUDY No.   [ ] [ ]   6–7
   CARD No.   [0] [5]   8–9

9 Have you ever received any of the following treatments for your drug use?
   1 Yes   2 No   9 Not known
   Through voluntary/self-help group   [ ]   –10
   Through your family doctor   [ ]   –11
   Private doctor   [ ]   –12
   Substance misuse team (outpatient/community)   [ ]   –13
   As inpatient   [ ]   –14
   As resident in rehabilitation   [ ]   –15
   Other (please specify): ....   [ ]   –16

   Please state when and where treatment took place, if known:

Date	Place		
[ ][ ]/[ ][ ]/[ ][ ]		[ ]	17–22
[ ][ ]/[ ][ ]/[ ][ ]		[ ]	23–28
[ ][ ]/[ ][ ]/[ ][ ]		[ ]	29–34
[ ][ ]/[ ][ ]/[ ][ ]		[ ]	35–40

10 How many cigarettes (tobacco) do you
smoke in a day? (number)   [   ] [   ] [   ]   41–43
   88   Does not smoke
   99   Not known

11 How soon after you wake up in the morning do   [   ]   –44
you smoke?
   1   Immediately   **5**   Within 6 hours
   2   Within the first hour   **8**   Not applicable
   3   Within 3 hours   **9**   Not known
   4   Evening only (i.e. 6.00 pm onwards)

12 *Assessment rating (drug use)*

> **1   Do you see your present 'drug use' as:**   [   ]   –45
>   1 No problem   2 Moderate problem
>   3 Serious problem   9 Not known
>
> **2   Do you think you need help because of your drug use**   [   ]   –46
>   1 No need   2 Moderate need
>   3 Serious need   9 Not known
>
> **3   Does interviewer think Client's drug use is:**   [   ]   –47
>   1 No problem   2 Moderate problem
>   3 Serious problem   9 Not known
>
> **4   Does interviewer assess client's need for help with**   [   ]   –48
>   **drug problem as:**
>   1 No need   2 Moderate need
>   3 Serious need   9 Not known

NOTES:

Section I(c): Summary of requests and requirements

INDEX No.	[ ] [ ] [ ] [ ] [ ] [ ]	1–5
STUDY No.	[ ] [ ]	6–7
CARD No.	[0] [6]	8–9

[1] What treatment is client asking for?
   1 Yes   2 No   9 Not known

OUT-PATIENT PROGRAMMES		
Programme	Client requests	Interviewer's initial recommendation
Out-patient detox programme		
Opiate	[ ]	[ ] 10–11
Sedative	[ ]	[ ] 12–13
Stimulants	[ ]	[ ] 14–15
Alcohol	[ ]	[ ] 16–17
Out-patient maintenance programme		
Opiate	[ ]	[ ] 18–19
Sedative	[ ]	[ ] 20–21
Stimulants	[ ]	[ ] 22–23
In-patient assessment prior to any of the above		[ ] –24
IN-PATIENT PROGRAMMES		
In-patient detox programmes		
Opiate	[ ]	[ ] 25–26
Sedative	[ ]	[ ] 27–28
Stimulants	[ ]	[ ] 29–30
Alcohol	[ ]	[ ] 31–32
In-patient treatment other (specify)..	[ ]	[ ] 33–34
Residential recovery/rehab	[ ]	[ ] 35–36

2 What is client asking for?
   1 Yes   2 No   9 Not known

Day care		
Programme	**Client requests**	**Interviewer's initial recommendation**
Day care	[ ]	[ ] 37–38
Other options		
Treatment for physical health (specify)	[ ]	[ ] 39–40
Treatment for psychiatric health problem (specify)	[ ]	[ ] 41–42
Naltrexone	[ ]	[ ] 43–44
Disulfiram	[ ]	[ ] 45–46
NET	[ ]	[ ] 47–48
Acupuncture	[ ]	[ ] 49–50
Needle exchange	[ ]	[ ] 51–52
HIV counselling/testing	[ ]	[ ] 53–54
Psychological interventions	[ ]	[ ] 55–56
Other (specify):	[ ]	[ ] 57–58
....	[ ]	[ ] 59–60
Social work assistance	[ ]	[ ] 61–62
Court report	[ ]	[ ] 63–64

3 At the time of this interview was the client: [ ]   –65
   1 Sober   2 Intoxicated   3 Withdrawing   9 Not known

4 *Assessment rating (general)*

1 **Does client perceive their present situation as:** [ ] −66
   1 Good   2 Fair
   3 Poor   9 Not known

2 **Does client perceive their present need for help as:** [ ] −67
   1 No need   2 Moderate need
   3 Serious need   9 Not known

3 **Does interviewer perceive Client's present situation as:** [ ] −68
   1 Good   2 Fair
   3 Poor   9 Not known

4 **Does interviewer perceive client's need for help as:** [ ] −69
   1 No need   2 Moderate need
   3 Serious need   9 Not known

NOTES:

Section II: Medical and mental health assessment

INDEX No.	[ ] [ ] [ ] [ ] [ ]	1–5
STUDY No.	[ ] [ ]	6–7
CARD No.	[0] [7]	8–9

Section II (a): Physical health

1 Have you any complaints about your present state [ ] –10
of physical health and/or do you suffer any disability?
1 Yes 2 No 9 Not known
If yes, specify: ....

2 What is your appetite like? [ ] –11
1 Good 2 Poor 9 Not known

3 How do you sleep? [ ] 12
1 Well 2 Poorly 9 Not known

4 Are you presently receiving any treatment for a
physical illness and/or disability?
1 Yes 2 No 9 Not known

From family doctor [ ] –13
From hospital, out-patient [ ] –14
From hospital, in-patient [ ] –15
Other (specify): .... [ ] 16

5 What is the illness/disability *[ ] [ ] [ ] [ ] 17–21
....

*Local coding system to be used

What is the treatment? *[ ] [ ] 22–23
....

*Local coding system to be used

If receiving prescribed drugs *[ ] [ ] [ ] [ ] 24–27
(apart from methadone) please give names:
....
....

*Local coding system to be used

6 Have you ever been hospitalized in
the last 2 years for a physical illness?
1 Yes   2 No   8 Not applicable   9 Not known   [ ]   28
If yes, specify:

Nature of illness	Age at which it occurred	Length of admission (months)

7 Have you ever injected?   [ ]   −29
   1 Yes   2 No   9 Not known

If No, go to question 12

8 Which method(s) of injecting do you use?
   1 Yes   2 No   9 Not known
   Intravenous (I.V.)   [ ]   −30
   Intramuscular (I.M.)   [ ]   −31
   Subcutaneous (skin-popping)   [ ]   −32

9 Which sites do you use?
   1 Yes   2 No   9 Not known
   Arm   [ ]   −33
   Groin   [ ]   −34
   Feet   [ ]   −35
   Neck   [ ]   −36
   Other (specify): ....   [ ]   −37

10 Have you ever shared?   [ ]   −38
   1 Yes   2 No   9 Not known

11 How long ago was most recent sharing?
      years   months   days
      [ ] [ ]   [ ] [ ]   [ ] [ ]   39–44

12 Has an HIV test ever been offered to you? [ ] −45
·1 Yes   2 No   9 Not known

13 Did you take up the offer of testing? [ ] −46
1 Yes   2 No   9 Not known

14 Have you ever completed a Hep. B vaccination course? [ ] −47
1 Yes   2 No   9 Not known

15 Have you ever had any of the following?
1 Yes   2 No   9 Not known

HIV [ ] −48
Hepatitis B [ ] −49
Hepatitis C [ ] −50
Septicaemia [ ] −51
Abscesses [ ] −52
Endocarditis [ ] −53
Over-dose (deliberate) [ ] −54
Over-dose (accidental) [ ] −55
Other (specify): .... [ ] −56

Female clients only
Amenorrhoea [ ] −57
Miscarriage/spontaneous abortion [ ] −58
Termination of pregnancy [ ] −59

16 Physical examination
(a) General physical examination
1 Yes   2 No   9 Not known

Poor dental care [ ] −60
Injection marks on skin [ ] −61
Tattoos [ ] −62
Abscesses [ ] −63
Anaemia [ ] −64
Malnutrition [ ] −65
Lymphadenopathy [ ] −66
Jaundice [ ] −67

16 Physical examination
   (b) Systems examination
      1 Normal   2 Abnormal (specify)   9 Not known

	Specify	Code	
Cardiovascular system		[ ]	−68
Respiratory		[ ]	−69
Alimentary		[ ]	−70
Urogenital		[ ]	−71
Endocrine		[ ]	−72
Nervous system		[ ]	−73
Locomotor		[ ]	−74

INDEX No.   [ ] [ ] [ ] [ ] [ ]   **1–5**
STUDY No.   [ ] [ ]   **6–7**
CARD No.   [0] [8]   **8–9**

17 Blood pressure:
   Systolic   [ ] [ ] [ ]   10–12
   Diastolic   [ ] [ ] [ ]   13–15
   Pulse   [ ] [ ] [ ]   16–18

18 Laboratory investigations:

(a) Hepatitis screen	1 Positive 2 Negative 8 Not done 9 Not known		
Type	Date of result	Code	
B antibody	[ ][ ] / [ ][ ] / [ ][ ]	[ ]	19–25
B antigen	[ ][ ] / [ ][ ] / [ ][ ]	[ ]	26–32
C antibody	[ ][ ] / [ ][ ] / [ ][ ]	[ ]	33–39
C antigen	[ ][ ] / [ ][ ] / [ ][ ]	[ ]	40–46

(b) HIV Screen	1 Positive 2 Negative 8 Not done 9 Not done	
	Date of result	Code
	[ ][ ] / [ ][ ] / [ ][ ]	[ ] 47–53

(c) Electrolytes and urea		
1 Normal 2 Abnormal 8 Not done 9 Not known		
Date of result	If abnormal, specify:	Code
[ ][ ] / [ ][ ] / [ ][ ]		[ ] 54–60

(d) Liver function test	1 Normal 2 Abnormal 8 Not done 9 Not known	
Date of result	If abnormal, specify:	Code
[ ][ ] / [ ][ ] / [ ][ ]		[ ] 61–67

(e) Full blood count	1 Normal 2 Abnormal 8 Not done 9 Not known	
Date of result	If abnormal, specify:	Code
[ ][ ] / [ ][ ] / [ ][ ]		[ ] 68–74

INDEX No.   [ ] [ ] [ ] [ ] [ ]   1–5
STUDY No.   [ ] [ ]   6–7
CARD No.   [0]   [9]   8–9

(f) X-rays	1 Normal 2 Abnormal 8 Not done 9 Not known	
Date of result	If abnormal, specify:	Code
[ ][ ] / [ ][ ] / [ ][ ]		[ ] 10–16

19 Urine results

1 Positive   2 Negative   8 Not done   9 Not known

Drug	Date: Result	Date: Result	Date: Result	Date: Result	
Morphine	[ ]	[ ]	[ ]	[ ]	41–44
Methadone	[ ]	[ ]	[ ]	[ ]	45–48
Other opiates	[ ]	[ ]	[ ]	[ ]	49–52
Amphetamines	[ ]	[ ]	[ ]	[ ]	53–56
Cocaine	[ ]	[ ]	[ ]	[ ]	57–60
Barbiturates	[ ]	[ ]	[ ]	[ ]	61–64
Benzodiazepines	[ ]	[ ]	[ ]	[ ]	65–68
Cannabis	[ ]	[ ]	[ ]	[ ]	69–72

INDEX No.	[ ] [ ] [ ] [ ] [ ]	1–5
STUDY No.	[ ] [ ] [ ]	6–7
CARD No.	[1] [0]	8–9

Drug					
Alcohol	[ ]	[ ]	[ ]	[ ]	10–13
Other (specify)	[ ]	[ ]	[ ]	[ ]	14–17

20 *Assessment rating (physical health)*

1	**How would you rate your physical health at present?**	[ ]	−18
	1 Good 2 Fair		
	3 Poor · 9 Not known		
2	**Do you think you need help with physical health problems?**	[ ]	−19
	1 No need 2 Moderate need		
	3 Serious need 9 Not known		
3	**How does interviewer rate client's physical health?**	[ ]	−20
	1 Good 2 Fair		
	3 Poor 9 Not known		
4	**Does interviewer think client needs help with physical health problems?**	[ ]	−21
	1 No need 2 Moderate need		
	3 Serious need 9 Not known		

NOTES:

Section II (b): Mental health

INDEX No.   [ ] [ ] [ ] [ ] [ ]   1–5
STUDY No.   [ ] [ ] [ ]   6–7
CARD No.   [1]   [1]   8–9

1 Are you presently receiving treatment for a mental
health problem? (Except drug/alcohol use)
1 Yes   2 No   9 Not known
From family doctor   [   ]   –10
Hospital (out-patient/day patient)   [   ]   –11
Hospital (in-patient)   [   ]   –12
Community mental health team   [   ]   –13
Other (specify): ....   [   ]   –14

(a) What is the illness/problem? * [   ] [   ] [   ] [   ] [   ]   15–19
....
....

Local coding system to be used

(b) What is the treatment?   * [   ] [   ]   20–21
....
....

Local coding system to be used

(c) If receiving prescribed drugs   [   ] [   ] [   ]   22–24
please give names:
....
....

Local coding system to be used

2 Have you ever been a hospital inpatient because   [   ]   –25
of mental illness?
1 Yes   2 No   9 Not known

If Yes, please specify:

Nature of illness	Age	Date	
	[ ] [ ]	[ ][ ] / [ ][ ] / [ ][ ]	26–33
	[ ] [ ]	[ ][ ] / [ ][ ] / [ ][ ]	34–41
	[ ] [ ]	[ ][ ] / [ ][ ] / [ ][ ]	42–49

3 What is your sexual orientation?   [   ]   −50
   1   Exclusively heterosexual
   2   Mainly heterosexual
   3   Mainly homosexual
   4   Bisexual
   5   Exclusively homosexual
   9   Not known

4 Do you consider you have any problem with
   your sexual functioning?   [   ]   −51
   1   Yes (secondary to drug/alcohol use)
   2   Yes (other reason)
   3   No
   9   Not known

   | If Yes, please specify: |

   ....

5 Mental state
   1 Normal   2 Abnormal (specify)   9 Not known

	Specify abnormality	Code	
Appearance		[ ]	−52
Behaviour		[ ]	−53
Mood		[ ]	−54
Talk		[ ]	−55
Thought		[ ]	−56
Perception		[ ]	−57
Insight		[ ]	−58
Cognitive function		[ ]	−59
Orientation		[ ]	−60
Concentration		[ ]	−61
Memory		[ ]	−62
Intelligence		[ ]	−63
Other		[ ]	−64

6 At the time of the mental state being carried out
was client   [   ]   −65
   1 Sober   2 Intoxicated   3 Withdrawing   9 Not known

7 *Assessment rating (mental health)*

1 **How would you rate your mental health at present?**   [   ]   −66
   1 Good   2 Fair
   3 Poor   9 Not known

2 **Do you think you need help with mental health**   [   ]   −67
  problems?
   1 No need   2 Moderate need
   3 Serious need   9 Not known

3 **How does interviewer rate client's mental health?**   [   ]   −68
   1 Good   2 Fair
   3 Poor   9 Not known

4 **Does interviewer think client needs help with**   [   ]   −69
  mental health?
   1 No need   2 Moderate need
   3 Serious need   9 Not known

NOTES:

Section III: Alcohol use

INDEX No.	[ ] [ ] [ ] [ ] [ ] [ ] 1–5
STUDY No.	[ ] [ ] 6–7
CARD No.	[1] [2] 8–9

1 Do you consider you have ever had problems with alcohol?   [   ]   –10
1 Yes   2 No   9 Not known

2 Do you consider you have current problems with alcohol   [   ]   –11
(within the last 12 months)?
1 Yes   2 No   9 Not known

3 Have you ever been convicted of alcohol related offences?   [   ]   –12
1 Yes   2 No   9 Not known

For example, drink/driving, drunk and disorderly, breach of the peace

4 Are you suffering financial hardship due to the amount   [   ]   –13
you spend on alcohol?
1 Yes   2 No   9 Not known

5 Do you think your relationships are suffering due to the   [   ]   –14
amount of alcohol you drink?
1 Yes   2 No   9 Not known

6 Have you been absent from work for more than two days   [   ]   –15
in the last month because of drink?
1 Yes   2 No   9 Not known

7 Number of standard drinks consumed in an average week:

grams	[ ]	[ ]	[ ]	16–18
or units	[ ]	[ ]	[ ]	19–21

Calculation formula:
1 Unit of alcohol = 8 g of absolute alcohol
No. of alcohol units =
% alcohol by volume (ABV) × amount of beverage (in ml)

8 | Have you experienced any of the following symptoms over
the last 6 months related to alcohol consumption?

1 Yes   2 No   9 Not known

Morning drinking	[ ]	−22
Morning nausea/vomiting	[ ]	−23
Shakes	[ ]	−24
Sweating	[ ]	−25
Anxiety/panic attacks	[ ]	−26
Depression	[ ]	−27
Loss of memory	[ ]	−28
Blackouts	[ ]	−29
Delirium tremens	[ ]	−30
Convulsions	[ ]	−31
Hallucinations	[ ]	−32

9 | On average how many days in a week do you
consume alcohol?   [ ]   −33
9 Not known

10 | What is your usual style of drinking?   [ ]   −34
1   Weekend/other short episodes
2   Bouts of more than 2 days
3   Steady, daily
4   Other (specify): ....
8   Not applicable
9   Not known

11 | If you drink in bouts what is their average duration?

days	weeks	months	
[ ] [ ]	[ ] [ ]	[ ] [ ]	35–40

12 | What is the average length of time between bouts?

days	weeks	months	
[ ] [ ]	[ ] [ ]	[ ] [ ]	41–46

13 | In the last year how many weeks have you
been alcohol free?   [ ] [ ]   47–48
88   Not applicable
99   Not known

14 How long do you think you have had a problem with alcohol?

	years	months	
	[ ] [ ]	[ ] [ ]	49–52

88   Not applicable
99   Not known

15 Have you ever had treatment for your problem
with alcohol?   [ ]   −53
1   Yes
2   No
8   Not applicable (i.e.. no alcohol problem)
9   Not known

> If the answer to question 15 is No treatment
> go to question 17

16 Treatment received:
1 Yes   2 No   9 Not known

Family Doctor treatment	[ ]	−54
As hospital out-patient	[ ]	−55
As hospital in-patient	[ ]	−56
Community Alcohol Team	[ ]	−57
Non-statutory/voluntary agency	[ ]	−58
Other (specify):	[ ]	−59

INDEX No.	[ ] [ ] [ ] [ ] [ ]	1–5
STUDY No.	[ ] [ ] [ ]	6–7
CARD No.	[1] [3]	8–9

Please state when and where treatment took place, if known:

Date	Place	
[ ][ ] / [ ][ ] / [ ][ ]	[ ]	10–16
[ ][ ] / [ ][ ] / [ ][ ]	[ ]	17–23
[ ][ ] / [ ][ ] / [ ][ ]	[ ]	24–30
[ ][ ] / [ ][ ] / [ ][ ]	[ ]	31–36

17 *Assessment rating (alcohol use)*

1 **How do you rate your alcohol use?**   [ ]   −37
   1 No problem   2 Moderate problem
   3 Serious problem   9 Not known

2 **Do you think you need help with an alcohol problem?**   [ ]   −38
   1 No need   2 Moderate need
   3 Serious need   9 Not known

3 **How does interviewer rate client's alcohol problem?**   [ ]   −39
   1 No problem   2 Moderate problem
   3 Serious problem   9 Not known

4 **Does interviewer think client needs help with alcohol problem?**   [ ]   −40
   1 No need   2 Moderate need
   3 Serious need   4 Not known

- -

NOTES:

Section IV: Forensic Assessment

INDEX No.	[ ] [ ] [ ] [ ] [ ]	1–5
STUDY No.	[ ] [ ]	6–7
CARD No.	[1] [4]	8–9

---

1 Have you ever been involved in any criminal activity?   [ ]   –10
1 Yes   2 No   9 Not known

If answer to this question is No: STOP HERE, leaving all
intervening boxes blank, and go to question 10

2 At what age did you first become involved in   [ ] [ ]   11–12
criminal activity?
99   Not known

3 Do you at present have any court cases pending?   [ ]   –13
1 Yes   2 No   9 Not known

If answer is Yes, please specify for what offence(s)   *[ ] [ ]   14–15

*Local coding system to be used

....

....

4 Are you at present on: .....
1 Yes   2 No   9 Not known

Condition of treatment	[ ]	–16
Probation	[ ]	–17
Suspended sentence	[ ]	–18
Deferred sentence	[ ]	–19
Parole	[ ]	–20
Other (specify):	[ ]	–21

If answer is yes, please specify for what offence(s)   *[ ] [ ]   22–23

....

....

*Local coding system to be used

5 Which of the following types of offences have you
ever committed, and number of convictions?
1 Yes   2 No   9 Not known

Offences	Committed before drug use began	Committed after drug use began	Number of convictions	
Drug related	[ ]	[ ]	[ ] [ ]	24–27
Driving	[ ]	[ ]	[ ] [ ]	28–31
Public disorder	[ ]	[ ]	[ ] [ ]	32–35
Violence against property	[ ]	[ ]	[ ] [ ]	36–39
Crimes of acquisition	[ ]	[ ]	[ ] [ ]	40–43
Sex offences	[ ]	[ ]	[ ] [ ]	44–47
Violence against the person	[ ]	[ ]	[ ] [ ]	48–51

6 Have you had any periods of imprisonment?   [ ] [ ]   52–53

If Yes, code number of times, i.e., three times   =   [0] [3]
If No go to question 9

99   Not known
88   Never been in prison

7 If you have been in prison, what was the longest sentence served?
                days   months   years
              [ ] [ ]   [ ] [ ]   [ ] [ ]   54–59
99   Not known

8 Whilst in prison did you continue to use drugs?   [ ]   –60
1 Yes, frequently   3 Yes, occasionally
2 No   9 Not known

9 Of the crimes committed since the onset of   [ ] [ ] [ ]   % 61–63
drug use, what percentage do you estimate
were committed whilst intoxicated?
99 Not known

10 *Assessment rating (forensic)*

1 **How severe would you rate your legal problem as**   [ ]   –64
being at the moment?
   1 No problems at all   2 Moderate problem
   3 Serious problem   9 Not known

2 **Do you think you need help with your legal problems**   [ ]   –65
at present?
   1 No need   2 Moderate need
   3 Serious need   9 Not known

3 **Does the interviewer think the client's present**   [ ]   –66
legal problems are:
   1 No problem at all   2 Moderate problem
   3 Serious problem   9 Not known

4 **How much help does the interviewer think the**   [ ]   –67
client needs with legal problems?
   1 No need   2 Moderate need
   3 Serious need   9 Not known

NOTES:

Section V: Psychosocial and family assessment
INDEX No.   [ ] [ ] [ ] [ ] [ ] [ ]   1–5
STUDY No.   [ ] [ ]   6–7
CARD No.   [1]   [5]   8–9

1 Do you have a social worker already involved with yourself or your family
                                                    [ ]   –10
   1 Yes   2 No   9 Not known
   Name and address   ....
   ....
   Tel: ....

2 Number of siblings
   Male   [ ] [ ]   11–12
   Female   [ ] [ ]   13–14
   88 None
   99 Not known

3 What position are you in birth order?   [ ] [ ]   15–16
   01 First
   02 Second (etc.)
   99 Not applicable (only child)

4 Are you a twin?   [ ]   –17
   1 Yes, identical twin
   2 Yes, non-identical twin
   3 No
   9 Not known

5 Father's occupation/last job   *[ ]   18–19
   Please specify:..................................

   *Local coding system to be used

6 Father's age/or age at death   [ ] [ ]   20–21
   10 Not applicable (i.e., father unknown)
   99 Not known

   Please delete as appropriate
   For example: ~~Father's age~~/or age at death

7 Mother's occupation/last job   *[   ]   [   ]   22–23
    Please specify:....................................

    | *Local coding system to be used |

8 Mother's age/or age at death   [   ]   [   ]   24–25
    10   Not applicable (i.e., mother unknown)
    99   Not known

    | Please delete as appropriate
    For example: mother's age/~~or age at death~~ |

9 Are members of the immediate family aware of drug use?
    1 Yes   2 No   8 Not applicable   9 Not known
    Parents   [   ]   −26
    Partner   [   ]   −27
    Children   [   ]   −28

10 Are members of the immediate family aware
    of alcohol problem?
    1 Yes   2 No   8 Not applicable   9 Not known
    Parents   [   ]   −29
    Partner   [   ]   −30
    Children   [   ]   −31

11 If you are married or have a regular partner,   *[   ]   [   ]   32–33
    what is partner's occupation
    Please specify:....................................

    | *Local coding system to be used |

12 Are you worried about your children in any
    of the following areas?
    1 Yes   2 No   8 No children   9 Not known

    Problems at work   [   ]   −34
    Problems at school   [   ]   −35
    Problems with police   [   ]   −36
    Using drugs/alcohol   [   ]   −37
    Physical health/handicap   [   ]   −38
    Mental health/handicap   [   ]   −39

13 Are any of your children, under the age of 16 years,
living away from you at present?
1 Yes   2 No   8 No children   9 Not known
With other parent/family member   [   ]   −40
Under the care of Statutory Supervision   [   ]   −41
Other reasons (please specify): .... [   ]   −42

> Include here, e.g., attending special school, children
> have left home, children in hostel, etc.

14 Are any of your children on a Statutory   *[   ]   [   ]   43–44
Protection Register (i.e., At Risk Register)
1 Yes   2 No   8 No children   9 Not known
If yes, please specify:...................................

> *Local coding system to be used

15 Do you usually use drugs: [   ]   −45
   1   Alone
   2   With others
   8   Not applicable (never uses drugs)
   9   Not known

16 What proportion of friends/associates take drugs?
                                            [   ] [   ] [   ]   %   46–48
   88   Not applicable (never uses drugs)
   99   Not known

17 What percentage of your time is spent in drug seeking/drug using?
                                            [   ] [   ] [   ]   %   49–51
   88   Not applicable (never uses drugs)
   99   Not known

18 Over the last 12 months have any of the following
caused you particular concern?
   1   Yes, serious concern   2   Yes, moderate concern
   3   Yes, slight concern   4   No concern   9   Not known

Problems at home	[ ]	−52
Financial hardship	[ ]	−53
Housing difficulties	[ ]	−54
Partners' drug/alcohol abuse	[ ]	−55
Ill health in the family	[ ]	−56
Relationship/marital discord	[ ]	−57
Violence in the family	[ ]	−58
Separation from children	[ ]	−59
Separation from partner/spouse	[ ]	−60
Bereavement	[ ]	−61
Other (specify)	[ ]	−62

INDEX No.   [ ] [ ] [ ] [ ] [ ]   1–5
STUDY No.   [ ] [ ]   6–7
CARD No.   [1] [6]   8–9

19 Have any members of your family suffered from a psychiatric illness/dependency on drugs and/or alcohol?
1 Yes   2 No   8 Not applicable   9 Not known

Member of family	Psychiatric illness	Dependency on drugs	Dependency on alcohol	
Father	[ ]	[ ]	[ ]	10–12
Mother	[ ]	[ ]	[ ]	13–15
Sibling(s)	[ ]	[ ]	[ ]	16–18
Children	[ ]	[ ]	[ ]	19–21
Partner	[ ]	[ ]	[ ]	22–24
Other (specify):	[ ]	[ ]	[ ]	25–27
If Yes, please give details	....	....	....	

20 Do any members of your family have a criminal record?

    1 Yes   2 No   8 Not applicable   9 Not known

	Criminal details	
Father	[ ]	−28
Mother	[ ]	−29
Sibling(s)	[ ]	−30
Partner	[ ]	−31
Children	[ ]	−32
Other (specify):		
....	[ ]	−33
....	[ ]	−34

21 During childhood or adolescence, was your family life disrupted
by any of the following events?

    1 Yes   2 No   3 Not known

Event	Childhood (10–12 years)	Adolescence (13–20 years)	
Client went into care/fostered/adopted	[ ]	[ ]	35–36
Frequent relocation	[ ]	[ ]	37–38
Financial hardship	[ ]	[ ]	39–40
Violence against Client	[ ]	[ ]	41–42
Sexual assault	[ ]	[ ]	43–44
Incest	[ ]	[ ]	45–46
Marital discord between parents	[ ]	[ ]	47–48
Violence between parents	[ ]	[ ]	49–50
Separation/divorce of parents	[ ]	[ ]	51–52
Imprisonment of parent	[ ]	[ ]	53–54
Hospitalization of parent for over 3/12	[ ]	[ ]	55–56
Death of sibling	[ ]	[ ]	57–58
Death of father	[ ]	[ ]	59–60
Death of mother	[ ]	[ ]	61–62
Family joined by step-parent/step-siblings	[ ]	[ ]	63–64

22 *Assessment rating (psychosocial/family)*

1 **How concerned are you about social/family problems?** [ ] −65
   1 No concern   2 Moderate concern
   3 Serious concern   9 Not known

2 **Do you think you need help with social/family problems?** [ ] −66
   1 No need   2 Moderate need
   3 Serious need   9 Not known

3 **How concerned is interviewer about client's social/family problems?** [ ] −67
   1 No concern   2 Moderate concern
   3 Serious concern   9 Not known

4 **Does interviewer think client needs help with social/family problems?** [ ] −68
   1 No need   2 Moderate need
   3 Serious need   9 Not known

NOTES:

Section VI: Assessment profile		
INDEX No.	[ ] [ ] [ ] [ ] [ ]	1–5
STUDY No.	[ ] [ ]	6–7
CARD No.	[1] [7]	8–9

1 Did the Client complete assessment?   [ ]   –10
   1 Yes   2 No   9 Not known
   If client failed to complete assessment,
   please state reason for dropping out:
   ....   [ ] [ ] [ ] [ ]   11–14
   ....
   ....
   ....

   *Local coding system to be used

2 Principle substance of misuse

   Please list in rank order, for example:
   1 = primary substance
   8 = not a problem now, or never used
   9 = not known

Opiates	[ ]	–15
Barbiturates	[ ]	–16
Benzodiazepines	[ ]	–17
Amphetamine	[ ]	–18
Cocaine	[ ]	–19
Other stimulants	[ ]	–20
Psychotropics (including LSD and cannabis)	[ ]	–21
Alcohol	[ ]	–22
Solvents/inhalants	[ ]	–23

3 Overall assessment rating scores
Insert corresponding scores from assessment ratings for each section.

	Clients' perceptions		Care workers' perceptions		Total	Box codes
	Problem	Need	Problem	Need		
Drug use	[ ]	[ ]	[ ]	[ ]		24–27
General	[ ]	[ ]	[ ]	[ ]		28–31
Physical health	[ ]	[ ]	[ ]	[ ]		32–35
Mental health	[ ]	[ ]	[ ]	[ ]		36–39
Alcohol use	[ ]	[ ]	[ ]	[ ]		40–43
Forensic	[ ]	[ ]	[ ]	[ ]		44–47
Psychosocial/family	[ ]	[ ]	[ ]	[ ]		48–51

The maximum problem/need score in each of the dimensions is 12.
Overall scoring is not deemed appropriate.
Code 9, i.e., Not known, should not be included in the total calculation in each sectional score.

4 Diagnosis

> Record as many co-existing mental disorders, general medical conditions
> and other factors that are relevant to the care and treatment of the
> individual. The primary diagnosis should be listed first. Please
> specify the classification system used (DSM-III-R/DSM-IV/ICD-9/ICD-10).

ICD.../DSM...Name	ICD.../DSM... CODE	Box code
	[ ] [ ] [ ].[ ] [ ]	52–56
	[ ] [ ] [ ].[ ] [ ]	57–61
	[ ] [ ] [ ].[ ] [ ]	62–66
	[.] [ ] [ ].[ ] [ ]	67–71

FOR EXAMPLE

ICD.../DSM...Name	ICD.../DSM... CODE	Box code
Alcohol Abuse (DSM-IV)	[3] [0] [5].[0] [0]	
Dependent personality		
disorder (DSM-III-R)	[3] [0] [1].[6] [0]	
Hypothyroidism (ICD-9-CM)	[2] [4] [4].[9] [ ]	

5 Client's requirements (as perceived by centre)

(a) Drug problem		
1 Requires in-patient treatment	[ ]	–72
2 Requires out-patient treatment	[ ]	–73
3 Requires in-patient treatment in DDU	[ ]	–74
4 Other (please specify):	[ ]	–75
8 Not applicable	[ ]	–76
9 Not known	[ ]	–77

INDEX No.	[ ] [ ] [ ] [ ] [ ]	1–5
STUDY No.	[ ] [ ]	6–7
CARD No.	[1] [8]	8–9

(b) Physical health problem		
1 Requires in-patient treatment in another hospital department	[ ]	−10
2 Requires in-patient treatment in drug treatment centre	[ ]	−11
3 Requires out-patient treatment in another hospital department	[ ]	−12
4 Requires out-patient treatment in drug treatment centre	[ ]	−13
5 Other (please specify):	[ ]	−14
8 Not applicable	[ ]	−15
9 Not known	[ ]	−16

(c) Mental health problem		
1 Requires formal inpatient psychiatric treatment	[ ]	−17
2 Requires formal outpatient psychiatric treatment in another hospital department	[ ]	−18
3 Requires outpatient treatment in this centre	[ ]	−19
4 Other (please specify):	[ ]	−20
8 Not applicable	[ ]	−21
9 Not known	[ ]	−22

(d) Social problems		
1 Requires referral to other agency	[ ]	−23
2 Requiring help from this centre	[ ]	−24
3 Other (please specify):	[ ]	−25
8 Not applicable	[ ]	−26
9 Not known	[ ]	−27

Section VII: Treatment profile
INDEX No.   [ ] [ ] [ ] [ ] [ ]   1–5
STUDY No.   [ ] [ ]   6–7
CARD No.   [1] [9]   8–9

1 | What type of treatment was offered to the client?   [ ]   –10
   1 Out-patient
   2 Community intervention
   3 In-patient
   4 Day care
   5 Residential rehabilitation

2 | Place of treatment   [ ] [ ]   11–12
   1 Specialized out-patient drug treatment centre
   2 General out-patient clinic
   3 Client's home
   4 Community health centre/family doctor's surgery
   5 Specialized in-patient drug treatment unit
   6 General in-patient psychiatric unit
   7 General medical/surgical in-patient unit
   8 Specialized drug day programme
   9 General day care programme
   10 Other (specify): ....

3 Was medication prescribed?
1 Yes   2 No
If Yes, please give details:

Dependency	Drug Prescribed	Dose in mg over a 24 hr period	Length of proposed detox*/maintenance*. Please indicate days*/weeks*/months* by deletion	Starting Date	Box codes
Opiate/opioid	Specify: .... [ ] [ ] [ ] [ ] [ ]	[ ] [ ] [ ] [ ]	[ ] [ ]	[II] / [II] / [II]	14–29
Benzodiazepines /sedative	Specify: .... [ ] [ ] [ ] [ ] [ ]	[ ] [ ] [ ] [ ]	[ ] [ ]	[II] / [II] / [II]	30–45
Alcohol	Specify: .... [ ] [ ] [ ] [ ] [ ]	[ ] [ ] [ ] [ ]	[ ] [ ]	[II] / [II] / [II]	46–61
Stimulant	Specify: .... [ ] [ ] [ ] [ ] [ ]	[ ] [ ] [ ] [ ]	[ ] [ ]	[II] / [II] / [II]	66–77

INDEX No.   [ ] [ ] [ ] [ ] [ ] [ ]   1–5
STUDY No.   [ ] [ ]   6–7
CARD No.   [2] [0]   8–9

| Other (specify): .... | Specify: .... [ ] [ ] [ ] [ ] [ ] | [ ] [ ] [ ] [ ] | [ ] [ ] | [II] / [II] / [II] | 10–25 |

*Local coding system to be used

Appendix 2

INDEX No.	[ ] [ ] [ ] [ ] [ ]	1–5
STUDY No.	[ ] [ ]	6–7
CARD No.	[2] [1]	8–9

4 Were any of the following general treatment measures offered?
1 Yes   2 No   9 Not known

Counselling   [ ]   –10
Individual psychotherapy   [ ]   –11
Behaviour therapy   [ ]   –12
Relaxation therapy   [ ]   –13
Family therapy   [ ]   –14
Joint marital therapy   [ ]   –15
Group therapy   [ ]   –16
Alcohol support group   [ ]   –17
Drug use support group   [ ]   –18
Other, please state: ....   [ ]   –19

5 Treatment Plan
A precis of the treatment plan agreed by the client and keyworker should be documented. It should include:
1 the nature of treatment
2 the order of interventions and their proposed duration
3 the ways in which treatment will be implemented

Section VII: Summary of assessment and treatment

This summary should provide an adequate basis for letters to family doctors, formal reports and referrals and should include:

1 reason and source of referral
2 date of assessment and discipline(s) of professionals involved
3 major substance(s) of use including the duration and pattern of use
4 previous treatment history and agencies involved
5 major problem areas and need for intervention
6 patient's personality, motivation and other psychological factors
7 treatment goals (short, medium and long-term) and plan of action
8 formulation of the case

....
....
....
....
....
....
....
....
....
....

Appendix 3

Narcotics Anonymous

The Twelve Steps*

1 We admitted that we were powerless over our addiction, that our lives had become unmanageable.
2 We came to believe that a Power greater than ourselves could restore us to sanity.
3 We made a decision to turn our will and our lives over to the care of God *as we understood God.*
4 We made a searching and fearless moral inventory of ourselves.
5 We admitted to God, to ourselves, and to another human being the exact nature of our wrongs.
6 We were entirely ready to have God remove all these defects of character.
7 We humbly asked God to remove our shortcomings.
8 We made a list of all persons we had harmed, and became willing to make amends to them all.
9 We made direct amends to such people wherever possible, except when to do so would injure them or others.
10 We continued to take personal inventory and when we were wrong promptly admitted it.
11 We sought through prayer and meditation to improve our conscious contact with God *as we understood God,* praying only for knowledge of God's will for us and the power to carry that out.
12 Having had a spiritual awakening as a result of these steps, we tried to carry this message to addicts, and to practice these principles in all our affairs.

The Twelve Traditions*

We keep what we have only with vigilance, and just as freedom for the individual comes from the Twelve Steps, so freedom for the group springs from our Traditions.

*Reprinted and adapted with permission of AA World Service Inc.

As long as the ties that bind us together are stronger than those that would tear us apart, all will be well.

1   Our common welfare should come first: personal recovery depends on NA unity.
2   For our group purpose there is but one ultimate authority – a loving God as He may express Himself in our group conscience. Our leaders are but trusted servants, they do not govern.
3   The only requirement for membership is a desire to stop using.
4   Each group should be autonomous except in matters affecting other groups or NA as a whole.
5   Each group has but one primary purpose – to carry the message to the addict who still suffers.
6   An NA group ought never to endorse, finance, or lend the NA name to any related facility or outside enterprise, lest problems of money, property or prestige divert us from our primary purpose.
7   Every NA group ought to be fully self-supporting, declining outside contributions.
8   Narcotics Anonymous should remain forever non-professional, but our service centres may employ special workers.
9   NA, as such, ought never be organized, but we may create service boards or committees directly responsible to those they serve.
10   Narcotics Anonymous has no opinion on outside issues; hence the NA name ought never be drawn into public controversy.
11   Our public relations policy is based on attraction rather than promotion: we need always maintain personal anonymity at the level of press, radio and films.
12   Anonymity is the spiritual foundation of all our Traditions, ever reminding us to place principles before personalities.

The Twelve Steps of Alcoholics Anonymous

1 We admitted we were powerless over alcohol – that our lives had become unmanageable   2 Came to believe that a Power greater than ourselves could restore us to sanity. 3 Made a decision to turn our will and our lives over to the care of God *as we understood Him.*   4 Made a searching and fearless moral inventory of ourselves.   5 Admitted to God, to ourselves, and to another human being the exact nature of our wrongs.   6 Were entirely ready to have God remove all the defects of character.   7 Humbly asked Him to remove our shortcomings.   8 Made a list of all persons we had harmed, and became willing to make amends to them all   9 Made direct amends to such people wherever possible, except when to do so would injure them or others.   10 Continued to take personal inventory and when we were wrong promptly admitted it.   11 Sought through prayer and meditation to improve our conscious contact with God *as we understood Him,*

praying only for knowledge of His will for us and the power to carry that out.   12
Having had a spiritual awakening as the result of these steps, we tried to carry this
message to alcoholics, and to practice these principles in all our affairs.

Reprinted and adapted with permission of AA World Services, Inc.

Appendix 4

Opiate Withdrawal

Opiate Withdrawal Symptom Questionnaire*

Patient's name: _____   Patient study no.[_____]

Please rate the absence or presence of the following symptoms over the past 24 hours using the following scale at approximately the same time each day.

Scale 0 = none/not at all   1 = slightly/little/occasionally
     2 = moderately   3 = very much/a great deal/continuously

Over the last 24 hours to   Enter date [_____]
what extent have you: Enter time [_____] am/pm

1	Been yawning		10	Felt sick
2	Had muscle cramp		11	Had stomach cramps
3	Had pounding heart		12	Had difficulty sleeping
4	Had a runny nose		13	Felt aches in bones or muscles
5	Been sneezing		14	Felt twitching and shaking
6	Experienced pins and needles		15	Felt irritable/bad tempered
7	Had hot/cold flushes		16	Been sweating
8	Had diarrhoea		17	Had runny eyes
9	Had gooseflesh		18	Felt craving *Total score* (leave blank)

*St George's Hospital, Department of Addictive Behaviour.

Opiate Withdrawal Scoring Sheet

Patient's name:_____   Patient study no. [_____]

Before each dose of opiate please complete a set of observations, filling in the results below.

At the same time give patient a symptom questionnaire to fill in.

Date and time of admission_____

Date								
Time (24 hour)								
*Signs**								
1 Yawning								
2 Lacrimation								
3 Rhinorrhoea								
4 Perspiration								
5 Tremor								
6 Piloerection								
7 Restlessness								
8 Pupil size (mm)								
9 Anorexia								
10 Vomiting								
11 Diarrhoea								
12 Insomnia								

Date								
Time (24 hour)								
*Signs**								
13 Drug seeking								
Observations†								
Temperature								
Respiration rate								
Pulse								
Blood pressure								
Weight								
Drugs								
Dose of opiates								
Other treatment								
Adverse effects								
Comments								
Other investigations								

*Sign 1–13 should be determined as either: present = 2; not sure = 1; or absent = 0.
†Observations (+ sign 8): record actual measurements.

Appendix 5

Attendance Record

Name: Key worker: Doctor:

Date							
Seen by							
Reason for attendance*							
Drug use in past 24 hours							
Clinical state: Intoxicated† ⌠sedated							
⌡elated							
Sober							
Withdrawing† ⌠opiate							
⌡sedative							
Urine result lab no.							
Amphetamine							
Barbiturate							
Benzodiazepine							
Cannabis							
Codeine							
Cocaine							
Methadone							
Morphine							
Other							

*e.g., follow-up (f/u); daily attendance (d/a); assessment, blood test; special visit.
†Score: +, ++, +++.

Note: This record is to be maintained at EVERY attendance. To be completed by member of team who formally sees the patient, e.g., key worker, doctor, clinic nurse, social worker, etc.

Index

Synanon 186
Syphilis 138
Syringe-exchange schemes 324–6

Talk assessment 136
  acute psychiatric disturbance 250
Tanzania 97
Telephone advisory services 34, 36
Temazepam 41
Temgesic *see* Buprenorphine
Teratogenicity 268–9
Teronac *see* Mazindol
Terrence Higgins Trust 242
Tetrahydrocannabinol (THC) 65, 68, 103, 104
  absorption/fate 104
  abstinence syndrome 106
  psychological effects 105
  tolerance 105
  toxic psychosis 105
Thailand 66, 69, 72
Therapeutic addicts 23, 25
  opiates 17
  sedative hypnotics withdrawal management 223–4
Therapeutic communities 185–8
  Christian-based 186
  community-based hostels 186, 188
  concept houses 186–7
  encounter-group therapy 186–7
  outcome evaluation 187, 307–8
  patient selection 187–8
Thin-layer chromatography (TLC) 142, 144
Thiopentone 87
Thioridazine, opiates detoxification 203, 284, 289
Thought content assessment 136–7
Tobacco, ICD-10 coding scheme 148
Tolerance
  ceiling effect 6
  definition 5–6
  DSM-III-R substance dependence criteria 159
  DSM-IV substance dependence criteria 161
  ICD-10 coding of dependence syndromes 152
  mechanisms 6
  physical dependence relationship 6–7
  specificity (cross-tolerance) 6
Toulene 109
Toxicology laboratories
  epidemiological data collection 58
  investigations 140–6
Traditional social controls 19
Treatment aims 329
Treatment centres
  historical aspects 25–6, 29
  notification of addicts 42
Treatment outcome *see* Follow-up

Treatment Outcome Prospective Study (TOPS) 308
Treatment plan 171
Trichloroethylene 109
Tricyclic antidepressants (TCAs) 7
  cocaine effects reduction 232
  stimulant drug abrupt cessation management 231
Tripelennamine pentazocine combination 82, 316
Tryptophan 231
Turkey 72

UK
  legislation 340–47
  treatment services 30–6
Unconsciousness 258–63
  accident and emergency department management 285
  chest X-ray following 140
  gastric lavage 260
  hypothermia 260
  laboratory investigations 260
  management 258–60
  mortality 304
  opiate overdose 260–1
  phencyclidine overdose 262–3
  physical examination 259
  resuscitation 259
  sedative hypnotics overdose 256, 262
United Nations Children's Fund (UNICEF) 340
United Nations Convention against Illicit Traffic in Narcotic Drugs and Psychotropic Substances (1988) 317, 333, 335
United Nations drug abuse control organs 336–40
United Nations Educational Scientific and Cultural Organization (UNESCO) 340
United Nations Funds for Drug Abuse Control (UNFDAC) 336, 338
United Nations International Drug Control Programme (UNDCP) 336, 338–9
Unlawful possession data 38, 39
Urine samples 141, 142
  accident and emergency department attendance 287
  driving licence bans 292, 293
  drug levels 143
  general practitioner patients 288, 289
  unconscious patient 260
USA 65
  historical aspects 23, 24
  illicit drugs availability 318

Veronal *see* Barbitone
Vidarabine 246
Viet Nam 66
Violent behaviour
  acute psychiatric disturbance 251